INFLAMMATORY BOWEL DISEASE

Executive Committee

Chairman	
Tsuneo Shiratori, M.D.	Professor, First Department of Surgery, Nara Medical University, Kashihara, Nara
Members	
Noboru Kobayashi, M.D.	Professor, Department of Pediatrics, Faculty of Medicine, University of Tokyo, Tokyo
Yoshio Mishima, M.D.	Professor, Department of Surgery, Tokyo Medical and Dental University, Tokyo
Shuji Tsuchiya, M.D.	Professor, Second Department of Surgery, Yokohama City University School of Medicine, Yokohama, Japan
Yutaka Yoshida, M.D.	Professor, First Department of Internal Medicine, Hirosaki University School of Medicine, Hirosaki, Aomori
Takashi Shimoyama, M.D.	Professor, Fourth Department of Internal Medicine, Hyogo Medical College, Nishinomiya, Hyogo
Haruki Wakasa, M.D.	Professor, Department of Pathology, Fukushima Medical College, Fukushima
Hikaru Watanabe, M.D.	Division of Gastroenterology, Sendai National Hospital, Sendai, Miyagi
Hiroshige Nakano, M.D.	Assistant Professor, First Department of Surgery, Nara Medical University, Kashihara, Nara

JAPAN MEDICAL RESEARCH FOUNDATION PUBLICATION No. 22

INFLAMMATORY BOWEL DISEASE

Proceedings of the International Symposium on Etiopathogenesis and Treatment of Inflammatory Bowel Disease, October 8-10, 1982, Nara, Japan

Edited by

TSUNEO SHIRATORI

HIROSHIGE NAKANO

UNIVERSITY OF TOKYO PRESS

JAPAN MEDICAL RESEARCH FOUNDATION
PUBLICATION NO. 22

8–2, Hirakawa-cho 2-chome, Chiyoda-ku, Tokyo 102, Japan

Published by
UNIVERSITY OF TOKYO PRESS
ISBN 4–13–068105–2 (UTP 69054)
ISBN 0–86008–364–0

Printed in Japan

Contents

II. IMMUNOLOGY

III. PATHOLOGY

IV. INCIDENCE

Foreword

The development of modern medicine has contributed to clarifying the etiology and treatment of various disease as well as to improving public health and welfare. However, there are many diseases of unknown etiology, which still leave large numbers of patients in a chronic incurable state. In order to promote research on the etiology and treatment of such intractable diseases, non-governmental funding, as well as governmental support, is very important. The Japan Medical Research Foundation has been in existence since October 1973 in order to meet this need with aid from non-governmental financial sources. One of the Foundation's main activities is to hold annual symposia and seminars on various diseases.

It is more than ten years since systematic studies on ulcerative colitis and Crohn's disease were begun in Japan under the sponsorship of the Ministry of Health and Welfare. Now the concept of inflammatory bowel disease is well diffused among clinicians, and many cases have been reported; however, the etiology is still unknown, and its elucidation is an urgent problem for researchers and clinicians.

This book is an outcome of the International Symposium on the Etiopathogenesis and Treatment of Inflammatory Bowel Disease, whose purpose was to share research results and discuss the present status of inflammatory bowel disease. Many investigators gathered and exchanged their knowledge on intestianl microflora of patients with inflammatory bowel disease, immunology, pathology, incidence, medical treatment, and surgical treatment. The Japan Medical Research Foundation is very pleased to sponsor this symposium, and I am hopeful that the publication of its proceedings will make its work available to a wide scientific readership.

June 18, 1984

Masayoshi Yamamoto
President
Japan Medical Research Foundation

Preface

Systematic studies on inflammatory bowel disease in Japan were initiated by two distinguished investigators, Dr. Fujio Matsunaga (internal medicine), now Professor Emeritus of Hirosaki University, and Dr. Tetsuo Maki (surgery), now Professor Emeritus of Tohoku University. In spite of their efforts, however, their investigations were not as fruitful as expected quantitatively and qualitatively, largely because of the scarcity of clinical cases during the 1958–1972 period.

However, in 1973, the Research Team for Ulcerative Colitis (headed by Shuji Tsuchiya) was organized under the sponsorship of the Ministry of Health and Welfare to begin organized, systematic research activities on inflammatory bowel diseases from the epidemiological, pathogenetic, and therapeutic aspects. In 1975, Crohn's disease was included in this Team's activities.

In 1976, the Team was divided into the Research Team for Crohn's Disease (headed by Shuji Tsuchiya) and the Research Team for Idiopathic Bowel Diseases (headed by Yutaka Yoshida); these continued their research activities until 1977 and 1978, respectively. The Research Team for Inflammatory Bowel Diseases (headed by Tsuneo Shiratori) was organized in 1979, and continued its research activities until 1982.

Thus research activities on inflammatory bowel diseases in Japan have been recorded over a period of one decade. During the period, the Team gradually accumulated data on approximately 5,000 cases. Considerable progress was, in the meantime, made on the etiological analysis and therapeutic guidelines as evolved on epidemiological, immunological, and bacteriological bases. However, the research in Japan still lagged behind that of Occidental countries quantitatively as well as qualitatively, and the Team participants felt the need of a direct interchange of research results in an international forum.

The International Symposium on Etiopathogenesis and Treatment of Inflammatory Bowel Disease was held in Nara from October 8 to 10, 1982, under the auspices of the Japan Medical Research Foundation. The Symposium was attended by approximately 150 Japanese workers and 7 invited foreign speakers: M. J. Hill (bacteriology), M. J. Hudson (bacteriology), and D. P. Jewell (immunological internal medicine) from England, and R. H. Ridell (pathology), R. G. Farmer (internal medicine), D. G. Jagelman (surgery), and K. A. Kelly (surgery) from the U. S. A. Significant intra- and inter-disciplinary discussions were held from the bacteriological, immunological, epidemiological, pathological, enterological, and surgical viewpoints. The work presented by Japanese investigators was comparable to the standard of the world and contained a great deal of valuable information.

The Japan Medical Research Foundation has compiled the research presented and discussions exchanged at this Symposium into a full publication. I wish to express my deep appreciation to the Foundation for supporting this very significant project.

June 11, 1984

Tsuneo Shiratori
Chairman of the Executive Committee

Opening Remarks

It is a great pleasure for us to convene this symposium sponsored by the Japan Medical Research Foundation, still more that we could invite seven experts of high renown from abroad and many specialists from Japan. I would like to express my gratitude to all of you.

First of all, let me introduce the structure of this symposium. We wanted to focus on *etiopathogenesis* and *treatment* of IBD. Moreover, we included *incidence* in order to clarify the actual conditions in Japan and a session on Crohn's disease to study the aspect of diagnosis.

The aims of this symposium are to develop the study of IBD to contribute to research in Europe and America by showing the recent progress of study in Japan, and to learn from the excellent work in foreign countries. To achieve this aim, I hope all of you will contribute to a lively exchange. I also hope the Japanese doctors will join the discussion using simultaneous interpretation.

I would like to end these words of opening with an earnest prayer for the great success of this symposium.

October 8, 1982

Tsuneo Shiratori
Chairman of the Executive Committee

I. INTESTINAL MICROFLORA

Intestinal Microflora in Inflammatory Bowel Disease

Michael J. Hill and Michael J. Hudson

SUMMARY

In this review, the data implicating bacteria in the causation of Crohn's disease and ulcerative colitis are discussed. Patients who have had IBD for more than 10 years are at high risk of colorectal carcinogenesis; the possible role of bacterial metabolites of bile acids in this progression is reviewed.

INTRODUCTION

Studies relating inflammatory bowel disease (IBD) to the gut flora have a long history. Acute IBD may result from enteric infection and it is plausible that the chronic disease may originate as one of the common enteric infections. It has also been suggested that acute infection only becomes chronic when the gut flora has certain characteristics and that the composition of the total flora has therefore, a role in maintaining the disease state.

Fresh impetus was given to these ideas following the successful introduction of salazopyrin (salicylazosulphapyridine, SASP) in the treatment of ulcerative colitis, since it was suspected that the success could be due to the sulphonamide released by the azo reductase action on SASP. However, to date it has proved to be extremely difficult to establish any link between the gut flora and either the initiation or the maintenance of the disease state in IBD.

In this paper we will review the evidence for a microbial etiology of IBD and present some new data of our own. As it is known that IBD of the large bowel carries a risk of malignancy, we will describe our studies of the mechanism of large bowel carcinogenesis in such patients.

PHLS-CAMR, Porton Down, Salisbury, England, UK

EVIDENCE RELATING THE GUT FLORA TO IBD

The study of the role of gut bacteria in IBD is complicated by the fact that they may be involved only in the initiation of the disease, or only in the maintenance of the disease, or in both the initiation and maintenance of the disease by the same or by different mechanisms. Further, chronic IBD has three major forms: ulcerative colitis (UC) is a mucosal disease confined to the large bowel; Crohn's disease (CD) affects all layers of the mucosal wall and affects the whole intestine (with the terminal ileum and cecum being most intensely affected); irritable bowel syndrome (IBS) is usually diagnosed by exclusion of the other two and by exclusion of a range of other bowel diseases. The definitions and differential diagnoses of these three, together with a host of minor forms, have been reviewed by Lockhart-Mummery and Morson[1] and more recently by Price[2] and by Lennard-Jones[3]; bacteria may play different roles in the different forms of IBD.

The original suggestion that these chronic diseases might have a microbial etiology arose by analogy with the acute bowel infections (food poisoning, cholera, dysentery, etc.) with similar symptoms and was supported by the apparent partial success of treatment with antimicrobial agents. It revived dramatically following the introduction of salazopyrine and took two main forms. One line of research was to search for specific pathogens on the assumption that the disease had a single causative organism (or small group of organisms) that was diagnostic of the disease and that its removal would result in the cure of the disease. The alternative approach was to study the whole flora and to look for differences in the overall "profile" of organisms. The rekindling of interest into the possibility of microbial involvement in IBD also coincided with greatly improved techniques for the study of the obligately anaerobic bacteria of the intestinal flora and interest in the microecology and metabolism of this flora.

A further alternative approach has been to look for raised antibody levels to fecal organisms in IBD patients, although it is widely believed that immune response to components of the flora may be manifest purely as a reflection of the increased permeability of a damaged mucosa to antigens and the differential host response to different antigens.

Specific organisms

The search for a single causative organism has a long history, and early studies of the role of bacteria in chronic UC implicated shigellae, diplostreptococci,[4] and bacteroides.[5] The early work was reviewed by Kirsner and Palmer[6] and by Weinstein[7] who concluded that there was no good evidence for the implication of any single organism in the causation of the disease. Later studies have been no more fruitful: Wiel-Korstanje and Winkler[8] reported increased numbers of enterococci and the presence of *Streptococcus mobilis* in the feces of colitics but not in those of normal healthy controls. The organism was capable of producing hyaluronidase, chondroitinase, mucinase, and other enzymes necessary for initiation of an epithelial lesion. *S. mobilis*, a phenon referring to the only motile enterococci, would not normally be detected among the other group D streptococci because motility is a property not usually looked for. However, following the first report of their association with colitis there have been no further confirmatory reports and we were unable to detect the organism in colitis patients.

Gorbach *et al.*[9] observed a significant increase in the number of coliforms (but not of other organisms) in patients with active colitis, and Cooke[10] reported the presence of increased numbers of hemolysin and necrotoxin-producing strains of *Escherichia coli*, which appeared to increase significantly during relapses of the disease.[11]

The search for a single causative organism of Crohn's disease has as long a history as that for colitis. Aluwihare[12] demonstrated intramural bacteria in the intact epithelia of six of eleven colon specimens from patients with CD, but these were not present in comparable specimens from patients with UC or non-IBD. More recently Cave and his colleagues have reported the existence of a transmissible agent from Crohn's disease.[13–15] When they took tissue from CD patients, homogenized it, and injected it intraperitoneally or intravenously into rabbits, a granulomatous lesion similar to those seen in CD resulted. The disease could be transmitted even by the filtered homogenate of a Crohn's lesion using 0.2-μ filters which would remove all conventional bacteria. The conclusion was that the transmissible agent was a virus or a bacterial L-form. Similar studies with tissue from UC patients also gave lesions, suggesting a common etiology.[16] There has been considerable controversy about this work and some groups have been unable to repeat the work.[17,18] The interpretation of such studies is plagued by variations in technique between laboratories and especially in the choice of species and strains of laboratory animals and the interpretation of histopathology of lesions.[19] Interestingly, one report suggests that the pre-incubation of CD tissue with ampicillin abolishes the ability to induce granulomatous changes in rabbit ileum,[20] suggesting that the transmissible factor is a bacterium rather than a virus or a chemotactic tissue macromolecule. The isolation of RNA viruses from CD material by Gitnick *et al.*[21,22] and Whorwell *et al.*[23] has not been confirmed by others.[24–26]

Two other candidates for filterable etiological agents have been reported, both cell-wall-deficient bacteria. Parent and Mitchell[27,28] describe the isolation and *in vitro* reversion of *Pseudomonas maltophila* and *Pseudomonas* Group Va cell-wall-deficient bacteria from CD tissue supported by demonstrable serum antibodies in CD patients but not in UC patients or controls,[29] but such organisms have not been isolated by other workers and have not been visualized by immunological staining in CD tissues.[30] Burnham *et al.*[31] and Stanford *et al.*[32] isolated cell-wall-deficient mycobacteria from CD and UC tissue, one strain of which reverted *in vitro* to a *Mycobacterium kansasii.* Although skin testing with this mycobacterium tended to support an etiologic role, other workers have not yet confirmed the presence of such bacteria in CD tissues by culture.

That mycobacterial cell-wall-deficient variants might be involved in the pathogenesis of CD is an attractive hypothesis due to the similarities of the mycobacterial disease of cattle—Johne's disease to CD and the recognized ability of mycobacterial cell wall material to elicit granuloma formation in experimental animals. When injected into mice, the revertant CD isolate of *M. kansasii* caused either septicemia or mycobacterial abscess according to dosage,[31] not mirroring the effects observed in the studies of Cave *et al.*[15] Whorwell *et al.*[30] were unable to visualize mycobacteria in CD tissue by immunofluorescence.

The observation made by Schuller and colleagues[33] that a high proportion of CD patients had serum antibody directed against chlamydia of the lymphogranuloma-venereum type have not been confirmed by others using both cultural and serological methods.[34–37]

Das and colleagues[38] have now increased the complexity of the CD puzzle by demonstrating a transmissible agent in the lymph nodes of each of four CD patients which, on intraperitoneal inoculation of athymic ("nude") mice produces lymphoma. This effect was absent from lymph nodes from two UC patients and five non-IBD patients. This most interesting observation awaits further study and confirmation by other groups.

Wensinck and his colleagues[39–41] have reported that the fecal flora of CD patients is characterized by the presence of three organisms, *Eubacterium* spp., *Peptostreptococcus* spp., and *Coprococcus* spp. The results were independent of the severity of the disease or duration; surprisingly, the organisms were also present in patients with ileocecal resection. Using these organisms as diagnostic indicators, Wensinck *et al.* are able to distinguish blind between CD patients and controls or patients with other IBD (UC, IBS, etc.). Their findings have had some support from other laboratories.[30]

There has been a number of reports that in CD patients the fecal flora is rich in the *Bacteroides fragilis* group,[42,43] a result that has not been observed consistently.[9,10,44]

Clostridium difficile, which has been associated with pseudomembranous colitis by many groups, was associated with acute relapse in IBD by Lamont *et al.*[45] and Bolton *et al.*,[46] but this has still to be confirmed by other laboratories. One unpublished series had found no such association (S. P. Borriello, personal communication), and Dorman *et al.*[47] concluded that it was unrelated to the activity of the disease.

Cytotoxins other than that of *C. difficile* have been noted in feces and tissues from patients with IBD by independent workers,[48,49] but may be present in normal tissues.[48] The differentiation of such cytotoxins from *C. difficile* cytotoxin reinforces the necessity for carefully controlled experiments in the search for IBD-associated agents.

Although there has been an impressive number of reports of specific organisms associated with IBD, the overall picture is similar to that in 1961 when Weinstein concluded that there was no good evidence which consistently implicated any particular organisms in either UC or CD. Many of the observations could have been due to the non-specific effects of diarrhea on the fecal flora, as noted by Weinstein.[7] However, a specific organism may be implicated in the initiation of IBD but not in maintenance of the disease state; if this is so, then the lack of consistent results may be due to the fact that all of the studies have been carried out on patients with established IBD and in whom the initiating lesion may have disappeared. The lack of consistent results implicating a single causal organism is therefore only an indication that a single organism is not responsible for the maintenance of the disease state and tells us nothing about the initiating lesion. Truelove,[50] De Dombal,[51] and many others have concluded that bacteria were unlikely to be among the prime causes of IBD.

Fecal bacterial profiles

The difficulties associated with the search for a single causal organism pale into insignificance when compared with those of looking at the total profile of organisms. Diarrhea causes a non-specific increase in the number of all organisms in feces, and this must be remembered in the interpretation of results; however, the biggest problem is the variation between normal healthy persons in their fecal flora.

Weijers and Van der Kamer[52] noted that it might be the metabolic products of the flora which gave rise to the disease, whereas Monteiro *et al.*[53] implicated the antigenic products; these two approaches have guided the studies of the fecal bacterial profile in IBD.

Most reports of studies of the fecal bacterial profile have shown differences between IBD patients and controls; the problem has been to determine their significance. An early study of the total flora was done by Seneca and Henderson[54] who found no significant differences in any genus. Gorbach *et al.*[9] compared patients with active disease with those in remission and with controls; they reported higher counts of *Bacteroides* spp. and of

E. coli in IBD patients. These results were not supported by West *et al.*[44] who could find no differences between patients with UC, CD, or no disease. In addition, they found no statistically significant differences between the flora of patients with acute disease and of patients in remission.

If the "bacterial profile" is important in maintenance of the disease state, then perhaps the fecal profile is not representative of that at the site of the lesion. Clearly, this latter profile is likely to be much more important if either of the two mechanisms (metabolic products or antigenic products) is valid. Attempts to overcome these problems will be discussed in Section II.

Serological studies

In 1971, Monteiro *et al.* reported higher mucosal antibody levels to fecal nonsporing anaerobic bacteria in UC patients than in controls. They suggested that the maintenance of the disease state might be due to an antibody-mediated hypersensitivity reaction of the Arthus type between the gut flora and the mucosal antibody. The mucosal antibody was IgG but did not react with the aerobic flora and so differed from the serum antibody (which only reacted with aerobic organisms). There had been previous reports of a role for autoimmune reactions[6,55] and for hypersensitivity reactions.[56] The hypothesis of an immune reaction explains the value of salazopyrine in the treatment of UC in that it would maintain a state of quiescence in the disease (by suppressing the antigen load) but would be less able to control the acute phase of the disease (since that would be the result of an immune reaction that had already taken place).

There have been similar studies of antibody levels in patients with Crohn's disease. In these patients there have been many reports of elevated titers of antibody to *Bacteroides fragilis* subspecies *vulgatus*.[57–59] Metronidazole is an antibiotic which is very active against all *B. fragilis* subspecies and has had some success in the treatment of Crohn's disease. Wensinck and Ven der Merwe[60] measured serum agglutinins to *Peptostreptococcus* spp. and to *Eubacterium* spp. in Crohn's disease patients and in controls. Using a set of three *Eubacterium* strains and one *Peptostreptococcus*, they developed a pattern of agglutinins which characterized 50% of CD patients and 0% of controls. They then applied the test to sera submitted for diagnosis: 97% of the positive sera were either CD (62%), UC (27%), or fistula and diarrhea (8%), but they did not report the number of cases of CD which were negative in their agglutinin test.

MORE RECENT STUDIES

The data presented above indicate that there may be a role for gut bacteria in the maintenance of the disease state in IBD, but the evidence in favor of any particular organisms or any particular mechanism is unconvincing. This may be because: a) bacteria play no part in the disease, or b) only those organisms at the site of the lesion are important (this would be particularly likely to be so if the hypothesis put forward either by Monteiro or by Weijers and Van der Kamer is true).

To test the importance of the local bacterial flora, two types of study have been carried out. The first type was to study the flora in the gut lumen at the site of the lesion; the second was to study the flora of the intestinal mucosa.

Lumenal flora by subsite in the gut

Studies of the lumenal flora at various subsites are beset by difficulties. It is very difficult to sample the colon by colonoscopy since the bowel is normally cleansed in order to carry out this procedure. It is also very difficult to sample the colon by naso-intestinal tube since ethical committees do not permit sampling beyond the ileocecal junction, and, in any case, the presence of the tube causes disturbances in the physiology of the gut.

It has been possible to sample the sigmoid colon using the snare of a sigmoidoscope; such samples had a bacterial composition identical to that of feces. It has also been possible to assay the flora of ileostomy fluid.[61-63] Finegold *et al.* studied patients with ileostomies for IBD (four for UC, two for CD), and all the aerobic bacteria outnumbered the anaerobes by at least 10 fold (Table 1). The principal aerobic organisms were *E. coli* and streptococci, with lactobacilli and micrococci carried by three persons each. The principal anaerobes were veillonella (carried by two of six) and bifidobacteria (two of six). The *Bacteroides fragilis* group was not isolated from

TABLE 1. Microbial Composition of Ileal Contents (Obtained by Aspiration from within the Stoma) and Ileostomy Effluent

	Ileostomy effluent		Ileal contents	
	Gorbach *et al.*[60]	Finegold *et al.*[63]	Gorbach *et al.*[61]	Hori *et al.*[62]
Aerobes				
Total		8.3	5.8	6.9
E. coli	7.0	7.5	3.6	5.4
Fecal streptococci		6.8		5.8
Streptococci	6.7	6.7	2.3	6.5
Micrococci and staphylococci	6.6	5.8	3.8	—
Lactobacilli	6.3	5.8	3.0	4.0
Anaerobes				
Total	7.8	6.5	6.0	5.1
Clostridia		3.3		4.2
Bacteroides		3.1		3.7
Bifidobacteria	6.7	6.3	3.3	3.2
Veillonella		6.5		4.6

any of the patients. A further patient with an ileoproctostomy had a richer flora with a greater variety of species (both anaerobic and aerobic) present. Gorbach *et al.*[61)] studied ileostomy fluid from 13 patients and found equal numbers of aerobes and anaerobes. The dominant organisms were coliforms, streptococci, lactobacilli, bifidobacteria, and micrococci. The results of Scarpino *et al.*[64)] and of Hori *et al.*[62)] were very similar to those of Finegold *et al.* The latter authors have offered a number of possible explanations (related to the techniques of quantitative bacteriology) for the differences between the results of Gorbach *et al.* and the other groups.

In addition to studying ileostomy fluid, Finegold *et al.* also studied the effluent from transverse colostomies in two patients (Table 2). There was a much richer anaerobic flora with large numbers of *B. fragilis*, bifidobacteria, and clostridia in both patients. Interestingly, *E. coli* was present only in small numbers in both patients. Again, the results of Finegold *et al.* are in agreement with those of Scarpino *et al.*

TABLE 2. Microbial Composition of Transverse Colostomy Fluid (from Finegold *et al.*[63)])

Organism			Mean $\log_{10}$ bacterial counts/g (two patients)
Aerobes			7.4
Coliforms:	*E. coli*	(2/2)	3.7
	Klebsiella	(1/2)	3.6
	Enterobacter	(1/2)	3.0
Streptococci		(2/2)	5.8
	S. faecalis		4.3
Lactobacillus		(1/2)	4.0
Anaerobes			8.3
B. fragilis		(2/2)	7.5
Bifidobacterium		(2/2)	7.6
Clostridium		(2/2)	4.9
Veillonella		(1/2)	1.0

A number of conclusions can be drawn from these results. The first is that the fecal flora is in no way representative of the flora of the right colon either qualitatively or quantitatively (Table 3). In Crohn's disease, the major site of the disease is the terminal ileum and the cecum; if *Bacteroides vulgatus* were responsible for the maintenance of the disease state by stimulating a local hypersensitivity reaction (for example), then we would expect to find the organism in the terminal ileum and right colon. Similarly, if the *Eubacterium* spp., *Peptostreptococcus* spp., and *Coprococcus* spp. reported by Wensinck were causally related to Crohn's disease, we would expect to find them at the site of the lesion.

TABLE 3. Microbial Flora of Ileum (from Ileostomy Fluid), Transverse Colon (from Transverse Colostomy Fluid), and Feces (Log_{10} Bacterial Counts/g)

	Ileostomy fluid	Transverse colostomy	Feces
Aerobes			
Total	8.3	7.4	8
E. coli	7.5	3.7	7
Streptococci	6.7	5.8	8
Lactobacilli	6.1	4.0	8
Micrococci/staphylococci	6.2	0	0
Anaerobes			
Total	7.1	8.3	11
B. fragilis	3.1	7.5	11
Bifidobacteria	6.5	7.6	11
Clostridia	3.34	4.9	7
Veillonella	6.5	1.0	4
Ratio: anaerobes/aerobes	1/10	10/1	1000/1

Intestinal mucosal flora

Most of the work on the intestinal mucosal flora has been carried out by Peach and her co-workers. To study the mucosal flora, it is necessary to use biopsy specimens or samples of intestinal material obtained at operation. The sample is washed carefully to remove lumenal contents adherent to the specimen, and it is then homogenized and bacterial flora assessed quantitatively in the usual manner. Since much of the sample is tissue, it is not possible to relate the number of organisms/g tissue to the population density of bacteria in the lumen, but it is possible to make quantitative comparisons between the flora associated with the gut mucosa at various subsites in the large bowel and to make qualitative comparisons with the lumenal flora.

Comparison between the lumenal and mucosal flora. Peach *et al.*[65)] studied the colonic mucosal flora of normal persons and, later,[66)] the mucosal flora of the jejunum, ileum, colon, and rectum in patients with Crohn's disease and in controls. They noted that the ratio between anaerobic and aerobic organisms in the mucosal flora of the rectum and colon was about 1, compared with 100 to 1,000 for the lumenal flora. Whereas the most numerous organisms in the lumen are the nonsporing anaerobic organisms (*Bacteroides* spp., *Bifidobacterium* spp., and *Eubacterium* spp.), with Gram-positive and Gram-negative rods being equally represented, in the mucosa not only were the anaerobic rods much less numerous but they were also much more dominated by the bacteroides organisms.

We have studied the mucosal flora of the rectum (Hudson, unpublished results) and obtained results essentially similar to those of Peach *et al.*[65,66] except that the dominant aerobic organisms were enterococci. This may be due to differences in patient preparation, this latter study being carried out on unprepared bowels.

The mucosal flora by subsite. The number of organisms per gram of mucosal tissue was higher in the large than in the small intestine and increased along the large intestine (Table 4). However, throughout the intestinal tract the qualitative flora remained constant, with equal numbers of anaerobic and aerobic organisms. Throughout, the aerobic flora was dominated by Gram-negative rod-shaped organisms (particularly enterobacteria), as was the anaerobic flora (particularly *Bacteroides* spp.).

TABLE 4. Log_{10} Bacterial Count per Gram of Mucosa at Various Subsites of Large Intestine (from Peach and Tabaqchali [67])

Subsite	Number of specimens	Log_{10} bacteria/g
Cecum	10	5.5
Ascending colon	9	5.8
Transverse colon	12	5.6
Descending colon	11	6.3
Rectum	8	6.4

Mucosal flora in Crohn's disease, colitis, and controls. Peach *et al.*[66] and Peach and Tabaqchali[67] compared the mucosal flora in patients with Crohn's disease and in controls. The mucosal flora of both the ileum and the colon was richer in the patients with CD (Table 5) and was more dominated by the Gram-negative rods (bacteroides and enterobacteria). The differences were not statistically significant.

Mucosal tissue from the distal ileum, transverse colon, and rectum of UC patients was assayed and compared with mucosal samples from similar sites in controls (Hudson, unpublished data). No significant differences were seen. Similarly, no consistent differences were seen between UC patients in remission and in relapse.

The effect of antibiotics. The mucosal flora of UC patients treated with various antibiotics has been studied in order to relate changes in the flora to changes in the patients' symptoms. Antibiotics have very little effect on the mucosal flora, even under circumstances when the lumenal flora is affected quite drastically. Marks *et al.*[68] showed that pre-operative treatment with phthalylsulphathiazole, which reduced the fecal flora by 10–100 fold, had no detectable effect on the mucosal flora.

However, when patients were treated with a combination of metronidazole and cotrimoxazole that has proved beneficial to patients with

TABLE 5. Mucosal Flora of Patients with CD and Controls (from Peach and Tabaqchali [67])

	Controls	Crohn's disease
Ileal mucosal flora		
Number of samples	10	10
Total aerobes	4.1 (2.4–4.9)	10–5.6 (3.2–6.1)
Total anaerobes	3.8 (2.8–5.5)	5.9 (2.3–6.4)
Colonic mucosal flora		
Number of samples	6	10
Total aerobes	6–5.6 (4.1–6.0)	10–6.7 (1.7–7.6)
Total anaerobes	6.1 (3.1–6.3)	6.6 (3.4–7.4)
Percentage distribution		
Aerobes: Gram⁻ rods	45%	59%
Gram⁺ rods	14%	9%
Gram⁺ cocci	40%	32%
Anaerobes: Bacteroides	64%	61%
Bifidobacteria	9%	14%
Clostridia	4%	6%

Crohn's disease, there was a large decrease in the number of mucosal bacteroides and coliforms,[69] whereas in the lumen only the bacteroides were significantly decreased (Table 6). Bacteriologically, these results can be rationalized since metronidazole is secreted into the colon (rather than reaching the colon from higher in the gastrointestinal tract) and so might have a much greater opportunity to interact with the mucosal flora. Clinically, there was no clear relation between the effect of the antibiotics on any component of the mucosal flora and on symptoms of the disease.

TABLE 6. Microbial Flora of Rectal Mucosa of Patients with Crohn's Disease, before and during Combination Treatment with Metronidazole and Cotrimoxazole

	Bacterial count before therapy (Mean ± SD)	Bacterial count during therapy (Mean ± SD)	*P* value
Total flora	6.4 ± 1.2	5.9 ± 0.9	NS
Total anaerobes	6.4 ± 1.3	5.2 ± 1.5	<0.05
B. fragilis group	5.6 ± 1.2	4.4 ± 1.6	<0.02
Veillonellae	3.3 ± 0.6	<3.0	<0.05
Sporing clostridia	3.1 ± 0.2	3.1 ± 0.3	NS
Total aerobes	5.3 ± 0.9	5.5 ± 0.6	NS
Coliforms	5.0 ± 1.1	4.1 ± 1.2	<0.05
Streptococci	4.4 ± 1.0	5.4 ± 0.6	<0.02
Lactobacilli	3.2 ± 0.5	3.3 ± 0.6	NS

Bacterial counts expressed as $\log_{10}$ colony forming units (cfu) per gram wet weight. SD = standard deviation; NS = not significant (Students' paired *t* test). (Taken from Hudson *et al.*[69])

Conclusions

To date there is no clear relationship between the gut bacterial flora and the initiation or maintenance of IBD, but there is enough inconclusive evidence to persuade many groups to keep looking. Perhaps it would be better to study the metabolic activities of the flora rather than the names assigned to them by classical bacteriology. In this respect, two studies can be used to illustrate the type of approach that might be useful.

Metabolic studies

To illustrate this approach, the report by Wiel-Korstanje and Winkler[8] and our own study will be described.

Wiel-Korstanje and Winkler followed up the lead given by Weijers and Van der Kamer[52] that the metabolic products of the gut flora might aggravate the symptoms of IBD and so prevent recovery. They studied the ability of the flora to degrade hyaluronic acid and chondroitin sulphate (and so facilitate tissue damage) and to degrade mucin (thereby exposing the mucosa). Since the enterococci were the organisms present in much greater numbers in the feces of their UC patients compared with controls, they concentrated their efforts on these organisms. Strains from both patients and controls produced mucinase and chondroitinase, but only those from the colitics produced hyaluronidase. Feces from colitics contains very high concentrations of lactic acid and they suggested that this might be due to the metabolism of the increased amount of mucin secreted by colitics and to the metabolism of the unprotected hyaluronic acid in the ulcers.

Gould[70] demonstrated that there was a higher concentration of prostaglandins in the feces of patients with ulcerative colitis than in those of control persons; their production could be inhibited *in vitro* by sulphasalazine and by 5-aminosalicyclic acid, and so it was postulated that they might be important in maintaining the disease state in UC. Several groups of workers have demonstrated increased prostanoid synthesis by colorectal mucosa of active UC patients, when assayed both *in vitro*[71-73] and *in vivo*[74] compared with controls or patients with quiescent UC. Not all inhibitors of prostaglandin synthesis have proved useful for disease management—indomethacin and flurbiprofen (both very powerful inhibitors of prostaglandin synthesis *in vitro* and *in vivo*) have been shown to be without effect when used as treatment in acute UC.[75,76] Moore and Hoult[77] suggest that this apparent paradox may be explained in terms of differential activity of prostaglandin inhibitors against synthesis and metabolism. We have shown[78] that colonic bacteria from both UC patients and controls were able to synthesize prostaglandins E_2 and $F_{2\alpha}$ from arachidonic acid (present in fecal fats) and that the ratio of E_2 to

$F_{2\alpha}$ (approximately 3 to 1) is similar to that observed in feces in acute UC. This synthesis was inhibited by salazopyrin and 5-aminosalicylic acid. The exact role played by colonic bacteria in prostaglandin synthesis within the colon is unknown, but suggests a role for bacterial metabolism in the pathogenesis of IBD.

CANCER IN INFLAMMATORY BOWEL DISEASE

Struthers first suggested that there was a link between ulcerative colitis and colon cancer in 1920, and since then there have been many studies confirming the link. The subject was studied systematically by McDougall[79)] who showed that the risk of malignancy in patients with UC increased with the duration of symptoms, the age of onset, and the amount of colon involved. Patients with subtotal involvement of the colon had only a slight excess risk, and there was no excess risk in patients whose symptoms had lasted less than 10 years. If the age of onset was less than 25 years, then the risk of malignancy was 2.5 fold greater than in persons with the same duration of symptoms but an older age of onset.

Although there have been few good studies, there are strong indications that Crohn's disease of the colon carries the same risk of malignancy as ulcerative colitis (for example, Weedon *et al.*[80)]; Greenstein *et al.*[81)]) with the same 10-year latency.

In general, a patient who has had ulcerative colitis with total colonic involvement for more than 10 years is happy to accept a prophylactic colectomy to prevent a malignancy (since it also cures the colitis), but there are more than 100 patients who attend the outpatient clinic at St. Mark's Hospital and have elected to retain their colon and have regular examintions for pre-cancer of the large bowel. We have studied these patients in order to determine whether we can predict which patients will develop a malignancy and which will remain free of cancer.

Study of the feces of these patients revealed that their flora was indistinguishable from that of healthy control persons. However, we have postulated that clostridia, which are able to produce unsaturated bile acids (referred to as NDC[82)]), are implicated in the causation of large bowel cancer[83)] and we have tested this hypothesis in patients at St. Mark's Hospital who have had ulcerative colitis for more than 10 years.

The patients attend the outpatient clinic regularly (and usually annually) for examination, and at these visits a fecal sample is collected and analyzed for the presence of NDC[84)] and for total fecal bile acid concentration.[85)] Since the patients have been followed for many years, a number of analyses is available for each patient and so a "running mean" value of the fecal bile acid concentration is obtained, together with a measure of the stability of the carriage of NDC. Carriage of NDC appears to be a very stable character in these patients (Table 7): of those for whom we have analyses for more than four years, 22/26 (85%) gave the same result on all occasions and only one (4%) gave a result different from the majority on more than one occasion.

TABLE 7. Stability of Carriage cf NDC in Patients with Chronic Ulcerative Colitis

Follow-up years	Number of patients	All samples agree	Number of patients in which		
			one sample differs[+]	two samples differ[+]	more than two differ[+]
6–8	10	7	3	0	0
5	5	4	0	1	0
4	11	11	0	0	–
3	30	24	6	–*	–
2	9	7	2	–	–

Serial specimens of feces collected at 12-month intervals were assayed for NDC and the patient then classified either as a carrier or as a non-carrier on the basis of the result most commonly obtained.
[+]The number of samples in which the result differs from that in the majority.
*Not applicable.

The proportion of colitis patients carrying NDC was lower than that in normal persons (Table 8). Of the 7 patients who had a colectomy because of severe relapse in their colitis, 4 were in the group where NDC status was unknown (and would not be determinable); the remaining 10 patients

TABLE 8. Carriage of NDC by Patients with Chronic Ulcerative Colitis

	NDC carriers	NDC non-carriers	Unknown NDC status
All chronic UC patients	26	66	14
Patients who died 1974–1981	0	3	0
Those given a colectomy for colitis	1	2	4
Those who developed severe dysplasia (SD) or carcinoma (Ca)	5	3	0
Those who developed mild or moderate dysplasia (MD)	2	9	0
Those with FBA concentration > 10mg/g	8 (31% of total)	14 (21% of total)	2
Those with D or Ca	5 (63%)	3 (21%)	0
Those with FBA concentration < 10mg/g	18	52	12
Those with SD or Ca	0	0	0

in whom the NDC status was unknown were poor attenders of the out-patient clinic and their NDC had not been assayed on the few samples (usually one) available because of antibiotics, insufficient sample size, etc. Of the 26 NDC carriers, 7 (27%) had dysplasia and 5 of those (19%) had developed an early carcinoma. Of the 66 non-carriers of NDC, 12 (18%) had dysplasia, 3 of whom (5%) had progressed to early carcinoma.

The mean fecal bile acid (FBA) concentration in the 106 patients was 7.9 mg/g dry weight, and 24 (23%) had an FBA concentration greater than 10 mg/g dry weight. There was no correlation between carriage of NDC and FBA concentration: of those with a high FBA concentration, 8 (33%) carried NDC and 14 (58%) did not. However, of those with a high FBA concentration who carried NDC, 5 (63%) have subsequently developed a carcinoma; of those with a high FBA concentration who did not carry NDC, 3 (21%) have subsequently developed a carcinoma; whereas of those 82 patients whose FBA concentration was less than 10 mg/g dry weight, none has developed a carcinoma.

These are of course preliminary results. However, if they are supported by subsequent findings, then they will give strong support to the hypothesis that metabolites of the bile acids produced by NDC are implicated in the causation of large bowel cancer.

Acknowledgments

The work from this laboratory described here was financially supported by the Cancer Research Campaign, the Wellcome Foundation, and the British Digestive Foundation, to all of whom we would like to express our thanks.

REFERENCES

1. Lockhart-Mummery, H. E. and Morson, B. C.: Crohn's disease (regional enteritis) of the large bowel and its distinction from ulcerative colitis. *Gut*, **1**: 87–105, 1960.
2. Price, A. B.: Difficulties in the differential diagnosis of ulcerative colitis and Crohn's disease. In: The Gastrointestinal Tract (ed. J. Yardley, B. Morson, and M. Abell), pp. 1–14. Williams and Wilkins, Baltimore, 1977.
3. Lennard-Jones, J. E.: Crohn's disease: definition, pathogenesis and aetiology. In: Recent Advances in Gastrointestinal Pathology (ed. R. Wright), pp. 173–189. W. Saunders, London, 1980.
4. Bargan, J. A.: The etiology of chronic ulcerative colitis. *J. Am. Med. Ass.*, **83**: 332–336, 1924.
5. Dack, G. M., Heinz, T. F., and Kirsner, J. B.: *Bacterium necrophorum* in chronic ulcerative colitis. *J. Am. Med. Ass.*, **106**: 7, 1936.
6. Kirsner, J. B. and Palmer, W. L.: Ulcerative colitis: consideration of its etiology and treatment. *J. Am. Med. Ass.*, **155**: 341–346, 1954.

7. Weinstein, L.: Bacteriologic aspects of ulcerative colitis. *Gastroenterology*, **40**: 323–330, 1961.
8. Wiel-Korstanje, J. A. A. and Winkler, K. C.: The faecal flora in ulcerative colitis. *J. Med. Microbiol.*, **8**: 491–501, 1975.
9. Gorbach, S. L., Nahas, L., Plaut, A. G., *et al.*: Studies of intestinal microflora. V. Fecal microbial ecology in ulcerative colitis and regional enteritis: relationship to severity of disease and chemotherapy. *Gastroenterology*, **54**: 575–587, 1968.
10. Cooke, E. M.: Properties of strains of *Escherichia coli* isolated from the faeces of patients with ulcerative colitis, patients with acute diarrhoea and normal persons. *J. Path. Bact.*, **95**: 101-113, 1968.
11. Cooke, E. M., Ewins, S. P., Hywel-Jones, J., *et al.*: Properties of strains of *Escherichia coil* carried in different phases of ulcerative colitis. *Gut,* **15**: 143–146, 1974.
12. Aluwihare, A. P. R.: Electron microscopy in Crohn's disease. *Gut*, **12**: 509–518, 1971.
13. Cave, D. R., Mitchell, D. N., Kane, S. P., *et al.*: Further animal evidence of a transmissible agent in Crohn's disease. *Lancet*, **2**: 1120–1122, 1973.
14. Cave, D. R., Mitchell, D. N., and Brooke, B. N.: Experimental animal studies of the etiology and pathogenesis of Crohn's disease. *Gastroenterology*, **69**: 618–624, 1975.
15. Cave, D. R., Mitchell, D. N., and Brooke, B. N.: Induction of granulomas in mice by Crohn's disease tissues. *Gastroenterology*, **75**: 635–637, 1978.
16. Cave, D. R., Mitchell, D. N., and Brooke, B. N.: Evidence of an agent transmissible from ulcerative colitis tissue. *Lancet,* **1**: 1311–1315, 1976.
17. Bolton, P. M., Owen, E., Heatly, R. V., *et al.*: Negative findings in laboratory animals for a transmissible agent in Crohn's disease. *Lancet*, **2**: 1122–1124, 1973.
18. Ahlberg, J., Bergstrand, O., Gillstom, P., *et al.*: Negative findings in search for a transmissible agent in Crohn's disease. *Acta Chir. Scand.* (*Suppl.*), **482**: 45–47, 1978.
19. Sachar, D. B. and Anslander, M. O.: Missing pieces in the puzzle of Crohn's disease. *Gastroenterology*, **75**: 745–748, 1978.
20. Donnelly, B. J., Delaney, P. V., and Healy, T. M.: Evidence for a transmissible factor in Crohn's disease. *Gut*, **18**: 360–363, 1977.
21. Gitnick, G. L., Arthur, M. H., and Shibata, I.: Cultivation of viral agents from Crohn's disease: a new sensitive system. *Lancet*, **2**: 215–217, 1976.
22. Gitnick, G. L. and Rosen, V. J.: Electron microscopic studies of viral agents in Crohn's disease. *Lancet*, **2**: 217–219, 1976.
23. Whorwell, P. J., Phillips, C. A., Beeken, W. L., *et al.*: Isolation of reovirus-like agents from patients with Crohn's disease. *Lancet*, **1**: 1169–1171, 1977.
24. Kapikian, A. Z., Barile, M. F., Wyatt, R. C., *et al.*: Mycoplasma contamination in cell culture of Crohn's disease material. *Lancet*, **2**: 466–467 (correpondence), 1979.
25. Phillpotts, R. J., Herman-Taylor, J., and Brooke, B. N.: Virus isolation studies in Crohn's disease: a negative report. *Gut*, **20**: 1057–1062, 1979.

26. Phillpotts, R. J., Herman-Taylor, J., and Teich, N. M.: A search for persistent virus infection in Crohn's disease. *Gut*, **21**: 202–204, 1980.
27. Parent, K. and Mitchell, P. D.: Bacterial variants: etiologic agents in Crohn's disease? *Gastroenterology*, **71**: 365–368, 1976.
28. Parent, K. and Mitchell, P.: Cell wall-defective variants of pseudomonas-like (Group Va) bacteria in Crohn's disease. *Gastroenterology*, **75**: 368–372, 1978.
29. Shafii, A., Sopher, S., Lev, M., *et al.*: An antibody against revertant forms of cell-wall-deficient bacterial variant in sera from patients with Crohn's disease. *Lancet*, **2**: 332–334, 1981.
30. Whorwell, P. J., Davidson, I. W., Beeken, W. L., and Wright, R.: Search by immunofluorescence for antigens of rotavirus, *Pseudomonas maltophila* and *Mycobacterium kansasii* in Crohn's disease. *Lancet*, **2**: 697–698, 1978.
31. Burnham, W. R., Lennard-Jones, J. E., Stanford, J. L., *et al.*: Mycobacteria as a possible cause of inflammatory bowel disease. *Lancet*, **2**: 693–696, 1978.
32. Stanford, J. L., White, S. A., and Burham, W. R.: Mycobacteria and inflammatory bowel disease. *Lancet*, **1**: 444 (correspondence), 1979.
33. Schuller, J. L., Piket-van Ulsen, J., Veeken, I. V. D., *et al.*: Antibodies against chlamydia of lymphogranuloma-venereum type in Crohn's disease. *Lancet*, **1**: 19–20, 1979.
34. Swarbrick, E. T., Kingham, J. G. C., Price, H. L., *et al.*: Chlamydia, cytomegalovirus, and yersinia in inflammatory bowel disease. *Lancet*, **2**: 11–12, 1979.
35. Taylor-Robinson, D., O'Morain, C. A., Thomas, B. J., *et al.*: Low frequency of chlamydial antibodies in patients with Crohn's disease and ulcerative colitis. *Lancet*, **1**: 1162-1163, 1979.
36. Munro, J., Mayberry, J. F., Matthews, N., *et al.*: Chlamydia and Crohn's disease. *Lancet*, **1**: 45–46 (correspondence), 1979.
37. Elliott, P. R., Forsey, T., Daroufor, S., *et al.*: Chlamydiae and inflammatory bowel disease. *Gut*, **22**: 25–27, 1981.
38. Das, K. M., Valenzuela, I., and Morecki, R.: Crohn's disease lymph node homogenates produce marine lymphoma in athymic mice. *Proc. Natl. Acad. Sci. USA*, **77**: 588–592, 1980.
39. Wensinck, F.: The faecal flora of patients with Crohn's disease. *Ant. v. Leeuwenhoek*, **41**: 214–215, 1975.
40. Wensinck, F.: Faecal flora of Crohn's patients. Serological differentiation between Crohn's disease and ulcerative colitis. In: The Management of Crohn's Disease (ed. I. Westerman, A. S. Pena, and C. Booth), pp. 103–105. Excerpta Medica, Amsterdam, 1976.
41. Wensinck, F., Custers-Van Lieshout, L. M., *et al.*: The fecal flora of patients with Crohn's disease. *J. Hyg.* (Camb.), **87**: 1–12, 1981.
42. Kieghley, M. R., Arabi, Y., Dimock, F., *et al.*: The influence of inflammatory bowel disease on intestinal microflora. *Gut*, **19**: 1099–1104, 1978.
43. Krook, A., Danielsson, D., Kjellander, J., *et al.*: The effect of metronidazole and sulfasalazine on the fecal flora in patients with Crohn's disease. *Scand. J. Gastroenterol.*, **16**: 183–192, 1981.

44. West, B., Lendrum, R., Hill, M. J., *et al.*: Effects of sulphasalazine (Salazopyrin) on faecal flora in patients with inflammatory bowel disease. *Gut*, **15**: 960–965, 1974.
45. LaMont, J. T. and Trika, Y. M.: Therapeutic implications of *Clostridium difficile* toxin during relapse of chronic inflammatory bowel disease. *Lancet*, **1**: 381–383, 1980.
46. Bolton, R. P., Sherriff, R. J., and Read, A. E.: *Clostridium difficile* associated with diarrhoea: a role in inflammatory bowel disease? *Lancet*, **1**: 383–384, 1980.
47. Dorman, S. A., Liggoria, E., Winn, W. C., *et al.*: Isolation of *Clostridium difficile* from patients with inactive Crohn's disease. *Gastroenterology*, **82**: 1348–1351, 1982.
48. Mórain, C. Ó., Prestage, H., Harrison, P., *et al.*: Cytopathic effects in cultures inoculated with material from Crohn's disease. *Gut*, **22**: 823–826, 1981.
49. McLaren, L. C. and Gitnick, G.: Ulcerative colitis and Crohn's disease tissue cytotoxins. *Gastroenterology*, **82**: 1381–1388, 1982.
50. Truelove, S.: Medical management of ulcerative colitis. *Brit. Med. J.*, **2**: 605–607, 1968.
51. De Dombal, F. T.: Ulcerative colitis. Epidemiology and etiology, course and prognosis. *Brit. Med. J.*, **1**: 649–650, 1971.
52. Weijers, H. A. and Van der Kamer, J. H.: Alteration of intestinal bacterial flora as a cause of diarrhoea. *Nutr. Abstr. Rev.*, **35**: 591, 1965.
53. Monteiro, E., Fossey, J., and Shiner, M.: Antibacterial antibodies in rectal and colonic mucosa in ulcerative colitis. *Lancet*, **1**: 249–251, 1971.
54. Seneca, H. and Henderson, E.: Normal intestinal bacteria in ulcerative colitis. *Gastroenterology*, **15**: 34–39, 1950.
55. Goldgraber, M. B. and Kirsner, J. B.: The histopathology of the experimental hypersensitive state in the gastrointestinal tract: a critical review. *Arch. Int. Med.*, **102**: 134–148, 1958.
56. Bendixen, G.: Cellular hypersensitivity to components of intestinal mucosa in ulcerative colitis and Crohn's disease. *Gut*, **10**: 631–636, 1969.
57. Helphingstine, C. J., Hentges, D. J., *et al.*: Antibodies detectable by counterimmunoelectrophoresis against *Bacteroides* antigens in serum of patients with inflammatory bowel disease. *J. Clin. Microbiol.*, **9**: 373–378, 1979.
58. Lindberg, A. A., Weinstraub, A., and Nord, C. E.: The humoral antibody response to *Bacteroides fragilis* infections in humans. *Scand. J. Inf. Dis.* (*Suppl.*), **19**: 46–51, 1979.
59. Persson, S. and Danielsson, D.: On the occurrence of serum antibodies to *Bacteroides fragilis* and serogroups of *E. coli* in patients with Crohn's disease. *Scand. J. Inf. Dis.* (*Suppl.*), **19**: 61–67, 1979.
60. Wensinck, F. and Van der Merwe, J. P.: Serum agglutinins to *Peptostreptococcus* and *Eubacterium* species in patients with Crohn's and other diseases. *Gut*, **20**: A932, 1979.
61. Gorbach, S. L., Nahas, L., and Weinstein, L.: Studies of intestinal microflora. IV. The microflora of ileostomy effluent: a unique microbial ecology. *Gastroenterology*, **53**: 874–880, 1967.
62. Hori, S., Berghouse, L., Hill, M. J., Hudson, M. J., *et al.*: The microbio-

logical and oligosaccharide content of ileostomy fluid in subjects taking an unrefined and a refined carbohydrate diet. *Gut*, 1984.
63. Finegold, S. M., Sutter, V. L., Boyle, J. D., *et al.*: The normal flora of ileostomy and transverse colostomy effluents. *J. Inf. Dis.*, **122**: 376–381, 1970.
64. Scarpino, P. V., Deters, L. E., and Niemeier, R. W.: Investigations of the types and numbers of aerobic and anaerobic bacteria occurring in intestinal specimens obtained from adult human ileostomy and colostomy subjects. *Bact. Proc.*, p. 103, 1969.
65. Peach, S. L., Drasar, B. S., Harley, P. R., *et al.*: Mucosal flora of the human colon. *Gut*, **16**: 824, 1975.
66. Peach, S., Lock, R., Katz, D., *et al.*: Mucosa-associated bacterial flora of the intestine in patients with Crohn's disease and in a control group. *Gut*, **19**: 1034–1042, 1978.
67. Peach, S. L. and Tabaqchali, S.: Mucosa-associated flora of the human gastrointestinal tract in health and disease. *Eur. J. Chemother. Antibiot.*, **2**: 41–50, 1982.
68. Marks, C. G., Hawley, P. R., Peach, S. L., *et al.*: The effects of phthalylsulphathiazole on the bacteria of the colonic mucosa as revealed by examintion of surgical samples. *Scand. J. Gastroenterol.*, **14**: 891–895, 1979.
69. Hudson, M. J., Hill, M. J., Elliott, P. R., *et al.*: The microbial flora of the rectal mucosa and faeces of patients with Crohn's disease before and during antimicrobial chemotherapy. (Submitted for publication.)
70. Gould, S. R. and Lennard-Jones, J.: Production of prostaglandins in ulcerative colitis and their inhibition by sulphasalazine. *Gut*, **17**: 828, 1976.
71. Harris, D. W., Smith, P. R., and Swan, C. H. J.: Determination of prostaglandin synthetase activity in rectal biopsy material and its significance in colonic disease. *Gut*, **19**: 875–877, 1978.
72. Sharon, P., Ligunsky, M., Rachmilewitz, D., *et al.*: Role of prostaglandins in ulcerative colitis: Enhanced production during active illness and inhibition by sulphasalazine. *Gastroenterology*, **75** 4: 638–640, 1970.
73. Ligunsky, M., Karemli, F., Sharon, P., *et al.*: Enhanced thromboxane A_2 and prostacyline production by cultured rectal mucosa in ulcerative colitis and its inhibition by steroids and sulfasalazine. *Gastroenterology*, **81**: 444–449, 1981.
74. Rampton, D. S., Sladen, G. E., and Youlten, L. J. F.: Rectal mucosal prostaglandin E_2 release and its relation to disease activity, electrical potential difference and treatment in ulcerative colitis. *Gut*, **21**: 591–596, 1980.
75. Gilat, T., Tatan, J., Rosen, P., *et al.*: Prostaglandins and ulcerative colitis. Indomethacin retention enemas given over 2 weeks period had *no* benefit. *Gastroenterology*, **76**: 1083 (correspondence), 1979.
76. Rampton, D. S. and Sladen, G. E.: Prostaglandin synthesis inhibitors in ulcerative colitis: flurbiprofen compared with conventional treatment. *Prostaglandins*, **21**: 417–425, 1981.
77. Moore, P. K. and Hoult, J. R. S.: Selective actions of aspirin- and sulphasalazine-like drugs against prostaglandin synthesis and breakdown. *Biochem. Pharm.*, **31** 6: 969–971, 1982.
78. Hudson, M. J., Hill, M. J., Gould, S. R., *et al.*: Bacteria, prostaglandins and

ulcerative colitis. *Gut*, **19** 10: A989 (abstract), 1978.
79. MacDougall, I. P. M.: The cancer risk in ulcerative colitis. *Lancet*, **2**:655–658, 1964.
80. Weedon, D. D., Shorter, R. G., and Ilstinp, D. M.: Crohn's disease and cancer. *N. Engl. J. Med.*, **289**: 1099–1102, 1973.
81. Greenstein, A. J., Sachar, D. B., Smith, H., *et al.*: A comparison of the cancer risk in Crohn's disease and ulcerative colitis. *Cancer,* **48**: 2742–2745, 1981.
82. Goddard, P., Fernandez, F., West, B., *et al.*: The nuclear dehydrogenation of steroids by intestinal bacteria. *J. Med. Microbiol.*, **8**: 429–435, 1975.
83. Cohen, B., Borriello, S. P., and Hill, M. J.: Carriage rates of nuclear dehydrogenating clostridia (NDC) in groups at various levels of risk of colorectal cancer. *Eur. J. Chemother. Antibiot.*, **2**: 162–163, 1982.
84. Borriello, S. P.: Clostridial flora of the gastrointestinal tract in health and disease. PhD. thesis (Univ. of London), 1981.
85. Cummings, J., Wiggins, H., Jenkins, D., *et al.*: The influence of different levels of dietary fat intake on faecal composition, microflora and gastrointestinal transit time. *J. Clin. Invest.,* **61**: 953–963, 1978.

Bacterial Groups of the Intestinal Microflora in Inflammatory Bowel Disease in Japan

Shinji Hori and Takashi Shimoyama

A possible role for the intestinal microflora in the etiology of various disease states has recently been suggested. It is generally understood that the intestinal microflora might play a role as a so-called functional unit and that an imbalance in it might be the more important aspect. It is thought that the existence of causative microorganisms is rather doubtful. In our department we have studied 93 ulcerative colitis and 13 Crohn's disease patients who were investigated bacteriologically for the past 8 years and were compared with 37 healthy subjects. Bacteriological data from the cases of ulcerative colitis were correlated with stool condition, stage, and distribution of the disease.

METHODS AND SUBJECTS

In this study, the microbiological methods used were those of Mitsuoka and were identified on either the family or genus level, except for the Enterobacteriaceae which were identified on the species level.

We studied 93 patients with ulcerative colitis (UC), 13 patients with Crohn's disease (CD), and 37 healthy controls. The age and sex distributions of each group are shown in Table 1. We chose healthy volunteer doctors

TABLE 1. Background Data on Study Subjects

	No.	Age (years)		Male	Female
		Mean	Range		
Ulcerative colitis	93	30.9	13–55	32	61
active	68	34.9	13–55	16	52
in remission	25	31.5	16–52	16	9
Crohn's disease	13	25.3	16–39	5	8
Healthy subjects	37	29.8	25–42	36	1

Fourth Department of Internal Medicine, Hyogo College of Medicine, Nishinomiya, Hyogo, Japan

from our department as a control group, and all but one were male. The age and sex distributions of each group were similar.

RESULTS

Fecal bacterial counts of 37 healthy subjects are shown in Table 2. Values are expressed as $\log_{10}$ bacterial count per gram of wet feces and the figures in parentheses indicate numbers of subjects in whom the bacterial groups were present. In this study, detectable bacterial counts were more than 200 per gram of wet feces. It is generally understood that total obligate anaerobes comprise approximately 10^{11} per gram of wet feces of healthy Japanese people, and our data have similarly shown approximately $10^{10.8}$. On the other hand, total facultative anaerobes comprise approximately 10^8 and consequently the ratio of total facultative anaerobes to total obligate anaerobes is about 1,000 to 1.

TABLE 2. Fecal Bacterial Counts of 37 Healthy Subjects

Bacterial groups	$\log_{10}$ bacterial count per gram of wet feces	No. of subjects harboring
Facultative anaerobes	8.1 ± 0.9	(37)
Enterobacteriaceae	7.7 ± 1.1	(37)
Streptococcus	7.3 ± 1.0	(37)
Micrococcaceae	3.4 ± 0.9	(26)
Yeasts	3.8 ± 1.2	(24)
Lactobacillus	6.5 ± 1.5	(35)
Obligate anaerobes	10.8 ± 0.4	(37)
Bifidobacterium	9.8 ± 0.7	(37)
Eubacterium	9.4 ± 0.7	(37)
Bacteroidaceae	10.4 ± 0.5	(37)
Peptococcaceae	9.7 ± 0.8	(37)
Clostridium	8.7 ± 1.3	(32)
Veillonella	7.4 ± 1.4	(20)

Of the facultative anaerobes, the Enterobacteriaceae and streptococci comprised the predominant bacterial groups, and Micrococcaceae, including staphylococci and yeasts, comprised the minor components; in addition their frequency of occurrence was low.

Corynebacteria and bacilli are omitted from Table 2 since they showed a wide variation from person to person and since the frequency of occurrence was low.

Lactobacilli tend to be isolated in most Japanese people. The bacterial counts were only 10^6–10^7/g, and they could not be isolated in some cases.

Of the obligate anaerobes, the Bacteroidaceae, bifidobacteria, eubacteria, and Peptococcaceae comprised the predominant bacterial groups, and they were isolated from all of the healthy controls.

Table 3 shows the genera of Enterobacteriaceae in the feces of 25 healthy subjects. *E. coli* were isolated from all of the subjects and were numerically predominant. This is said to be characteristic of the fecal flora of Japanese adults. *Citrobacter, Enterobacter*, and *Klebsiella* were isolated occasionally, but *Proteus* was not isolated from healthy controls.

TABLE 3. Genera of Enterobacteriaceae in Feces of 25 Healthy Subjects

Bacterial genera	Log_{10} bacterial count		No. of subjects harboring
	Range	Mean	
Escherichia	5.2–9.1	7.4	25
Citrobacter	4.3–7.7	6.5	3
Enterobacter	6.6–7.1	6.8	3
Klebsiella	3.0–8.9	6.1	12
Serratia	6.4	6.4	1
Proteus	ND	ND	0

ND: none detected (less than 200 organisms per gram of wet feces).

Fecal flora and stool condition of UC patients

Fecal flora of 68 patients with active ulcerative colitis were compared with those of healthy controls, separating the results for the patients according to stool condition and obvious presence of blood (Table 4).

Total facultative anaerobes tended to increase regardless of stool condition or presence of blood, although they were significantly increased in formed stool. Of the bacterial groups, streptococci were significantly increased regardless of stool condition, and the Enterobacteriaceae were significantly increased in cases with formed bloody stool. Total obligate anaerobes were decreased in active ulcerative colitis regardless of stool condition, and, therefore, it should be noted that the fall in total obligate anerobes was not due to diarrhea. Bifidobacteria, Bacteroidaceae, and Peptococcaceae were significantly decreased independent of stool condition, although bifidobacteria were not isolated in one third of the active cases.

Eubacteria were not isolated in about 10% of the active cases with loose stool, and their absence was more remarkable in the cases with loose stool and diarrhea.

In the Enterobacteriaceae, *E. coli* tend to become a minor component in the active cases, and this tendency was more remarkable in the cases with bloody stool (Table 5). In addition to this tendency, it should be emphasized that *Proteus*, which were not isolated from feces of healthy controls, were isolated surprisingly often in active ulcerative colitis, in

TABLE 4. Fecal Bacterial Counts in Patients with Ulcerative Colitis—Correlation with Stool Condition in Active Stage

Bacterial groups \ Stool condition	Loose stool, diarrhea		Formed stool	
	Bloody stool ($n = 24$)	Not bloody ($n = 6$)	Bloody stool ($n = 31$)	Not bloody ($n = 7$)
Facultative anaerobes	8.5 ± 1.0 (24)	8.7 ± 0.3 (6)	8.8 ± 0.8* (31)	9.3 ± 0.4* (7)
Enterobacteriaceae	8.0 ± 0.9 (24)	8.3 ± 0.4 (6)	8.2 ± 0.7* (31)	8.6 ± 0.8* (7)
Streptococcus	8.3 ± 1.0* (24)	8.3 ± 0.5* (6)	8.3 ± 1.1* (31)	9.1 ± 0.3* (7)
Micrococcaceae	3.5 ± 1.5 (23)	8.3 ± 0.5 (5)	3.9 ± 1.9 (16)	3.6 ± 0.7 (7)
Yeasts	4.2 ± 1.3 (19)	4.3 ± 1.4 (6)	4.6 ± 1.5 (20)	5.1 ± 1.5* (7)
Lactobacillus	6.0 ± 2.3 (21)	5.5 ± 1.5 (6)	5.8 ± 1.8 (25)	5.8 ± 2.5 (6)
Obligate anaerobes	9.4 ± 1.2* (24)	9.5 ± 0.8* (6)	10.1 ± 0.5* (31)	10.3 ± 0.3* (7)
Bifidobacterium	8.7 ± 1.7* (17)	9.0 ± 0.3* (4)	9.3 ± 0.6* (21)	8.8 ± 0.9* (5)
Eubacterium	8.6 ± 1.7* (21)	8.6 ± 1.0* (5)	9.0 ± 0.8* (31)	9.0 ± 0.9 (7)
Bacteroidaceae	9.2 ± 1.1* (23)	8.2 ± 2.9* (6)	9.6 ± 1.0* (30)	9.9 ± 0.7* (7)
Peptococcaceae	8.2 ± 1.9* (19)	8.7 ± 0.6* (6)	8.8 ± 0.6* (29)	8.4 ± 2.0* (6)
Clostridium	6.9 ± 2.1* (19)	7.1 ± 2.5* (5)	7.5 ± 2.0* (29)	9.0 ± 1.0 (7)
Veillonella	7.4 ± 1.6 (11)	6.5 ± 1.7 (5)	6.6 ± 1.6* (15)	7.7 ± 0.4 (3)

Log_{10} bacterial counts per gram of wet feces.
*Significantly different from the healthy control group ($p < 0.05$).
( ): No. of subjects in whom the bacterial groups were present.

TABLE 5. Genera of Enterobacteriaceae in Feces of Patients with Ulcerative Colitis—Correlation with Stool Condition in Active Stage

Stool condition / Bacterial genera	Loose stool, diarrhea				Formed stool			
	Bloody stool (n = 24)		Not bloody (n = 6)		Bloody stool (n = 31)		Not bloody (n = 7)	
	Range	Mean	Range	Mean	Range	Mean	Range	Mean
Escherichia	6.7–8.9	7.9 (16)	7.9–8.9	8.3 (4)	6.5–9.4	8.1 (21)	7.7–9.7	8.1 (7)
Citrobacter	5.2–7.3	6.3 (2)		ND		ND		ND
Enterobacter	6.1–7.3	6.8 (3)	6.3–7.3	6.8 (2)	4.2–6.6	5.4 (2)		6.3 (1)
Klebsiella	4.4–9.0	6.9 (10)	6.0–8.4	7.3 (3)	4.3–7.4	6.0 (9)	6.3–9.2	8.0 (5)
Serratia		6.7 (1)		6.3 (1)		ND		ND
Proteus	3.8–8.9	6.9 (12)	7.0–7.5	7.3 (2)	4.4–8.0	6.9 (12)	6.3–8.9	7.6 (3)

Log_{10} bacterial counts per gram of wet feces.
ND: none detected (less than 200 organisms per gram of feces).
( ): No. of subjects in whom the bacterial groups were present.

about half of the cases with loose bloody stool, bloody diarrhea, and formed bloody stool; among them the ratio of strains producing H_2S was relatively high.

Moreover, *Proteus* were isolated in about one third of the cases without bloody stool and *Klebsiella* in more than half of the cases without bloody stool.

Fecal flora and type of clinical course of UC

We have grouped the patients with active ulcerative colitis into three: first-attack type, relapsing type, and continuous type (Table 6). The total number of facultative anaerobes had a tendency to increase and was significantly increased in both the relapsing and continuous types. Specifically, the bacterial counts in the relapsing type were significantly higher than in those in the first-attack type.

Streptococci were also significantly increased in the relapsing and continuous types, and in addition they were significantly increased in these two types compared with those in the first-attack type.

In the relapsing type, the Enterobacteriaceae were significantly increased. Moreover, the frequencies of occurrence of Micrococcaceae and yeasts in both first-attack and relapsing patients were higher than those in the healthy control groups; and in the relapsing type, counts of those two groups were significantly higher than those with a first attack of colitis.

TABLE 6. Fecal Bacterial Counts in Patients with Ulcerative Colitis—Correlation with Clinical Course in Active Stage

Bacterial groups \ Type of clinical course	First-attack ($n = 14$)		Relapsing ($n = 27$)		Continuous ($n = 27$)	
Facultative anaerobes	8.5 ± 0.6	(14)	9.0 ± 0.6*,#	(27)	8.7 ± 0.9*	(27)
Enterobacteriaceae	8.3 ± 0.5	(14)	8.4 ± 0.7*	(27)	7.9 ± 0.9	(27)
Streptococcus	7.7 ± 1.4	(14)	8.6 ± 0.8*,#	(27)	8.6 ± 0.8*,#	(27)
Micrococcaceae	3.6 ± 0.7	(13)	4.1 ± 1.6#	(21)	3.8 ± 0.8	(16)
Yeasts	3.8 ± 1.1	(10)	4.7 ± 1.5	(20)	4.8 ± 1.3*	(22)
Lactobacillus	5.2 ± 2.0	(11)	6.4 ± 1.9	(22)	5.7 ± 2.1	(25)
Obligate anaerobes	9.4 ± 0.9*	(14)	9.7 ± 0.9*	(27)	10.1 ± 0.8*	(27)
Bifidobacterium	8.8 ± 0.8*	(8)	8.9 ± 1.6*	(20)	9.2 ± 0.7*	(19)
Eubacterium	8.7 ± 1.0*	(13)	8.4 ± 1.4*	(25)	9.3 ± 0.8#	(26)
Bacteroidaceae	9.2 ± 0.7*	(13)	9.2 ± 1.3*	(26)	9.8 ± 0.8*	(27)
Peptococcaceae	8.1 ± 1.2*	(12)	8.8 ± 1.3*	(22)	8.6 ± 1.4*	(26)
Clostridium	7.2 ± 2.1*	(13)	7.3 ± 2.4*	(24)	7.6 ± 1.9*	(23)
Veillonella	7.1 ± 1.3	(10)	7.1 ± 1.8	(17)	6.3 ± 1.6	(7)

Log_{10} bacterial counts per gram of wet feces.
( ): No. of subjects in whom the bacterial groups were present.
*Significantly different from the healthy control group ($p < 0.05$).
#Significantly different from the first-attack type.

TABLE 7. Genera of Enterobacteriaceae in Feces of Patients with Ulcerative Colitis—Correlation with Clinical Course in Active Stage

Bacterial genera \ Type of clinical course	First-attack ($n = 14$) Range	Mean	Relapsing ($n = 27$) Range	Mean	Continuous ($n = 27$) Range	Mean
Esherichia	6.5–8.8	8.0 (13)	7.3–9.7	8.5 (12)	5.9–9.0	7.9 (23)
Citrobacter	ND		ND		5.2–7.3	6.3 (2)
Enterobacter	4.2–6.3	5.3 (2)	6.6–7.3	6.9 (3)	6.1–7.3	6.6 (3)
Klebsiella	5.5–8.8	7.0 (7)	4.3–9.0	7.0 (10)	4.6–9.2	6.7
Serratia	ND			6.7 (1)		6.3 (1)
Proteus	5.3–7.6	6.1 (8)	3.8–8.9	7.4 (14)	4.4–7.9	6.2 (10)

Log_{10} bacterial counts per gram of wet feces.
ND: none detected (less than 200 organisms per gram of feces).
( ): No. of subjects in whom the bacterial groups were present.

Total obligate anaerobes were significantly decreased independently of clinical course. Bifidobacteia were not isolated in about 40% of the first-attack patients and in about 25–30% of both relapsing and continuous types. Moreover, the counts in those cases in which it was detected were significantly decreased compared with controls.

Eubacterium spp. were significantly decreased in the first-attack and relapsing types, and in some cases of all three types they were not isolated at all.

Bacteroidaceae were significantly decreased independently of clinical course. This tendency was more marked in the first-attack and relapsing types.

Peptococcaceae were also significantly decreased independent of clinical course, and in the first-attack type this tendency was especially remarkable. The frequency of occurrence of clostridia was similar to that in healthy control groups, but the bacterial counts in those cases where they were detected were significantly decreased independently of clinical course.

Genera of Enterobacteriaceae in feces of patients with active ulcerative colitis are shown in Table 7. *E. coli* were isolated in the first-attack type, but they were not isolated in 15 out of 27 cases of the relapsing type.

Klebsiella were isolated in 7 out of 14 of the first-attack type and in 10 each out of 27 of the relapsing and continuous types, respectively. *Proteus* were isolated in about half of the cases of the first-attack and relapsing types and in 10 out of 27 cases of the continuous type.

Fecal flora and distribution and stage of UC

We have grouped patients with active ulcerative colitis into two types according to distribution of the disease—total colitis, left-sided colitis, and proctitis—and also compared active cases with cases in remission (Table 8).

TABLE 8. Fecal Bacterial Counts in Patients with Ulcerative Colitis—Correlation with Distribution and Stage of the Disease

Bacterial groups \ Distribution and stage of disease	Active: Total colitis and left-sided colitis ($n = 54$)		Active: Proctitis ($n = 14$)		In remission ($n = 25$)	
Facultative anaerobes	8.8 ± 0.8*	(54)	8.7 ± 0.9*	(14)	8.6 ± 0.7*	(25)
Enterobacteriaceae	8.2 ± 0.8*	(54)	8.0 ± 0.7	(14)	8.1 ± 0.9	(25)
Streptococcus	8.4 ± 1.1*	(54)	8.4 ± 0.9*	(14)	8.4 ± 0.7*	(25)
Micrococcaceae	3.8 ± 1.8	(40)	3.5 ± 0.7	(10)	3.9 ± 2.0	(16)
Yeasts	4.7 ± 1.4*	(42)	3.9 ± 1.3	(10)	4.5 ± 1.2	(20)
Lactobacillus	6.4 ± 2.0	(44)	4.3 ± 1.1	(10)	7.0 ± 2.1	(21)
Obligate anaerobes	9.7 ± 1.0*	(54)	10.2 ± 0.5*	(14)	10.3 ± 0.4*	(25)
Bifidobacterium	9.0 ± 1.3*	(35)	8.9 ± 0.7*	(12)	9.6 ± 0.5*	(24)
Eubacterium	8.8 ± 1.3*	(50)	9.0 ± 1.0*	(14)	9.2 ± 0.8	(25)
Bacteroidaceae	9.3 ± 1.1*	(52)	9.6 ± 2.0*	(14)	9.9 ± 0.5*	(25)
Peptococcaceae	8.4 ± 1.3*	(47)	8.9 ± 1.4*	(13)	8.8 ± 0.8*	(23)
Clostridium	7.1 ± 2.2*	(46)	8.4 ± 1.3	(14)	6.7 ± 2.7*	(23)
Veillonella	7.2 ± 1.5	(27)	6.2 ± 1.9	(7)	6.7 ± 2.3	(14)

Log_{10} bacterial counts per gram of wet feces.
*Significantly different from the healthy control group ($p < 0.05$).
( ): No. of subjects in whom the bacterial groups were present.

Total facultative anaerobes were significantly increased independently of distribution and stage of the disease. Streptococci were similarly significantly increased. Enterobacteriaceae also had a tendency to increase compared to controls, and this tendency was more marked in the total and left-sided colitis type in active-stage patients.

Yeast also had a tendency to increase independently of stage of the disease, and in the total and left-sided colitis type, they were isolated in 42 out of 54 cases, where they were significantly increased.

Lactobacilli were not isolated in 4 out of 14 cases of proctitis, and bacterial counts were low. The percentage of frequency of cases in which lactobacilli were not isolated in the total and left-sided colitis type and cases in remission was higher than that of healthy control groups.

Total obligate anaerobes were significantly decreased independently of distribution and stage of the disease. In particular, the tendency was remarkable in the total and left-sided colitis type.

Bacteroidaceae and Peptococcaceae were also significantly decreased independently of distribution and stage of the disease. This decrease in bifidobacteria was marked in the active stage, and 19 out of 54 cases of total and left-sided colitis had no bifidobacteria detectable. Bacteroidaceae and Peptococcaceae showed a more remarkable decrease in total and left-sided colitis and they were not isolated in 2 and 7 cases, respectively.

Eubacteria were significantly decreased in active-stage patients, and clostridia were significantly decreased in the total and left-sided colitis type and in cases in remission.

Table 9 shows the genera of the Enterobacteriaceae in feces of patients with ulcerative colitis correlated with distribution and stage of the disease. *E. coli* were not isolated in 18 out of 54 cases of total and left-sided colitis in the active stage. Moreover they were not isolated in 2 out of 14 cases of proctitis or in 4 out of 25 cases in remission.

TABLE 9. Genera of Enterobacteriaceae in Feces of Patients with Ulcerative Colitis—Correlation with Distribution and Stage of the Disease

Bacterial genera \ Distribution and stage of disease	Active				In remission ($n = 25$)	
	Total colitis and left-sided colitis ($n = 54$)		Proctitis ($n = 14$)			
	Range	Mean	Range	Mean	Range	Mean
Escherichia	6.5–9.7	8.1 (36)	5.9–8.7	7.9 (12)	6.9–8.9	8.1 (21)
Citrobacter	5.2–7.3	6.1 (2)		ND	4.2–6.9	5.7 (3)
Enterobacter	6.1–7.4	6.8 (9)		7.3 (1)	4.8–6.4	5.6 (2)
Klebsiella	4.6–9.2	7.3 (19)	4.3–7.4	5.8 (8)	4.3–8.1	6.3 (10)
Serratia		6.7 (1)		6.3 (1)		ND
Proteus	3.8–8.9	7.0 (22)	4.4–7.9	6.7 (7)	5.3–8.1	6.6 (8)

Log_{10} bacterial counts per gram of wet feces.
ND: none detected (less than 200 organisms per gram of feces).
( ): No. of subjects in whom the bacterial groups were present.

Enterobacter were isolated in 9 out of 54 cases of total and left-sided colitis in the active stage. *Klebsiella* were isolated in 19 out of 54 of the total and left-sided colitis type, in 8 out of 14 of the proctitis type, and in 10 out of 25 cases in remission. The percentage frequencies of occurrence of each group were higher than that of the healthy control group. *Proteus* were isolated in 22 out of 54 of total and left-sided colitis, in 7 out of 14 of the proctitis type, and in 8 out of 25 cases in remission.

Fecal flora in CD patients

We have so far had 13 cases of Crohn's disease. Since the number of samples is so small, we have gathered all the data in one table regardless of distribution of disease and compared the fecal bacterial counts with those of the healthy control group (Table 10).

Total facultative anaerobes, in particular the Enterobacteriaceae and streptococci, were significantly increased. Yeasts were isolated in 11 of the 13 cases, and their numbers were significantly increased. Lactobacilli

TABLE 10. Fecal Bacterial Counts in 13 Patients with Crohn's Disease

Bacterial groups	Log_{10} bacterial count per gram of wet feces
Facultative anaerobes	9.3 ± 0.9* (13)
Enterobacteriaceae	8.6 ± 0.7* (13)
Streptococcus	9.0 ± 0.4* (13)
Micrococcaceae	3.2 ± 1.3 (8)
Yeasts	5.3 ± 1.4* (11)
Lactobacillus	6.1 ± 2.0 (11)
Obligate anaerobes	9.9 ± 0.6* (13)
Bifidobacterium	8.7 ± 1.0* (7)
Eubacterium	8.8 ± 1.0 (8)
Bacteroidaceae	9.4 ± 1.3* (13)
Peptococcaceae	8.6 ± 0.8* (11)
Clostridium	6.9 ± 2.5* (9)
Lecithinase⁺, Cl	3.3 ± 1.0* (5)
Veillonella	7.4 ± 1.9 (7)

Genera of Enterobacteriaceae	Bacterial count Range	Mean
Escherichia	6.7–9.6	8.4 (12)
Citrobacter	6.3–7.3	6.8 (2)
Enterobacter		7.8 (1)
Klebsiella	6.7–9.0	8.0 (9)
Serratia		ND
Proteus	5.5–8.6	7.7 (7)

*Significantly different from the healthy control group ($p < 0.05$).
( ): No. of subjects in whom the bacterial groups were present.

were isolated also in 11 of the 13 cases, although their bacterial counts were similar to those of healthy controls.

Of the Enterobacteriaceae, *E. coli* were isolated in 12 cases, *Klebsiella* in 9 cases, and *Proteus* in 7 cases.

Total obligate anaerobes were significantly decreased. Bifidobacteria were isolated in only 7 cases, and the bacterial counts were also significantly decreased. Eubacteria were isolated in only 8 cases. Bacteroidaceae were isolated in all cases, but the bacterial counts were significantly decreased. Peptococcaceae were isolated in 11 cases and their bacterial counts were significantly decreased. Clostridia were isolated in 9 cases, and of these, lecithinase-positive clostridia were isolated in 5 cases. Bacterial counts of these two groups were significantly decreased.

SUMMARY

In this study we have demonstrated certain changes in the fecal bacterial flora in IBD of the major bacterial groups investigated. The predominant obligate anaerobes were significantly decreased, whereas facultative anaerobes were significantly increased.

More specifically, *E. coli* tended to be less dominant and other Enterobacteriaceae tended to increase in IBD. This tendency indicates the presence of abnormal fermentation in the gut, and this could be involved in the etiology of IBD.

Furthermore, this tendency is consistently seen in cases in remission and also in cases with formed stool in the active stage. Therefore, these changes cannot be caused by diarrhea. Of the various components of the normal fecal bacterial flora which were shown to be changed, further studies are necessary to discover whether any particular organism is involved in the etiology of IBD.

Bacterial Species of Intestinal Microflora of Patients with Inflammatory Bowel Disease

*Tomotari Mitsuoka**,** *and Yoshimi Benno***

SUMMARY

The bacteria recovered from the feces of 10 normal healthy subjects, 10 untreated patients with ulcerative colitis (UC), 8 patients with UC treated with Salazopyrin, and 8 patients with Crohn's disease were identified on the species level. In all the patients, especially in treated patients with UC and those with Crohn's disease, the total bacterial counts and the counts and the frequencies of occurrences of anaerobic species, especially ***Bifidobacterium adolescentis, B. longum, B. bifidum, Eubacterium aerofaciens, Lactobacillus acidophilus***, and ***L. reuteri***, were remarkably decreased. Furthermore, some increases in ***Escherichia coli*** were also noted in patients with inflammatory bowel disease.

INTRODUCTION

Ulcerative colitis is a serious gastrointestinal disease which is associated with hypersecretion, inflammation, and hemorrhage of the large intestine. The serious changes may result in abnormality of the intestinal microflora. Van der Wiel-Korstanje *et al.*[1)] have reported that the fecal flora in patients with ulcerative colitis showed a dysbiotic flora with increase of enterobacteria and streptococci and with reduction of anaerobes, especially bifidobacteria, in comparison with the fecal flora of normal healthy subjects. However, previous reports[2–4)] have failed to identify a specific bacterial pathogen associated with the disease process.

Salazopyrin is commonly used to treat patients with ulcerative colitis. West *et al.*[5)] reported that the fecal flora of patients treated with Salazopyrin caused decrease of the counts of total bacteria, anaerobes, and

*Department of Biomedical Science, Faculty of Agriculture, University of Tokyo, Tokyo, Japan

**The Institute of Physical and Chemical Research, Wako, Saitama, Japan

enterobacteria. The present study was carried out to compare the bacterial species of the fecal flora in untreated patients with ulcerative colitis, patients with ulcerative colitis receiving Salazopyrin, patients with Crohn's disease, and normal healthy subjects.

MATERIALS AND METHODS

Subjects

Ten untreated patients with ulcerative colitis, 8 patients with ulcerative colitis receiving Salazopyrin, 8 patients with Crohn's disease, and 10 healthy control subjects were used in this study (Table 1).

TABLE 1. Subjects

		Control subjects	Patients with ulcerative colitis		Patients with Crohn's disease
			Untreated	Treated with Salazopyrin	
Sex:	Male	8	3	6	2
	Female	2	7	2	6
Age:	Range	21–34	16–62	13–49	21–48
	Mean	23.1	36.7	25.9	29.9

Bacteriology

The fecal specimens from all the subjects were collected in a pre-reduced transport medium[6] and transported to the laboratory at 4° C. Then they were homogenized by kneading under gassing with oxygen-free CO_2. Culture techniques and media used were the same as those previously described.[6,7]

Isolates were divided into genera on the basis of Gram's stain, cell morphology, colony morphology, and aerobic growth. Anaerobic isolates were further classified into species by biochemical tests.[6,7] Aerobic bacteria were identified according to Cowan and Steel's manual.[9]

RESULTS AND DISCUSSION

Changes in bacterial groups of fecal flora

The mean counts per gram of wet feces and standard deviations, as well as the frequencies of occurrences (%) of a given bacterial group for normal healthy subjects, untreated patients with ulcerative colitis, patients with ulcerative colitis receiving Salazopyrin, and patients with Crohn's disease are presented in Table 2.

In the untreated patients with ulcerative colitis, the total bacterial counts and the counts and the frequencies of occurrences of anaerobes, including bifidobacteria, Peptococcaceae, eubacteria, Bacteroidaceae,

TABLE 2. Comparison of Fecal Flora of Control Subjects, Untreated with Ulcerative Colitis, Patients Receiving Salazopyrin, and Patients with Crohn's Disease

Organism(s)	Control subjects	Patients with ulcerative colitis		Patients with Crohn's disease
		Untreated	Treated with Salazopyrin	
Total counts	11.1 ± 0.2[a] (100)[b]	10.4 ± 0.3 (100)	8.2 ± 1.3 (100)	8.8 ± 1.5 (100)
Bacteroidaceae	10.7 ± 0.3 (100)	9.6 ± 1.0 (90)	7.4 ± 2.1 (87.5)	9.2 ± 1.7 (75)
Peptococcaceae	10.2 ± 0.3 (100)	8.8 ± 0.8 (50)	7.8 ± 1.7 (50)	7.0 ± 2.7 (37.5)
Eubacterium	10.0 ± 0.4 (100)	8.9 ± 0.5 (60)	6.0 (12.5)	8.0 ± 1.8 (37.5)
Bifidobacterium	10.3 ± 0.5 (100)	8.3 ± 1.9 (60)	2.8 (12.5)	8.4 ± 0.8 (25)
Veillonella	6.1 ± 1.5 (90)	6.9 ± 2.5 (50)	3.9 ± 0.3 (25)	6.8 ± 1.2 (25)
Megasphaera	8.7 ± 0.8 (50)			
C. perfringens	4.3 ± 1.5 (70)	3.5 ± 1.4 (30)	5.6 ± 1.8 (25)	
Clostridium, other	8.9 ± 1.1 (100)	8.0 ± 2.1 (100)	6.5 ± 1.2 (37.5)	8.4 ± 1.8 (50)
Lactobacillus	6.8 ± 1.1 (80)	3.4 ± 1.9 (50)	4.3 ± 0.1 (25)	6.3 (12.5)
Enterobacteriaceae	7.2 ± 1.3 (100)	8.0 ± 1.2 (100)	6.6 ± 2.8 (87.5)	7.2 ± 0.9 (87.5)
Streptococcus	6.2 ± 1.7 (100)	6.6 ± 1.5 (100)	6.5 ± 1.9 (100)	6.3 ± 0.9 (62.5)
Micrococcaceae	3.5 (10)	2.4 ± 0.3 (60)	4.3 ± 1.3 (25)	
Yeasts	4.1 ± 1.0 (50)	3.6 ± 0.9 (40)		
Bacillus	4.0 ± 2.2 (90)	3.0 ± 0.7 (30)		

[a]Mean ± SD of $\log_{10}$ bacterial counts (when present).
[b]Frequency of occurrence (%).

lactobacilli, and Megasphaerae, were remarkably decreased. Since anaerobes constitute the largest part of the fecal flora, a concomitant decrease in the total bacterial counts was also present. Conversely, the counts of aerobes, including Enterobacteriaceae and streptococci, were increased over that of normal subjects.

In the patients with ulcerative colitis treated with Salazopyrin and those with Crohn's disease, the fecal flora changed more markedly. The tendency was nearly the same as that in untreated patients.

Changes in bacterial species of fecal flora

Altogether over 101 different species of bacteria were recovered from all the groups: these are over 17 *Bacteroides* spp., over 7 *Fusobacterium* spp., 7 *Lactobacillus* spp., over 3 *Peptococcus* spp., over 5 *Peptostreptococcus* spp., over 4 *Ruminococcus* spp., over 2 *Coprococcus* spp., 1 *Veillonella* sp., 1 *Megasphaera* sp., over 4 *Bifidobacterium* spp., over 7 *Eubacterium* spp., over 18 *Clostridium* spp., and over 24 miscellaneous aerobic spp. Although over 99 distinct species were recovered from 10 normal subjects, the species recovered from the patients with ulcerative colitis or with Crohn's disease were remarkably decreased. The corresponding figure for those of the 10 untreated patients with ulcerative colitis was over 58, for the patients with ulcerative colitis receiving Salazopyrin over 30, and for the patients with Crohn's disease over 33.

Details on the specific bacteria recovered, together with the mean counts per gram wet feces and standard deviations and the frequencies of occurrences of a given bacterial species, are presented in Tables 3 through 6.

TABLE 3. *Bacteroides* and *Fusobacterium*

Organism(s)	Control subjects	Patients with ulcerative colitis		Patients with Crohn's disease
		Untreated	Treated with Salazopyrin	
Bacteroides				
B. multiacidus	8.6 ± 0.6[a] (40)[b]			
B. melaninogenicus ss. *intermedius*		8.3 (10)		
B. asaccharolyticus	8.6 (10)			
B. thetaiotaomicron	9.4 ± 1.2 (70)	8.1 ± 1.5 (40)	5.6 ± 3.3 (25)	6.4 ± 0.1 (25)
B. uniformis	10.1 ± 0.7 (30)	7.7 ± 1.1 (30)		
B. distasonis	9.9 ± 0.4 (90)	8.7 ± 1.2 (90)	7.2 ± 3.0 (50)	6.9 ± 0.8 (50)
B. vulgatus	10.5 ± 0.6 (100)	9.1 ± 1.1 (70)	8.1 ± 0.8 (37.5)	7.9 ± 1.6 (50)
B. fragilis	9.9 ± 0.3 (80)	8.9 ± 1.2 (60)	6.5 ± 1.9 (50)	8.4 ± 1.6 (62.5)
B. eggerthii	9.5 (10)			
B. ruminicola/oralis group	10.0 ± 0.3 (60)	9.6 ± 0.6 (40)	6.7 (12.5)	9.0 ± 0.9 (25)
B. bivius	8.3 (10)	7.6 (10)		
B. putredinis	9.4 ± 0.1 (20)			
B. coagulans	8.3 (10)			
B. furcosus	9.4 ± 0.1 (20)			
B. capillosus	9.3 (10)			
B. ureolyticus	9.3 (20)			
Bacteroides spp.	9.4 ± 0.6 (70)	8.0 ± 0.7 (30)	7.9 (12.5)	7.3 ± 1.0 (25)
Fusobacterium				
F. russii	8.5 ± 0.2 (20)	8.3 ± 1.3 (30)	8.7 (12.5)	
F. mortiferum	9.3 ± 0.7 (50)	8.4 ± 1.1 (30)		
F. varium	9.3 ± 0.3 (40)			
F. nucleatum	8.3 (10)	9.1 ± 1.1 (20)		10.2 (12.5)
F. necrophorum	8.3 (10)			
F. prausnitzii	9.8 (10)			
Fusobacterium spp.	8.0 (10)	9.3 ± 1.2 (20)	10.9 (12.5)	

[a]Mean ± SD of $\log_{10}$ bacterial counts (when present).
[b]Frequency of occurrence (%).

TABLE 4. *Bifidobacterium, Eubacterium,* and *Clostridium*

Organism(s)	Control subjects	Patients with ulcerative colitis		Patients with Crohn's disease
		Untreated	Treated with Salazopyrin	
Bifidobacterium				
B. adolescentis	10.3 ± 0.5[a] (100)[b]	7.8 ± 2.7 (40)		6.2 (12.5)
B. longum	9.9 ± 0.4 (70)	7.0 ± 1.7 (30)	2.8 (12.5)	3.9 ± 1.3 (25)
B. bifidum	9.7 ± 0.4 (60)	7.4 ± 0.5 (20)		
Bifidobacterium spp.	9.5 ± 0.6 (20)	9.0 (10)		9.0 (12.5)
Eubacterium				
E. aerofaciens	9.6 ± 0.9 (100)	8.7 ± 0.4 (20)		8.3 (12.5)
E. rectale	9.4 ± 0.2 (30)	7.3 ± 0.6 (30)		7.8 ± 0.8 (25)
E. lentum	9.2 ± 0.7 (50)	8.5 ± 1.2 (30)		
E. biforme	8.2 (10)			
E. contortum	8.6 (10)			
E. moniliforme	8.8 (10)			
E. alactolyticum		8.8 (10)		
Eubacterium spp.	9.3 ± 0.3 (70)	8.7 ± 1.3 (20)	6.0 (12.5)	6.4 ± 4.6 (25)
Clostridium				
C. perfringens	5.0 ± 1.7 (70)	3.5 ± 1.4 (30)	5.6 ± 1.8 (25)	
C. bifermentans	6.9 (10)			
C. gohni	5.4 (10)			
C. difficile	3.2 (10)			
C. tertium	7.4 ± 2.3 (30)			
C. sphenoides	6.3 (10)			
C. clostridiiforme	9.4 ± 1.3 (40)	5.5 ± 3.0 (70)		10.2 (12.5)
C. coccoides	5.2 ± 2.5 (30)			
C. nexile	5.3 ± 1.5 (20)			
C. butyricum	4.7 ± 1.7 (30)	3.0 ± 1.0 (40)		
C. beijerinkii	4.9 ± 1.8 (50)			
C. paraputrificum	5.3 ± 1.0 (50)	3.7 ± 2.1 (60)	5.5 (12.5)	
C. innocuum	8.7 ± 0.4 (70)	8.2 ± 0.8 (40)		7.3 (12.5)
C. cochleariuum	5.3 ± 0.3 (30)			
C. tyrobutyricum	4.3 (10)			
C. ramosum	8.3 ± 0.5 (40)	7.9 ± 1.9 (50)	7.0 ± 1.9 (25)	6.4 ± 1.7 (37.5)
C. sartagoformum	3.1 (10)	4.5 ± 1.6 (40)		
Clostridium spp.	7.4 ± 1.8 (100)	6.7 ± 2.9 (60)		6.4 (12.5)

[a]Mean ± SD of $\log_{10}$ bacterial counts (when present).
[b]Frequency of occurrence (%).

A few strains could not be fit into any of the established species: these were designated as "spp."

The specific bacterial species in the patients with inflammatory bowel

TABLE 5. *Lactobacillus* and Anaerobic Cocci

Organism(s)	Control subjects	Patients with ulcerative colitis		Patients with Crohn's disease
		Untreated	Treated with Salazopyrin	
Lactobacillus				
L. acidophilus	6.7 ± 1.2[a](70)[b]		3.8 ± 0.6 (25)	
L. salivarius	6.8 ± 0.3 (40)	2.3 ± 0.1 (30)		
L. fermentum	6.1 ± 1.6 (30)	6.8 (10)	4.3 (12.5)	6.3 (12.5)
L. reuteri	5.8 ± 1.0 (50)	2.1 (10)		
L. casei	6.8 (10)			
L. plantarum	5.3 (10)			
L. brevis	5.3 (10)			
Peptococcus				
P. asaccharolyticus	9.3 ± 0.5 (10)			4.0 (12.5)
P. prevotii	9.5 ± 0.1 (10)	8.3 (10)		
P. magnus		8.4 ± 0.2 (30)		
Peptococcus spp.	9.2 ± 0.7 (40)			7.8 (12.5)
Peptostreptococcus				
P. anaerobius	8.8 (10)	7.7 (10)	6.6 (12.5)	8.8 (12.5)
P. productus	9.5 ± 0.7 (50)	8.6 ± 1.2 (40)	10.3 (12.5)	8.0 (12.5)
P. parvulus	8.8 (10)			
P. micros	9.1 ± 0.7 (30)	8.6 ± 0.1 (20)	7.1 (12.5)	8.0 (12.5)
Peptostreptococcus spp.	9.9 ± 0.4 (20)	8.5 ± 0.2 (20)	7.0 (12.5)	7.0 ± 2.7 (37.5)
Ruminococcus				
R. albus	9.7 (10)			
R. lactaris	9.7 (10)			
R. gnavus	8.9 ± 0.1 (20)			
Ruminococcus spp.	8.7 ± 0.8 (30)			
Coprococcus				
C. comes	9.7 (10)			
Coprococcus spp.	9.6 (10)			
Veillonella parvula	6.1 ± 1.5 (90)	6.9 ± 2.5 (50)	3.9 ± 0.3 (25)	6.8 ± 1.2 (25)
Megasphaera elsdenii	8.7 ± 0.8 (50)			

[a]Mean ± SD of $\log_{10}$ bacterial counts (when present).
[b]Frequency of occurrence (%).

disease could not be recognized: almost all the species isolated from the patients were also isolated from normal control subjects. In the untreated patients with ulcerative colitis, the counts and the frequencies of occurrences of anaerobic species, especially *Bifidobacterium adolescentis*, *B. longum*, *B. bifidum*, *Eubacterium aerofaciens*, *Lactobacillus acidophilus*, and *L. reuteri*, were remarkably decreased, while some increases in

TABLE 6. Aerobic Bacteria

Organism(s)	Control subjects	Patients with ulcerative colitis: Untreated	Patients with ulcerative colitis: Treated with Salazopyrin	Patients with Crohn's disease
Escherichia coli	7.2 ± 1.3[a] (100)[b]	7.8 ± 1.4 (100)	7.0 ± 3.0 (62.5)	7.4 ± 0.8 (87.5)
Arizona hinshawii	5.3 (10)			
Citrobacter freundii	6.5 ± 0.8 (40)	7.2 ± 0.6 (20)	5.6 ± 2.8 (25)	
Citrobacter sp.	6.3 (10)	4.9 (10)		
Enterobacter aerogenes	6.6 ± 1.0 (20)			
Klebsiella pneumoniae	6.8 ± 0.6 (50)	7.0 ± 0.9 (60)	6.5 ± 1.8 (50)	7.8 ± 1.0 (25)
Pseudomonas aeruginosa	4.0 ± 1.2 (40)	2.6 (10)	6.9 (12.5)	3.3 ± 1.0 (25)
Streptococcus				
S. faecalis	5.7 ± 1.7 (90)	5.7 ± 1.7 (90)	8.3 (12.5)	4.4 ± 1.8 (62.5)
S. faecium	4.8 ± 1.8 (70)	6.3 ± 2.3 (40)	6.9 ± 2.4 (37.5)	4.4 ± 1.5 (25)
S. durans	4.6 ± 1.7 (40)	5.6 ± 2.1 (30)	7.0 ± 0.5 (25)	7.0 (12.5)
S. bovis	5.8 ± 2.1 (20)	5.1 ± 0.3 (30)		
S. avidum	4.3 (10)			
S. intermedius	8.0 ± 1.2 (40)	7.9 ± 0.9 (50)	5.8 (25)	7.2 ± 0.1 (25)
Streptococcus spp.	6.0 ± 2.1 (50)		4.0 ± 1.6 (25)	6.2 ± 1.6 (25)
Staphylococcus				
S. aureus	2.3 (10)	2.7 (10)		
S. epidermidis	2.3 (10)	2.4 ± 1.8 (30)	4.3 ± 1.3 (25)	
Micrococcus spp.	3.5 (10)	2.5 ± 0.2 (20)		
Bacillus				
B. subtilis	4.2 ± 1.8 (90)	3.2 ± 0.3 (20)		
Bacillus spp.	3.7 ± 2.2 (40)	3.0 ± 0.3 (10)		
Candida				
C. albicans	4.1 ± 1.0 (50)	3.2 ± 1.0 (30)		
C. tropicalis	3.5 (10)			
Candida spp.	3.0 ± 0.9 (20)	3.4 ± 1.6 (20)		
Corynebacterium spp.	5.1 ± 0.1 (20)			
Filamentous fungi	2.2 ± 0.2 (20)	2.3 (10)		

[a]Mean ± SD of $\log_{10}$ bacterial counts (when present).
[b]Frequency of occurrence (%).

Escherichia coli were noted. The counts of most of the other aerobic species maintained nearly the same levels as normal subjects. Since the total bacterial counts were remarkably decreased in the untreated patients, these changes resulted in an abnormal composition of the fecal flora.

In the patients with ulcerative colitis receiving Salazopyrin and the patients with Crohn's disease, however, the counts and the frequencies of occurrences of anaerobic species were further decreased.

Our results are somewhat different from the previous reports.[1–5,10] Why this discrepancy occurred is unknown. In the paper by Wensinck *et al.*,[10] the fecal samples from the patients with Crohn's disease were noted to contain significantly higher counts of *Eubacterium contortum*, *E. rectale*, and *Peptostreptococcus productus* than specimens from normal subjects. This was not noted in the present study. Additional studies are certainly needed to investigate further the interrelationships among the extent of the severity of disease, the part of the lesions, and intestinal bacteria.

REFERENCES

1. Van der Wiel-Korstanje, J. A. A. and Winkler, K. C.: The faecal flora in ulcerative colitis. *J. Med. Microbiol.*, **8**: 491, 1975.
2. Cooke, E. M.: A quantitative composition of the faecal flora of patients with ulcerative colitis and that of normal persons. *J. Path. Bacteriol.*, **9**: 439, 1967.
3. Gorbach, S. L., Nahas, L., Plaut, A. G., Weinstein, L., Patterson, J. F., and Levitan, R.: Studies on intestinal microflora. V. Fecal microbial ecology in ulcerative colitis and regional enteritis: relationship to severity of disease and chemotherapy. *Gastroenterology*, **54**: 575, 1968.
4. Weinstein, L.: Bacteriological aspects of ulcerative colitis. *Gastroenterology*, **40**: 323, 1961.
5. West, B., Lendrum, R., Hill, M. J., and Walker, G.: Effects of sulphasalazine (Salazopyrin) on faecal flora in patients with inflammatory bowel disease. *Gut*, **15**: 960, 1974.
6. Mitsuoka, T.: A Color Atlas of Anaerobic Bacteria. Sobunsha, Tokyo, 1980 (in Japanese).
7. Mitsuoka, T., Sega, T., and Yamamoto, S. : Eine verbesserte Methodik der qualitativen und quantitativen Analyse der Darmflora von Menschen und Tieren. *Zentralbl. Bakteriol. Parasit. Infekt. Hyg.*, Abt. I. Orig. **195**: 455, 1965.
8. Holdeman, L. V., Cato, E. P., and Moore, W. E. C.: Anaerobic Laboratory Manual, 4th ed. Anaerobe Laboratory, Virginia Polytechnic Institute and State University, Blacksburg, 1977.
9. Cowan, S. T.: Cowan and Steel's Manual for the Identification of Medical Bacteria. Cambridge University Press, New York, 1974.
10. Hazenberg, M. P., Bakker, M., Both-Patoir, H. C., Ruseler-van Embden, J. G. H., and Schröder, A. M.: Effect of sulphasalazine on the human intestinal flora. *J. Appl. Bacteriol.*, **52**: 103, 1982.
11. Wensinck, F., Custers-van Lieshout, L. M. C., Poppelaars-Kustermans, P. A. J., and Schröder, A. M.: The faecal flora of patients with Crohn's disease. *J. Hyg.* (Camb.), **87**: 1, 1982.

Bacterial Species from Mesenteric Lymph Nodes in Inflammatory Bowel Disease

Rintaro Nakaya, Toshio Chida, Kiyoshi Hasegawa, Harumi Shibaoka, and Noboru Okamura

SUMMARY

The mesenteric lymph nodes resected from patients with ulcerative colitis (UC; 22 cases, 25 specimens), Crohn's disease (CD; 9 cases, 9 specimens), and noninflammatory bowel diseases (controls; 21 cases, 24 specimens) were examined for the presence of aerobic and anaerobic bacterial species to investigate the possible role of bacteria in the etiopathogenesis of inflammatory bowel disease. A significantly higher incidence of positive culture was observed in UC (77%) than in CD (44%) and controls (48%). It was, however, found that the bacterial isolates belonged to various species, and none of the species could be assigned as the etiologic agent. The viable counts of bacteria were generally small, and most of the isolates belonged to the indigenous microbes usually found in human intestinal flora. *Bacteroides vulgatus* was found in two cases of UC and one case of Behçet's syndrome. Various members of the intestinal flora may have a more frequent opportunity to enter the mesenteric lymph nodes in UC.

To investigate the possible role of bacteria in the etiopathogenesis of inflammatory bowel disease, we examined the mesenteric lymph nodes resected from patients with ulcerative colitis (UC), Crohn's disease (CD), and noninflammatory bowel diseases (control) for the presence of aerobic and anaerobic bacterial species.

A significantly higher incidence of positive culture was observed in UC than in CD and controls. It was, however, found that the bacterial isolates belonged to various species, and none of the species could be assigned as the etiologic agent.

Department of Microbiology, Tokyo Medical and Dental University School of Medicine, Tokyo, Japan

MATERIALS AND METHODS

Bacteriology

Isolation, identification, and enumeration of aerobic and anaerobic organisms were carried out by the methods described previously.[1)]

Specimens tested were the mesenteric lymph nodes resected aseptically from the affected regions of the colon upon surgical operation. Sections of the intestinal wall and mucous membrane, and the intestinal contents of the same subjects were also taken to compare the bacteriological findings with the lymph nodes. All of the specimens taken were kept in an anaerobic condition until bacteriological examinations were made.

Cases and specimens

Cases and specimens subjected for bacteriological examinations are listed in Table 1. We examined the mesenteric lymph nodes resected from the patients with UC (22 cases, 25 specimens), CD (9 cases, 9 specimens), and controls (21 cases, 24 specimens). The ages of the patients ranged from 12 to 68 years.

TABLE 1. Number of Cases and Specimens Examined for the Presence of Bacteria in the Mesenteric Lymph Nodes

Disease	No. of cases	No. of specimens
Ulcerative colitis	22	25
Crohn's disease	9	9
Control	21	24

RESULTS

Incidence of bacteria

The ratio of positive cases for bacterial culture were 77, 44, and 48% in UC, CD, and controls, respectively (Table 2). The incidences of positive specimens for bacteria were almost the same as those of the positive cases. A significantly higher incidence of positive isolation of bacteria from the lymph nodes was observed in UC as compared with CD and controls.

TABLE 2. Positive Incidence of Bacteria in the Mesenteric Lymph Nodes

Disease	Case Positive/total	(%)	Specimen Positive/total	(%)
Ulcerative colitis	17/22	(77)	19/25	(76)
Crohn's disease	4/9	(44)	4/9	(44)
Control	10/21	(48)	12/24	(50)

Bacterial species of the isolates

From the 19 specimens of the lymph nodes of the UC patients, 23 different bacterial species were recovered (Table 3). Among those, *Bacteroides* spp., *Streptococcus faecalis*, and *Escherichia coli* were the most frequent

TABLE 3. Bacterial Species of the Isolates from the Mesenteric Lymph Nodes of Ulcerative Colitis

Bacterial species	Incidence
Bacteroides distasonis	2
vulgatus	2
fragilis	4
spp.	3
Eubacterium lentum	1
spp.	2
Clostridium butyricum	1
innocuum	1
Propionibacterium acnes	2
Peptococcus asaccharolyticus	1
Peptostreptococcus anaerobius	1
spp.	1
Escherichia coli	6
Citrobacter freundii	1
Klebsiella pneumoniae	2
Alcaligenes faecalis	1
Pseudomonas putida	1
Staphylococcus epidermidis	1
Streptococcus faecalis	8
faecium	3
intermedius	1
durans	1
spp.	1
Total	47

TABLE 4. Bacterial Species of the Isolates from the Mesenteric Lymph Nodes of Crohn's Disease

Bacterial species	Incidence
Bacteroides fragilis	1
Clostridium spp.	1
Propionibacterium acnes	1
Pseudomonas maltophilia	1
Acinetobacter calcoaceticus	1
Staphylococcus spp.	1
Bacillus spp.	1
Corynebacterium spp.	1
Yeast	1
Total	9

isolates. A total of 9 species were detected from the cases of CD, but none of the species was common to all the specimens examined (Table 4).

In the control group, we found 30 bacterial species from the lymph nodes (Table 5). The most frequent isolates were *Bacteroides* spp. and *E. coli*. The noninflammatory bowel diseases of the controls were composed of adenomatosis coli, Behçet's disease, and others; and the incidence of cases positive for the presence of bacteria are summarized in Table 6. It should be noted that the two cases of Behçet's syndrome showed 100% positive for the presence of bacteria in their mesenteric lymph nodes.

TABLE 5. Bacterial Species of the Isolates from the Mesenteric Lymph Nodes of Controls

Bacterial species	Incidence
Bacteroides distasonis	1
vulgatus	2
fragilis	3
ruminicola/oralis	2
Bifidobacterium longum B	1
Clostridium innocuum	1
Propionibacterium acnes	2
Escherichia coli	5
Klebsiella pneumoniae	1
Staphylococcus epidermidis	3
Streptococcus faecalis	2
faecium	3
sanguis	1
Bacillus spp.	1
Corynebacterium spp.	1
Gram-positive aerobic rod	1
Total	30

TABLE 6. Diseases of Controls and the Cases Positive for Bacterial Cultures from the Mesenteric Lymph Nodes

Disease	No. of cases tested	Positive for bacteria No.	%
Adenomatosis coli	14	6	43
Behçet's disease	2	2	100
Malignant lymphoma	1	1	100
Multiple ulcer of the small intestine	1	1	100
Colon cancer	1	0	0
Rectum cancer	1	0	0
Ulcerative colitis (normal site)	1	0	0
Total	21	10	48

Versatility of bacterial species

Since many species of bacteria were isolated from the mesenteric lymph nodes from the cases of UC, CD, and controls, the incidence of different species was compared between the specimens taken from these cases. As shown in Table 7, the incidences per specimen positive for bacteria were almost the same among the disease groups. It was shown that two to three different species of bacteria were detected from the lymph nodes on the average. This indicates that no simple bacterial species could be assigned as the etiopathogenetic agent for each disease.

TABLE 7. Versatility of Bacterial Species Isolated from the Mesenteric Lymph Nodes of Ulcerative Colitis, Crohn's Disease, and Controls

Disease (n)[a]	Specimens positive for bacteria		Bacterial species isolated		Incidence of presence of different species	
	No.	(%)[b]	No.	Mean[c]	No.	Mean[d]
Ulcerative colitis (25)	19	(76)	23	1.2	47	2.5
Crohn's disease (9)	4	(44)	9	2.3	9	2.3
Control (24)	12	(50)	16	1.3	30	2.5

[a]n = Number of specimens tested.
[b]Percent positive.
[c]Number of bacterial species per specimen positive for bacteria.
[d]Incidence of the presence of different bacterial species per specimen positive for bacteria.

Viable counts

The mean viable counts of organisms per gram of lymph node were $10^{3.40}$, $10^{3.10}$, and $10^{3.14}$ in UC, CD, and controls, respectively (Table 8). The maximum viable counts were $10^{6.7}$, $10^{3.8}$, and $10^{5.5}$ per gram of lymph node in UC, CD, and controls, respectively, but generally the numbers were small.

TABLE 8. Viable Counts of Bacteria in the Mesenteric Lymph Nodes from Ulcerative Colitis, Crohn's Disease, and Controls

Disease	No. of bacteria ($\log_{10}$/g)	
	Mean	Range
Ulcerative colitis	3.40	1.8–6.7
Crohn's disease	3.10	2.3–3.8
Control	3.14	1.0–5.5

Identity of bacterial species from the lymph nodes to those from the intestinal wall

The incidences of the cases in which identical bacterial species were found commonly between the mesenteric lymph nodes and the intestinal wall of the affected colon were 11/16 (69%), 2/3 (67%), and 5/5 (100%), in UC, CD, and controls, respectively.

Cases positive for Bacteroides vulgatus

Two cases of UC and one case of Behçet's disease in the controls showed the presence of *B. vulgatus* in their mesenteric lymph nodes. The bacterial species and the viable counts in each of these cases are shown in Tables 9, 10, and 11 in comparison with the corresponding findings on the intestinal wall and the mucous membrane.

TABLE 9. A Case of Ulcerative Colitis in Which *Bacteroides vulgatus* was Isolated from the Mesenteric Lymph Nodes (K. N., male, 44 y.)

Bacterial species isolated	No. of bacteria ($\log_{10}$/g) Lymph nodes	Intestinal wall
Bacteroides vulgatus	2.6	3.4
Eubacterium spp.	2.6	0
Streptococcus faecalis	3.2	4.8
Others	0	5.3
Total count	3.4	5.5

TABLE 10. A Case of Ulcerative Colitis in Which *Bacteroides vulgatus* was Isolated from the Mesenteric Lymph Nodes (A. S., male)

Bacterial species isolated	No. of bacteria ($\log_{10}$/g) Lymph nodes	Intestinal wall
Bacteroides vulgatus	3.1	2.9
fragilis	2.9	0
Others	0	3.1
Total count	3.1	3.1

TABLE 11. A Case of Behçet's Disease in Which *Bacteroides vulgatus* was Isolated from the Mesenteric Lymph Nodes (N. A., male, 45 y.)

Bacterial species isolated	No. of bacteria ($\log_{10}$/g)		
	Lymph nodes	Intestinal wall	Mucous membrane
Bacteroides vulgatus	5.5	6.4	6.8
fragilis	3.8	0	5.4
ruminicola/oralis	4.4	0	0
Others	0	0	2.5
Total count	5.5	6.4	6.8

DISCUSSION

There has been no conclusive evidence that ulcerative colitis is caused by a specific infection.[2] Nevertheless, it seems very probable that the microflora of the gut may influence the pathogenesis of the disease. Our findings, presented in this communication, also suggest that there is no justification for ascribing etiological significance to any one of the bacterial species detected from the mesentric lymph nodes of UC and CD. It is, however, probable that various members of indigenous intestinal microflora have more frequent opportunity to enter the regional mesenteric lymph nodes in UC. It is possible that, once mucosal inflammation has occurred, bacterial antigens may initiate immune responses within the colonic mucosa which may cause further mucosal damage by hypersensitivity reactions.

The production of toxic substances by some of the bacteria, such as hemolysins and necrotoxins, has also been mentioned.[2] Recently, Onderdonk *et al.*[3] reported that experimental ulcerative colitis can be produced in gnotobiotic guinea pigs associated with a certain simplified intestinal microflora originating from conventional guinea pigs that had developed ulcerations of their ceca and large intestines after the oral administration of a solution of 5% degraded carrageenan. They have further shown that cecal ulcerations develop in germ-free animals mono-associated with a strain of *B. vulgatus* isolated from one of the pools of microflora, suggesting a bacterial involvement in disease development in the absence of carrageenan treatment. Onderdonk *et al.*[4] also described that concurrent treatment of conventional guinea pigs with metronidazole and carrageenan prevents the development of intestinal ulcerations. In the present study we have paid special attention to the presence of *B. vulgatus* in the mesenteric lymph nodes resected from patients of UC. *B. vulgatus* was detected in 2 out of 17 cases which were positive for bacteria. The etiologic relationship of *B. vulgatus* and other related species with the development of human ulcerative colitis should be further investigated.

Acknowledgment

We thank Dr. T. Mitsuoka for providing us with the experimental results obtained in his laboratory for inclusion in this communication.

REFERENCES

1. Mitsuoka, T.: A Color Atlas of Anaerobic Bacteria. Sobunsha, Tokyo, 1980 (in Japanese).
2. Thomas, H. C. and Jewell, D. P.: Ulcerative Colitis. Clinical Gastrointestinal

Immounology, pp. 137–163. Blackwell Scientific Publications, Oxford, England, 1979.

3. Onderdonk, A. B., Franklin, M. L., and Cisneros, R. L.: Production of experimental ulcerative colitis in gnotobiotic guinea pigs with simplified microflora. *Infect. Immun.*, **32**: 225, 1981.
4. Onderdonk, A. B., Hermos, J. A., Dzink, J. L., and Bartlett, J. G.: Protective effect of metronidazole in experimental ulcerative colitis. *Gastroenterology*, **74**: 521, 1978.

IgA Protease Activity of the Intestinal Flora in Inflammatory Bowel Disease

Tadao Bamba, Yoshihide Fujiyama, Noriko Kutani, and Shiro Hosoda

The secretory IgA (sIgA) system plays an important role as a first-line defense mechanism, existing independently of the systemic immune system, in the bowel, which is constantly exposed to various microorganisms or heteroprotein antigens. The impairment of the sIgA system is assumed to be a key factor in the establishment and the development of various intestinal diseases. The authors have reported that the impairment of the secretion of sIgA exists in malabsorption syndrome and ulcerative colitis, based on the observations by the immune fluorescent antibody technique in their intestinal biopsied specimens.[1] We have already postulated that the mechanisms of secretion and production in the sIgA system are based on eight factors[2] : 1) recognition of antigen, 2) number of IgA-containing cells, 3) IgA synthesis ability, 4) secretory component (sc) production in the epithelial cells, 5) binding between IgA and sc, 6) intraluminal transport of sIgA, 7) secretion of sIgA from the epithelial cell to the intestinal lumen, and 8) cleavage of sIgA by microorganisms.

It is suggested that the impairment of the first-line defense mechanism of sIgA on the intestinal surface may be induced by IgA1 protease-producing strains. From this viewpoint, it is interesting to regard IgA1 protease-producing strains as a background factor modifying the pathophysiology of the inflammatory bowel diseases (IBD).

METHODS

Preparation of the bacterial enzyme

IgA1 protease production was done according to the method of Plaut *et al.*[3] with some modification. Each strain was purely cultured in 50 ml Todd-Hewitt broth and incubated under anaerobic conditions at 37°C for 24–72 hr; then the cell-free supernatant was obtained by centrifugation

Second Department of Internal Medicine, Shiga University of Medical Science, Otsu, Japan

at 10,000 rpm for 30 min and lyophilized. The enzyme was resuspended with 5 ml of distilled water and dialyzed against 0.1 M phosphate buffer (pH 7.0).

Analysis of IgA1 protease production

Each bacterial enzyme was reacted with the same volume of myeloma IgA1, IgA2, sIgA, or serum polyclonal IgA (5 mg/ml) at 37° C for 4–8 hr. Immunoelectrophoresis was performed against anti-human α chain and unabsorbed anti-human IgA or sIgA rabbit serum. Digested myeloma IgA1 with bacterial enzyme was analyzed by SDS polyacrylamide gradient gel electrophoresis.

Blastoid formation of peripheral lymphocytes to IgA1 protease-producing strains

Twenty microliters of each strain treated at 80° C for 30 min was added to 0.2 ml of lymphocyte suspension (5×10^5/ml, 20% FCS, RPMI 1640 mixed with 100 μg of Streptomycin and 100 U of penicillin), and cultured under 5% CO_2 for five days. At 5 hr before the end of the culture, ^{3}H-thymidine (final concentration 1 μCi/ml) was added and ^{3}H-thymidine uptake was measured by liquid scintillation counter for stimulation index after the lymphocytes were collected by cell harvester.

RESULTS

The bacterial composition of the intestinal flora isolated from the feces and the jejunal fluid of a volunteer without any intestinal disorders except for fatty liver are shown in Table 1. The identification of each strain was performed by Professor Osawa, Department of Microbiology, Tokai University Medical School. IgA1 protease was examined in 84 strains of 36 species. The IgA1 protease activity was found in only one strain of *Bifidobacterium infantis*. No other strain of *B. infantis* nor any of three strains of *Streptococcus sanguis* produced IgA1 protease.

IgA1 protease production of the intestinal bacterial composition was examined in patients with IBD. The bacterial composition of the intestinal flora from the feces and biopsied rectal mucosa of the patients with ulcerative colitis is shown in Table 2. The isolation of the intestinal flora was performed by Professor Shimoyama, Department of Internal Medicine, Hyogo College of Medicine. Out of 86 strains of 14 genera of *Bifidobacterium*, two strains produced IgA1 protease. Three isolates of Bacteroidaceae caused IgA1 fragmentation. Thus, the following studies were designed to investigate IgA1 protease production in the strains of tentatively classified genus *Bifidobacterium* as well as Bacteroidaceae isolated from the patients with IBD.

TABLE 1. The Jejunal and Fecal Bacterial Composition of the Patient with Fatty Liver (N. S., male, 42 y.o.)

	Fecal bacterial composition	No. of isolates	Jejunal bacterial composition	No. of isolates
Anaerobic:	*Clostridium innocum*	1	*Clostridium cochlearium*	2
	putrifaciens	1	*innocum*	2
	tyrobutyricum	1	*Eubacterium aerofaciens*	2
	melanominatum	1	*lentum*	2
	ramosum	1	*Bacteroides corrodens*	2
	sardiniensis	1		
	Bifidobacterium bifidum	1		
	infantis	2[a]		
	Lactobacillus plantarum	1		
	minutus	2		
	ruminis	2		
	rogosae	3		
	Eubacterium aerofaciens	1		
	lentum	2		
	contortum	1		
	Fusobacterium mortiferum	1		
	plauti	1		
	Bacteroides multiacidus	1		
	furcosus	1		
	Streptococcus magnus	1		
	morbillorum	1		
	Peptococcus magnus	1		
	Veillonella parvula	2		
Aerobic:	*Escherichia coli*	7	*Escherichia coli*	4
	Citrobacter freundii	1	*Citrobacter freundii*	4
	intermedius A	1	*intermedius* A	4
	Klebsiella pneumoniae	1	*Klebsiella ozaenae*	2
	Enterobacter cloacae	4	*pneumoniae*	4
	Staphylococcus epidermidis	1	*Staphylococcus epidermidis*	2
	aureus	1		
	Streptococcus faecalis	4		
	sanguis	3		
	anginosus	2		

[a]IgA1 protease was found in one strain.

In total, 165 strains of tentative Bacteroidaceae and 23 strains of tentative *Bifidobacterium* were isolated from the feces of 15 patients with IBD, as shown in Table 3. The IgA1 protease-producing strains were not found in all cases, but only in two cases, that is, *Clostridium* sp. in Case 9 and *Bifidobacterium* in Case 17.

The immunoelectrophoresis of myeloma IgA1 digested with the bacterial enzyme is shown in Fig. 1. The two IgA1 proteases found in this study were both EDTA-sensitive and did not cleave other classes of immunoglobulin,

TABLE 2. The Fecal Bacterial Composition and the Isolates from the Inflamed Mucosa of the Patient with Ulcerative Colitis (C. F., female, 23 y.o.)

	Fecal bacterial composition	No. of isolates examined	Isolates from the inflamed mucosa	No. of isolates examined
Anaerobic:	Clostridium	6	*Clostridium perfringens*	1
	Lactobacillus	5	Lactobacillus	4
	Bacteroidaceae	21	*Escherichia coli*	3
	Veillonella	2	Bacteroidaceae	17
	Escherichia coli	2	Eubacterium	5
	Bifidobacterium	7[a]	Megasphaera	1
	Eubacterium	1	Peptococcus	2
	Peptococcus	1		
	Streptococcus	1		
Aerobic:	*Escherichia coli*	1	*Escherichia coli*	1
	P. morganii	1	Streptococcus	2
	Streptococcus	1		
	Staphylococcus	1		

[a]IgA1 protease was found in two isolates.

TABLE 3. IgA1 Protease Production of the Isolates from the Intestinal Bacterial Flora of IBD Patients

Case	No. of isolates (positive/examined)	
	Bacteroidaceae[a]	Bifidobacterium[a]
1[b]	0/7	
2[b]	2[c]/86	
3	0/10	0/3
4	0/12	
5	0/17	
6	0/5	0/6
7	0/13	
8	0/9	
9	1[d]/2	
10	0/8	0/1
11	0/24	
12	0/14	
13	0/16	
14	0/11	
15	0/6	0/3
16	0/5	0/2
17	0/13	1/8
Total (Cases 3–17)	1/165	1/23

[a]Tentatively classified tribe and genus.
[b]All isolates.
[c]*Bifidobacterium* sp.
[d]*Clostridium* sp.

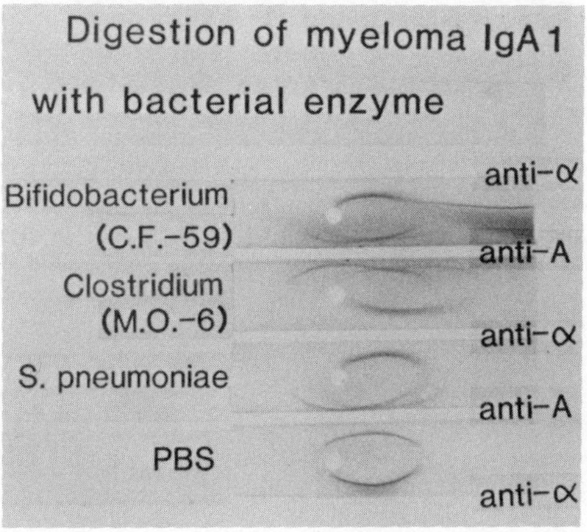

FIG. 1. Immunoelectrophoresis of the digested myeloma IgA1 with the bacterial enzyme. anti-α: anti-human α-chain rabbit serum; anti-A: unabsorbed anti-human IgA rabbit serum.

including IgA2 and albumin. Immunoelectrophoretic analysis of digestants showed two precipitin arcs crossing the anti-human α chain and anti-human κ chain.

Therefore, these findings strongly suggested that IgA1 was cleaved to Fc_α and Fab_α by IgA1 protease.

SDS polyacrylamide gradient gel electrophoresis of digested IgA1 is shown in Fig. 2. Digested myeloma IgA1 with the bacterial enzyme of *Bifidobacterium* is shown in panel 2, *Clostridium* in panel 3, *Streptococcus pneumonia* in panel 4, control of IgA1 (which was inactivated in the presence of EDTA) in panel 1, and Pharmacia low molecular weight standard in the right panel. Although we have not yet determined the exact site of cleavage for these two IgA1 proteases, the cleaved products were different from each other.

Blastoid formation of lymphocytes of peripheral blood to *Clostridium* sp. with IgA1 protease production was obviously noted in 4 of 10 patients with IBD, as shown in Fig. 3. However, there was no difference between the patients with IBD and controls. Furthermore, there was no difference between IgA1 protease and non-IgA1 protease strains.

DISCUSSION

Selective IgA deficiency causes the impairment of the production and secretion of sIgA in the intestinal local immunity of host, and occasionally

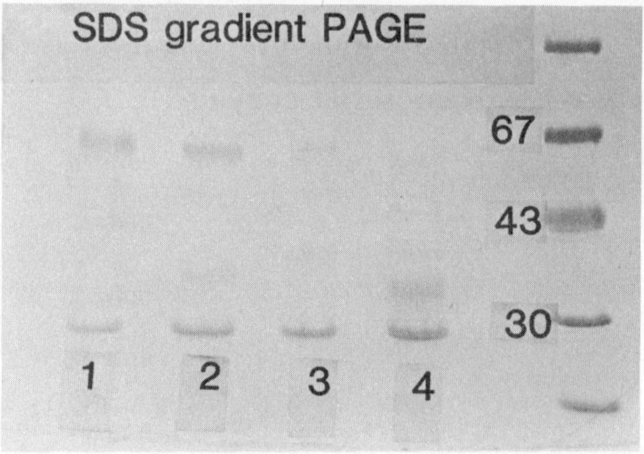

FIG. 2. SDS polyacrylamide gradient gel electrophoresis of the digested myeloma IgA1. 1. IgA + PBS; 2. IgA1 + enzyme (*Bifidobacterium*, Case 2); 3. IgA1 + enzyme (*Clostridium*, Case 9); 4. IgA1 + enzyme (*Streptococcus pneumoniae*).

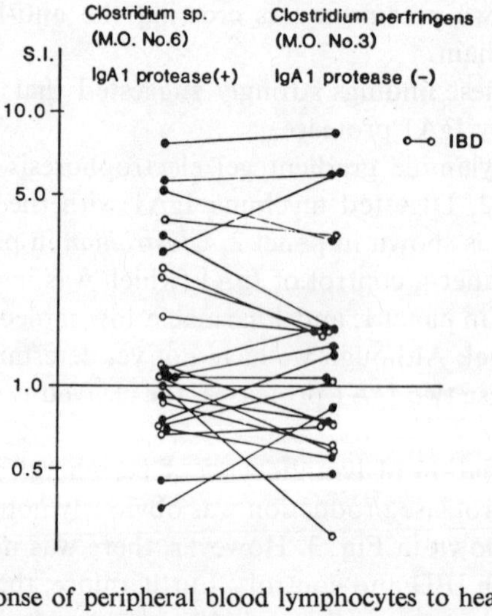

FIG. 3. Response of peripheral blood lymphocytes to heat-inactivated bacterium isolated from feces of the patient with IBD.

results in intestinal infection. We have also reported that the impairment of the sIgA system in the host exists in intestinal diseases.[1,2] This study was undertaken to evaluate the significance of the intestinal flora against the host sIgA system by examining the IgA1 specific-producing strains among the intestinal flora in IBD. It was previously reported that IgA1 protease-producing strains were *Streptococcus sanguis*,[3] *S. mitior*,[4] *S. pneumoniae*,[5] *Hemophilus influenzae*,[6] *Neisseria meningifidis*,[6] and *N. gonorrheae*.[6] All of them are specific to IgA1, but irresponsive to IgA2.

IgA1 protease in the intestinal bacteria may be involved as one of the aggressive factors against sIgA on the surface of the intestinal mucosa, a host-protective mechanism, and in the development of systemic infection. The antibody activity of IgA1 myeloma protein was markedly reduced or eliminated after treatment with IgA1 protease.[7] Leucocyte chemotaxis inhibitory activity of polymeric IgA or sIgA was also reported to be inactivated by IgA1 protease.[8] These results can be attributed to the cleavage of mutivalent bonds in the IgA antibody by IgA1 protease. IgA1 protease is regarded as a direct aggressive factor against a protective function produced by the antibody activity of the sIgA system.

IgA1 protease-producing strain was found in only one strain of *Bifidobacterium infantis* in the healthy controls. In order to investigate the involvement of IgA1 protease-producing strains in the manifestation and the development of chronic inflammatory bowel diseases such as ulcerative colitis and Crohn's disease, we examined the components of the intestinal bacterial flora in 17 patients with IBD and found IgA1 protease-producing strains in two strains of *Bifidobacterium* and in one strain of genus *Clostridium* and genus *Bifidobacterium*. However, intestinal bacteria recognized as IgA1 protease-producing strains remain minor components in this study. Furthermore, no difference was observed between the patients with IBD and healthy controls in the reactivity of lymphocytes of peripheral blood to lipopolysaccharide obtained from IgA1 protease-producing strains. There was no particular tendency in the relation with the IgA protease-nonproducing strain.

Although the IgA1 protease-producing strain arouses interest as a symptom-modifying factor, there has been no evidence suggesting a direct involvement of the IgA1 protease-producing strain in the pathophysiology of IBD.

SUMMARY

1) IgA1 protease production was investigated in 281 strains isolated from the intestinal bacterial flora of 17 patients with IBD, and IgA1 protease production was proved in three isolates of *Bifidobacterium* spp. and one isolate of *Clostridium* sp.

2) There was no specific reactivity of peripheral blood lymphocytes of the patients with IBD to the LPS obtained from the IgA1 protease-producing strain.

REFERENCES

1. Bamba, T., Aki, H., Kinugasa, K., Kashima, K., Yamaguchi, N., and Hosoda, S.: The role of the secretory IgA system on the establishment of the intestinal disorders. In: Proceedings of the 5th Asian Pacific Congress of Gastroenterology, p. 871. Stamford College Press, Singapore, 1976.
2. Hosoda, S., Bamba, T., and Fujiyama, Y.: The role of local immune system of gastrointestinal tract and the mechanism of s-IgA secretion. Presented at 6th World Congress of Gastroenterology, Madrid, 1978.
3. Plaut, A. G., Genco, R. J., and Tomasi, T. B.: Isolation of an enzyme from *Streptococcus sanguis* which specifically cleaves IgA. *J. Immunology*, **113**: 289, 1974.
4. Kilian, M. and Holmgren, K.: Ecology and nature of immunoglobulin A_1 protease producing streptococci in human oral cavity and pharynx. *Infect. Immun.*, **31**: 868, 1981.
5. Male, C. J.: Immunoglobulin A_1 protease production by *Hemophilis influenzae* and *Streptococcus pneumoniae*. *Infect. Immun.*, **26**: 254, 1979.
6. Plaut, A. G., Gilbert, J. V., Artenstein, M. S., and Capra, J. D.: *Neisseria gonorrheae* and *Neisseria meningifidis*: Extracellular enzyme cleaves human immunoglobulin A. *Science,* **190**: 1103, 1975.
7. Plaut, A. G., Gilbert, J. V., and Wister, R., Jr.: Loss of antibody activity in human immunoglobulin A exposed to extracellular immunoglobulin A protease of *Neisseria gonorrhoae* and *Streptococcus sanguis*. *Infect. Immun.*, **17**: 130, 1975.
8. Van Epps., D. E., Plaut, A. G., Bernier, G. M., and Williams, R. C., Jr.: IgA paraprotein inhibition of human neutrophil chemotaxis: Reduced activity following treatment with IgA-specific protease from *Neisseria gonorrhoae*. *Inflam.*, **4**: 137, 1980.

Fecal Bacteria and Short-Chain Fatty Acid in Patients with Ulcerative Colitis

Tsuneo Fukushima, Masaru Kawamoto, Akira Kubo, Hiroshi Takemura, and Shuji Tsuchiya

Short-chain fatty acid (SCFA) and bacterial flora were investigated in patients with ulcerative colitis followed at Yokohama City University Hospital. SCFA is one of the bacterial end products degraded mainly from unabsorbed carbohydrates, e.g., cellulose, hemicellulose, and pectin. Structurally, it is a mono-carbonic acid and the number of carbon molecules ranges from one to six.

Changes in fecal SCFA and bacterial flora were correlated with each clinico-pathological stage of ulcerative colitis.

SUBJECTS

Thirty-one patients with ulcerative colitis were studied. They included 6 cases with proctitis, 5 left-sided colitis, 9 total colitis, and 11 postoperative cases which included 10 total colectomy with ileoproctostomy and one proctocolectomy with ileostomy. Clinically, 16 patients were in the active stage and the remaining 14 patients were in remission. Except for the patient with ileostomy, they were given sulphasalazine in a dose of 3.0–4.5 g/day and in the active stage, prednisolone suppository in a dose of 5–30 mg/day.

METHODS

SCFA was measured by a modified method of Collin *et al.*[1] Five milliliters of 0.2 N of HCl was added to 1 g of stool specimen and ultrafiltrated. Then cation-exchanging resin was added to the ultrafiltrate. An aliquot of 2-methyl valeric acid was added to the supernatant as an internal standard. Volatile fatty acids were measured by gas chromatography and lactic acid was measured enzymatically using lactic dehydrogenase.

Second Department of Surgery, Yokohama City University, Yokohama, Japan

Fecal bacteria were cultured according to the method of Mitsuoka,[2)] in which 13 selective and nonselective culture media were used and aerobic and anaerobic cultures were performed and identified.

RESULTS

The mean concentration of SCFA in ulcerative colitis was lowered compared to that of healthy controls. In left-sided colitis and total colitis, it was approximately one half of the value for healthy controls. In the ileostomy effluent, it was less than one tenth of the control value. Acetic, propionic, and butyric acids predominated in the fecal fraction of healthy controls. However, the percentage of these volatile fatty acids decreased as the mucosal lesion extended proximally, and lactic acid increased as the mucosal lesion extended proximally (Fig. 1).

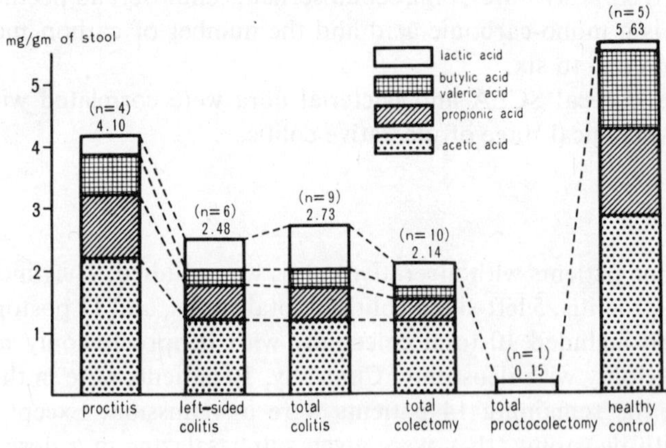

FIG. 1. Mean concentration of SCFA in UC patients and healthy controls.

Dividing the patients into active and inactive stages for each anatomic type of ulcerative colitis by presence or absence of fresh blood per rectum, volatile fatty acids—such as acetic, propionic, butylic, and valeric acids—were decreased in the active stage of every anatomic type of ulcerative colitis. On the other hand, nonvolatile fatty acid—lactic acid—was increased in the active stage of every anatomic type of ulcerative colitis. The increase in lactic acid was more prominent in total colitis compared to left-sided colitis and proctitis (Fig. 2).

From this evidence, the fecal volatile/nonvolatile SCFA ratio was cal-

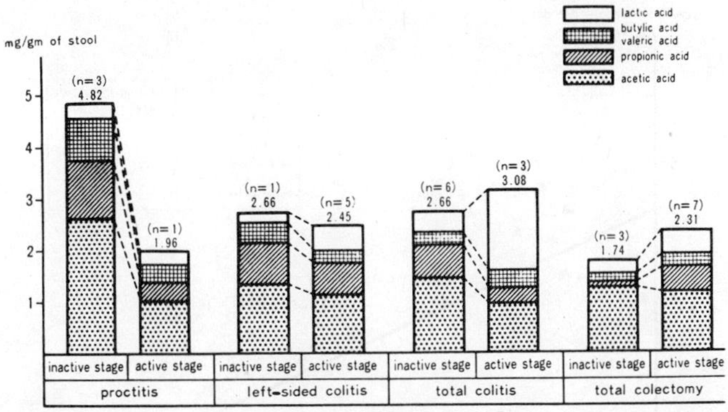

FIG. 2. Mean concentration of SCFA in UC patients by anatomic type.

culated and is shown in Fig. 3. The ratio was 45 in the healthy controls; however, it decreased in ulcerative colitis.

Interestingly, the ratio decreased with extension of mucosal lesion and also decreased in the active compared to the inactive stage of every anatomic type.

The relationship between the frequency of daily bowel movements and volatile/nonvolatile SCFA ratio in ulcerative colitis was analyzed (Fig. 4). As the ratio decreased, daily bowel movements increased. The inverse re-

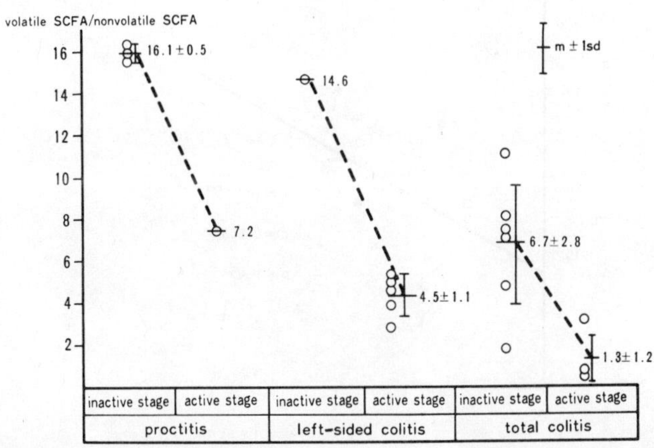

FIG. 3. Fecal volatile/nonvolatile SCFA ratio in UC patients by anatomic type.

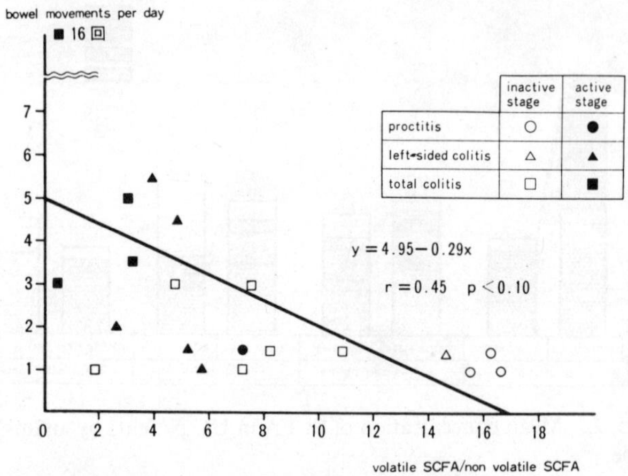

FIG. 4. Relationship between daily bowel movements and volatile/nonvolatile SCFA ratio in UC patients by anatomic type.

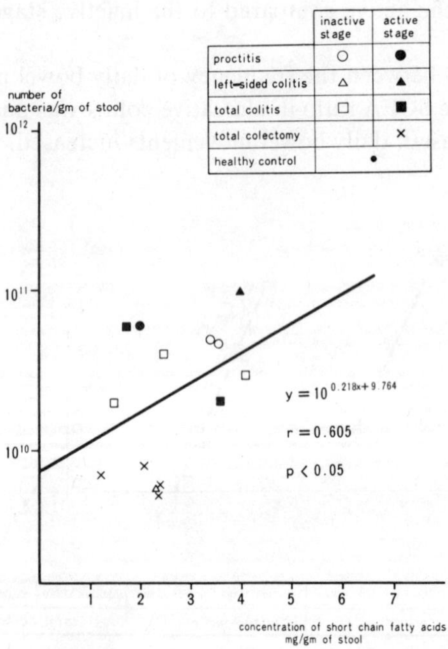

FIG. 5. Fecal bacterial count and concentration of SCFA in UC patients and healthy controls.

lationship was statistically significant. The composition of SCFA was recognized as an important factor regulating the frequency of bowel movements in ulcerative colitis.

The number of fecal bacteria and concentration of SCFA is plotted on the graph in Fig. 5. They were positively correlated and the concentration of SCFA was found to be dependent on the total number of fecal bacteria. Changes of fecal bacteria in various anatomic types and in the active and inactive stages of ulcerative colitis were analyzed. Compared to healthy controls, fecal bacteria were decreased in proctitis, left-sided colitis, and total colitis. The decrease in bacteria was more marked in the active stage than in the inactive stage.

Bacterial species of ulcerative colitis were compared to those of healthy controls. Anaerobic bacteria, such as Bacteroidaceae, *Eubacterium*, and Peptococcaceae were significantly decreased.

DISCUSSION

Fecal bacteria and SCFA were found to be closely related to the clinical picture of ulcerative colitis.[3] In the human colon, SCFA has been reported to be constant regardless of diet.[4] Thus the change in fecal SCFA in ulcerative colitis was not due to diet but due to other intraluminal changes such as inflammatory exudate, colonic motility, pH, and potential difference.

Large amounts of SCFA have been known to be absorbed from the normal human colon. Increased absorption of SCFA in ulcerative colitis would be one factor in lowered SCFA. Montgemery[5] and Shimoyama[6] reported increases of daily excreted SCFA, especially in the nonvolatile fraction, in ulcerative colitis.

Roediger[7] reported lowered utilization of butyrate using isolated colonic epithelial cells of ulcerative colitis and suggested that ulcerative colitis is an energy-deficiency disease. He also found an increase of lactate production in the cells prepared from acute colitis in which colonic cells instead of colonic bacteria produced lactate. The increase in lactate in the stool specimens of our patients could be derived from the colonic epithelium. Lactate may be formed from pyruvate by many gut anaerobes but is not a key intermediate in fermentation. Significant amounts are rarely found in the human gut; however, when large quantities of readily fermentable soluble carbohydrate are available, lactate production is favored.

Increased fermentation rate also results in a lowering of pH which in turn inhibits the metabolism of organisms which utilize lactate. Thus, lactate levels may become significant, but the exact mechanism of increased lactate in ulcerative colitis is unknown.

Metabolic studies of colonic bacteria and colonic epithelium are as important as immunologic and pathologic studies in order to resolve the etiology of ulcerative colitis.

REFERENCES

1. Collin, D. P., *et al.*: Quantitative gas-chromatographic determination of short chain fatty acid in aqueous samples. *Clin. Chem.*, **20**: 1235, 1974.
2. Mitsuoka, T.: Normal enteric flora. *Rinsho-kensa,* **23**: 320, 1979 (in Japanese).
3. Kawamoto, M., *et al.*: Fecal bacteria and short chain fatty acid in ulcerative colitis. *Nippon Shokakibyo Gakkai Zasshi,* **79**: 193, 1982 (in Japanese).
4. Cummings, J. H.: Short chain fatty acids in the human colon. *Gut,* **22**: 763, 1981.
5. Montgomery, R. D., *et al.*: Studies of intestinal fermentation in ulcerative colitis. *Gut,* **9**: 521, 1968.
6. Shimoyama, T., *et al.*: Enteric microflora and its pathogenicity. *Saishin Igaku,* **33**: 2047, 1968 (in Japanese).
7. Roediger, W. E. W.: The colonic epithelium in ulcerative colitis: An energy-deficiency disease? *Lancet,* **2**: 712, 1980.

Experimental Ulcerogenecity of Bacteroides

Atsuo Kitano and Kenzo Kobayashi

INTRODUCTION

The authors and co-workers have induced lesions similar to human ulcerative colitis in the rabbit colon by applying immunological techniques using carrageenan.[1] The relationship between bacteria in the intestine and ulcerative colitis has drawn much recent attention, and we have frequently reported on results obtained in experiments to induce similar lesions by using an enterobacterial common antigen (ECA) and *E. coli* 014 LPS.

In this experiment, we studied whether or not anaerobic bacterium could become an antigen using *Bacteroides fragilis* as antigen in addition to colon antigen and ECA, and made a comparative study between the lesions thus induced and the colon lesions induced by the antigens employed previously.

MATERIALS AND METHODS

Bacteroides fragilis. *B. fragilis* was cultured on semi-fluid GAM medium supplied by Nissui Gas Pack System. After mass-culturing in 4 *l* of GAM bouillon, the culture was sterilized in an autoclave. After washing, it was dried by acetone and the entire strain was used for immunization.
Lipopolysaccharide (*LPS*). LPS was extracted from *E. coli* 014 by the Westphal method and the warm phenol-water method.
Freund's complete adjuvant (FCA). FCA of Difco Corp. was used.
Animals. Female Hartley guinea pigs weighing 450–550 g were used for immunization.
Method of immunization and intracutaneous reaction. After 0.1 ml of physiological saline and 0.1 ml of FCA were added to *B. fragilis* and *E.*

Third Department of Internal Medicine, Osaka City University Medical School, Osaka, Japan *coli* 014 LPS, 0.2 ml of each was hypodermically injected at the sole of the foot of the animal. In the first and second immunizations, 5 mg of bacteroides was used; while in the third and fourth immunizations, 1 mg each was used. For *E. coli* 014 LPS, 0.05 mg was used at each immunization. Six weeks after the initial immunization, the first booster was applied, and thereafter three boosters were applied at an interval of two weeks between each. Twelve weeks after the initial immunization, an intracutaneous reaction was tested using various antigens to confirm cellular immunity. One week later, the colon of the animal was removed and tissue specimens were prepared.

RESULTS

Intracutaneous reaction caused by various antigens after immunization by B. fragilis *and* E. coli *014 LPS*

In the case of guinea pigs immunized by *B. fragilis*, the intracutaneous reaction caused by bacteroides was on the average 12.4 ± 4.1 mm in diameter, which was significantly more pronounced than in the case of immunization by ECA, colon antigen, or small intestinal antigen. Retarded hypersensibility caused by bacteroides was clearly observed.

In the animals immunized by *E. coli* 014 LPS, a medium degree of intracutaneous reaction was observed for each antigen. The presence of cross-reactivity between *E. coli* 014 LPS and these antigens was suggested.

Tissue image of guinea pig colon immunized by B. fragilis

Contrary to our expectation, the histological image of the mucous membrane of the colon after four immunizations by *B. fragilis* indicated roughly a normal image showing no marked difference from those of the control animals or the animals immunized by *E. coli* 014 LPS.

However, it indicated infiltration of round cells at the propria in the vicinity of the muscular tunic of the mucous membrane, which suggested the time of approaching tissue destruction.

DISCUSSION

We have reported on the effects of different combinations of antigen, adjuvant, immunization method, etc., as the methods to induce lesions similar to human ulcerative colitis in the colon of guinea pigs immunologically.[2,3]

As antigens, ECA, colon mucous membrane antigen, and bacteroides were used; for adjuvant, phospholipids and LPS combined with FIA were used. For some systems, a booster was applied to reinforce immunity.

The combination of ECA and FIA only or colon mucous membrane antigen and FIA only was used not for the purpose of inducing cellular immunity but for the control of other experimental systems.

In fact, with these systems, it was confirmed by intracutaneous reaction that retarded hypersensibility to ECA had not been established.[2] In terms of histological degeneration, disturbance of linear structure, decrease of mucus-producing cells, degeneration of linear cells, and a medium degree of cellular infiltration (mainly by monocytic cells) were observed.

In the system in which FIA was added to the combination of ECA and colon mucous membrane antigen or the system used in this experiment in which bacteroides antigen was combined with FCA, the histological changes in mucous membrane of the colon were generally moderate. The results generally indicated induction of a medium degree of histological degeneration.

Among the systems, that system using ECA, phospholipids, and FIA indicated relatively strong histological degeneration of the colon, and unlike the systems in which FCA or LPS was blended, it did not generate necrosis or ulcer at the injection point at the sole of the guinea pig foot; it was therefore a preferable system as allowed booster injections over an extended period.

Many reports on the adjuvant action of phospholipids have been published recently.[4,5] We reported that phospholipids induce retarded hypersensibility to protein antigen[6,7] and a report was also made that similar effects are observed with ECA.[8]

The influence of phospholipids on antibody production and the reinforcement of cellular immunity are also drawing attention. Having studied the relation between bacteroides and ulcerative colitis, Monteiro *et al.*[9] and William *et al.*[10] made the interesting observations that antibodies to auto-anaerobic bacterium or *B. fragilis* had increased in the mucous membrane of the colon or serum of patients. In the present experiments made by the authors, retarded hypersensibility to bacteroides was found to be established but histological changes in the colon were very small.

However, in this experiment, the entire strain was used for immunization and therefore it would be necessary to further check the results of this test by using extracted and purified LPS instead of the whole body of the strain.

REFERENCES

1. Kitano, A., Kobayashi, K., Murai, M., Tanaka, Y., Katayama, T., Yamaguchi, K., Kuwajima, S., and Yamamoto, S.: Study of experimental ulcerative colitis induced by carageenan in rabbit. *Jap. J. Gastroenterol.*, **75**: 1719–1726, 1978.

2. Tanaka, Y., Kobayashi, K., Murai, M., Katayama, T., Yamaguchi, K., Kawajima, S., Kitano, A., Yamamoto, S., Yano, I., and Masui, M.: Immunoadjuvant activity of phospholipids extracted from animal tissues (intestine, liver and brain) to ovalbumin and enterobacterial common antigen (ECA), and their possible role in the chronic inflammatory bowel disease. *Jap. J. Gastroenterol.*, **77**: 361–367, 1980.
3. Kobayashi, K., Kitano, A., Oka, S., Murai, M., Tanaka, Y., Kuwajima, S., Kamata, T., and Yamamoto, S.: Experimental colitis induced by enteral antigen and antigen of *E. coli*. *Digest. Org. Immunol.*, **5**: 85–91, 1980.
4. Allison, A. C. and Cregorladis, G.: Liposomes as immunological adjuvants. *Nature*, **252**: 252, 1974.
5. Heath, T. D., Edwards, D. C., and Ryman, B. E.: The adjuvant properties of liposomes. *Biochem. Soc. Trans.*, **4**: 129–133, 1976.
6. Masui, M., Yano, I., Yanagida, G., Tanaka, Y., Kuwajima, S., and Yamamoto, S.: Immunoadjuvant activity of negatively charged phospholipids on delayed hypersensitivity. *FEBS Letters*, **83**: 237–240, 1977.
7. Tanaka, Y.: Immunoadjuvant activity of synthetic and animal phospholipids on delayed hypersensitivity. *J. Osaka City Med. Center*, **28**: 347–364, 1979.
8. Sanchez, Y., Ionescu-matiu, I., Dressman, G. K., Kramp, W., Six, H. R., Hollinger, F. B., and Melnick, J. L.: Humoral and cellular immunity to hepatitis B virus-derived antigens: Comparative activity of Freund's complete adjuvant, alum, and liposomes. *Infect. Immun.*, **30**: 729–733, 1980.
9. Monterio, E., Fossey, J., Shiner, M., Drasar, B. S., and Allison, A. C.: Antibacterial antibodies in rectal and colonic mucosa of ulcerative colitis. *Lancet*, **6**: 249–251, 1971.
10. William, R., Brown, M. D., and Lee, E.: Radioimmunological measurements of bacterial antibodies. *Gastroenterology*, **66**: 1145–1153, 1974.

Discussion: Intestinal Microflora

Michael J. Hill and Takashi Shimoyama, Chairmen

Dr. Shimoyama: I would like to ask Dr. Hill as to whether the microflora of IBD is different from the microflora of healthy subjects.

Dr. Hill: We heard in England that ulcerative colitis and Crohn's disease are becoming more common in Japan. Also, the fact that Dr. Hori can study 93 ulcerative colitis patients and the numbers of patients that the other workers have been able to study testify to that fact that ulcerative colitis is now becoming a problem in Japan. It does great credit to the Japanese Medical Research Association that you are actually studying colitis now while the problem is developing. In the West we are very used to waiting until the medical problem has arisen, and then we tackle it. It is good to see it being done this way round.

It is very impressive to see the quality of the bacteriology that is being done in these various centers. The whole world is assisted by Dr. Mitsuoka in its bacteriology. He is one of the world leaders in this field and we all learn from him. You are very lucky to have him in Japan as your leader in this field.

It was good to see the breadth of the studies going on. I think that you are reaching the same conclusions as we are. This is not an easy problem, and there is no single organism we are going to be able to blame for the causation of ulcerative colitis. It is a two-stage process: initiation of the disease is probably very different from the maintenance of the disease. Perhaps initiation takes place all the time and if you do not have the right flora or the right conditions to maintain the disease, then you have a case of diarrhea which goes away, and then you do not recognize the initiation stage. Similarly there must be many people who have the right condition in their gut for maintenance of the disease but never had the disease initiated. This is again going to make it very difficult for bacteriologists trying to look for differences between patients and controls. These are problems that we have to live with in these studies and have to overcome. As Dr. Hudson said, we believe that the flora which is actually associated with the mucosa and appears to be different from the flora in the lumen is probably very important, and I think it is likely that bacteria are involved either in stimulating immune response, introducing toxins, or in some other way maintaining the disease state. It is more likely that those organisms closely associated with the mucosa are more important in these diseases. I am sure these are ways that studies will develop, but it has been very impressive listening to the range of work going on.

Dr. Shimoyama: Dr. Hill mentioned mucosal flora and luminal flora. Related to this point, I would like to invite Dr. Mitsuoka to comment.

Dr. Mitsuoka: In our laboratory, we have still not looked at the differences between mucosal flora and luminal flora, and we have not really looked at the exact relationship between these two. I think it is necessary to differentiate these to distinguish them very clearly. For example, perhaps there is a higher concentration of some species in the mucosal flora; perhaps there is a great concentration of the mucosal flora compared to the luminal flora. I am sure there is very good material to study. Also, as Dr. Hill has just mentioned, we have to look at the first step and the maintenance, the flora of the time of initiation, what is related to that flora, and which flora is concerned with the maintenance. I have always believed that it is necessary to separate these two, the flora of initiation and the flora of maintenance.

In our laboratory, we are looking at the flora after treatment and untreated flora, and I think it is very necessary to look at the flora of untreated patients. After treatment the flora becomes much more complicated and in the lesion itself we see very complex interactions and interrelationships with the results of the treatment and results of the lesion, depending on the treatment itself. We have to really look at these differences and identify very clearly the mucosal flora from the luminal flora and see whether it is possible to differentiate between these two kinds of flora. I think this is a question which we must pursue. I think we can look at the genus level of bacterial groups and at the same sample at the species level, and then see what is contributing to the lesion. I think this is the path we must pursue.

Dr. Hill: We have done some studies of patients who are being treated with antibiotics or various regimens to look at the differences between the flora in patients during relapse and during remission hoping that this will give us some clues. One of the problems here of course is that when you treat with antibiotics you get many coincidental effects of the antibiotics. Lots of organisms are killed, in a vain attempt to kill the causative organism, and it is difficult to see which of the dead bodies was once firing the gun. We did a study of Salazopyrin in much less detail than Dr. Mitsuoka's study, but which gave us many similar conclusions. There was a general decrease in all organisms, but we could not see which way to go further. We did not pursue the study and it would be very interesting to see the extra information Dr. Mitsuoka has got by his much more detailed analysis of these patients.

Dr. Nakaya: I showed a slide of three cases in which *Bacteroides vulgatus* was detected in the lymph nodes. It was also detected in the intestinal wall. So it did affect the walls but not the mucosa. In the intestinal walls and the mucosa they were detected but not in other lesions. We have lot of other data but we have not analyzed it in the way that Dr. Hill has pointed out, so we would like to look at the existing data in the way that he has mentioned.

Dr. Hudson, I think you showed that the initiation factor of ulcerative colitis or Crohn's disease might be an RNA virus. Is that correct?

Dr. Hudson: Yes.

Dr. Nakaya: Would you give us some evidence to support this?

Dr. Hudson: My evidence is purely that of published work by Professor Gitnick and his colleagues in America who have for many years been attempting isolation of filterable agents from inflammatory bowel disease tissue. Some three or four years ago, Professor Gitnik reported that Crohn's disease tissue yielded a probable RNA virus of unusual type from Crohn's disease tissue and from some cases of colitis tissue. These agents are extremely difficult to grow even in very specialized tissue culture systems. Their work has been plagued with problems of contamination with adventicious agents, laboratory mycoplasmas, other viruses, and so on, but recently he has shown that it is possible serologically to differentiate the agents from colitis tissue from that of Crohn's disease tissue. He has raised antibodies to both agents in rabbits and shown that neutralization can be attained. These viruses grow to very low titers in tissue culture, 10^2 to 10^3 infective units/ml of tissue culture, which makes normal viral neutralization tests and other studies very difficult; but inasmuch as they are slow growing, difficult to grow, and yet persistent and found very commonly in most inflammatory bowel disease tissue, they are the best candidates we have of transmissible agents of Crohn's disease and ulcerative colitis at the moment.

Dr. Nakaya: Did you say that diseases clustered in some populations?

Dr. Hudson: Yes.

Dr. Nakaya: Do you have any familial clusters of ulcerative colitis or Crohn's disease?

Dr. Hill: The person who has studied this clustering in Britain is Dr. Maybury, who has studied clusters of Crohn's disease especially in South Wales. He has presented a number of papers at gastroenterology meetings and published a few papers describing familial clusters of Crohn's disease which indicates quite strongly an infective agent. In ulcerative colitis, I think the evidence is much weaker. There are odd reports of clusters which probably to my mind do not mean anything. I think that evidence for infective agents from clustering disease cases is weak, but I think it is stronger for Crohn's disease.

Dr. Shimoyama: I am sure that the changes in the microflora actually do take place, but I think that we must differentiate between the mucosal flora and luminal flora and we must also differentiate between the flora of time of initiation of the disease and that of time of maintenance of the disease. I think there is much of such research that has to be redone in the light of research and new suggestions. I would like to ask either Dr. Nakaya or Dr. Hudson how and what you can actually get as a mucosal flora. This may be a simple question but we always seem to be plagued by contamination. How can you get specimens so that you can really say definitely that this is mucosal flora, this is such a method, or this is such a specimen?

Dr. Nakaya: The surgeons take the specimens, so we do not know specifically once they are sent to our research group. We use anaerobic buffer by Dr. Mitsuoka and we wash slightly three times. Some we can take by that method and others we cannot. This is the only differentiation. As to the question of whether those are definitely from mucosal flora (or those which adhere to the mucosa) or not, we have not checked. In our research group, we took a certain standard method and we abided by it. I would be very happy to hear Dr. Hudson's response.

Dr. Hudson: The methods that I use I have adapted from studies conducted using the pig colon as a model. This has certain advantages from the point of view of obtaining experience in this field. There are certain types of bacteria found on the mucosal surface of the pig colon that one does not find in the luminal flora, so one can use these as indicator strains as to the purity of the flora one is obtaining. In these studies we took the colon, and we washed it very thoroughly in several changes of reduced buffer and monitored the loss of fecal-type organisms and the appearance of the mucosal-type flora. We found it very difficult to overwash the mucosa and from this, and from histological evidence, we think that the mucosal flora in the pig, and probably in man as well, is not necessarily lying on the surface but it is trapped beneath, deep in the crypts and attached specifically to goblet cell mucous, not on the overlying mucous itself because this is lost in the washings.

We no longer use surgical specimens of the mucosa for studies of the mucosal flora because we found that the mechanical and antimicrobial preparations that the patient was subjected to did cause certain nonspecific alterations to the flora. We now use colonoscopic or rectal biopsies by sigmoidoscopy from unprepared patients. These are washed thoroughly in four or five changes of reduced buffer in an anaerobic chamber, and homogenized with a stomacher. I do not know if you use a stomacher in this country—this causes maceration by squeezing action rather than a blender type of homogenization. This yields very high counts of the mucosal flora. As to the composition of the flora, it is qualitatively similar to the fecal flora in man, and although quantitatively there are differences in the rectal mucosa in colitis and Crohn's disease, there are far fewer anaerobes than aerobes.

Although there are reports of unique morphological types of bacteria in human mucosa in the rectum, spiral forms and so on, we have not been able to culture them; however, another group in Dr. Barnes' laboratory in England has had some success using more specialized procedures. The mucosal flora of the human colonic mucosa does not form a so-called pallisade layer that is seen in rodent ileal and colonic mucosal floras. This is a thick mat which one can use in talks such as this to demonstrate the presence of a mucosal flora. In man it is about two orders of magnitude less in density; one just does not see very many organisms histologically.

Dr. Hill: The streptococci that we have isolated from the mucosal flora did not subclassify; they were fecal streptococci but they did not fit standard classification patterns when examined by the Streptococcal Reference Laboratory. In fact, for a time the reference laboratory denied that they were streptococci, and they were returned with a variety of different names on them. Similarly, Dr. Hudson, clostridia that you isolated do not belong to major species you find in the lumen, do they?

Dr. Hudson: They are certainly not usual sporing clostridia; rather, they are reluctant to sporulate.

Dr. Shimoyama: I believe cancer risk should also be included in this discussion. I think you had a question for Dr. Hill.

Dr. Nakaya: Dr. Hill, I would like to have your further detailed comment on the NDC group of clostridia.

Dr. Hill: We have been studying the production of unsaturated bile acids and ability to remove hydrogen from the steroid nucleus. This is not an easy reaction. It is a reaction which is carried out by a wide range of soil organisms and it is very important to the pharmaceutical industry in producing anti-inflammatory steroids and so on. Those organisms introduce double bonds using oxygen as the acceptor of hydrogen. Of course the gut is very anaerobic—there is no oxygen, and so you need bacteria that can utilize different acceptors for hydrogen.

As a biochemist I believe clostridia can do anything; if you find the right clostridium then you can persuade it to do any reaction you are interested in; we are not surprised to find some clostridia that can produce unsaturated bile acids. However, these clostridia did not belong to a particular species so that, for example, we find that a high proportion of strains of *Clostridium paraputrificum* and *C. butyricum* are able to carry out this reaction although there are some strains of those species that cannot. About two thirds of the strains of *C. tertium* can carry out this reaction, but a proportion cannot. Some strains of *C. indolis* can carry out the reaction, but some cannot, and so on. We screened more than a thousand strains of clostridia and found about 19 different species of clostridia, representatives of those species, that could carry out the reaction. But we found no species where every strain could carry out the reaction. There were always some strains that could not carry out the reaction.

This meant that in studying the clostridial flora there was no value, in this respect, in identifying the clostridia. It was much simpler to just test their ability to carry out this reaction, and the test is a very simple one. You simply grow the organisms and incubate them with a substrate, a suitable steroid substrate, and then the product fluoresces under UV light. After incubating overnight in the presence of menaquinone, bacterial vitamin K, which we believe is the hydrogen acceptor, you can simply do thin-layer chromatography and look for the fluorescent spot with the right mobility. It is much easier to do this than to identify clostridia. We simply take the clostridia plate that we do a first isolation on and we pick the colonies from that plate and go directly to testing for the ability to dehydrogenate the steroid nucleus.

NDC means nuclear dehydrogenating clostridia—there are many dehydrogenating reactions which most clostridia can do. Dehydrogenating the steroid nucleus is a very specific and difficult reaction but these clostridia can do it. We find that we have a crude assay for carriage of these organisms. We find that about 30 to 35 percent of English people carry organisms which are able to carry out this reaction. The rest of the people carry clostridia, of course, but they carry related clostridia which cannot carry out the reaction. In Scotland where the incidence of colon cancer is higher, we found that carriage of these clostridia is more common as well; and in Nigeria, for example, where colon cancer is extremely rare, carriage of these clostridia is virtually unknown—we cannot find any carriage of these clostridia. So carriage of clostridia varies between populations. People seem to carry either these clostridia or related clostridia which cannot carry out the reaction.

Dr. Nakaya: Do you think that the NDC group has a direct relationship to bile acid metabolism in subjects of high concentration of fecal bile acids?

Dr. Hill: We have done simple statistical correlations between the numbers of NDC per gram of feces and the concentration of bile acids in the fecal sample, and there is no correlation at all. So a high bile acid concentration does not favor the growth of these clostridia at all. The two are totally unrelated, but of course when the clostridia are present that must affect the metabolism of bile acids. The amount of metabolism undergone by bile acids in the colon is somewhat related to the concentration of bile acids but not totally, so you can have a high concentration of bile acids in stool which has not undergone very much metabolism. The concentration of bile acids is determined by some factor unrelated to bacterial metabolism.

Dr. Shimoyama: I would like a comment from Dr. Hill on Dr. Fukushima's report about short-chain fatty acids and also on the IgA protease study given by Dr. Bamba.

Dr. Hill: I found Dr. Fukushima's paper on short-chain fatty acids very interesting indeed because I have been following the work of Dr. Roediger very closely. Dr. Roediger worked at Oxford and was studying the role of the short-chain fatty acids produced in the lumen of the gut as energy sources for the intestinal mucosal cells. He was able to show that the butyrate produced by the bacterial flora was much more important than glucose as an energy source to the intestinal mucosal cells. He published a hypothesis in the *Lancet* in 1980 in which he suggested that ulcerative colitis may be simply a disease of energy deficiency of the intestinal mucosal cells. If one did not produce enough short-chain fatty acids to keep mucosal cells healthy, then colitis resulted. The study by Dr. Fukushima is a very nice study in this respect. It fits in beautifully with this hypothesis of Dr. Roediger. Dr. Roediger proposed his hypothesis with very little data and it is very nice to see some data which support it. This again illustrates how important our bacteria are to us. We depend on the bacterial flora in our gut to keep our intestinal mucosal cells healthy. Bacteria are not bad; they are usually very good for us. We concentrate on the disease and we always talk about the harmful effect of bacteria, but most effects of bacteria are very beneficial and they are very good for us.

I was also interested in the paper by Dr. Bamba because bacteriologists are very familiar with proteolysis and with how highly proteolytic intestinal bacteria are, particularly the clostridia and bacteroides; we do tests in cooked meat broth to see how rapidly they can destroy all of the meat in the broth, and it is frightening. You realize if you did not have good protective systems in the gut against these bacteria, they would dissolve you very rapidly. It is very impressive, therefore, how resistant the IgA is to all of these proteolytic enzymes that bacteria produce, and particularly interesting that it should be bifidobacteria of all organisms producing the proteolytic enzyme that breaks down IgA, because we tend not to think of bifidobacteria as being very active in proteolysis. I normally consider them to be rather mild in comparison with bacteroides and clostridia. Amongst the hundreds of strains he tested, including many bacteroides and very many clostridia which between them must have produced a very wide range of extremely active proteolytic enzymes, IgA is resistant to all of them except to just three strains. I wonder whether Dr. Bamba could comment on the great resistance of IgA to bacterial proteolysis. He has given his paper on the breakdown of IgA by proteolysis. I wonder if he could comment on the reverse: why is it so resistant to proteolysis by the enzymes of other organisms?

Dr. *Bamba*: Usually IgA occurs as secretory IgA or sIgA. It is secreted as sIgA. If it is IgA alone then proteolysis occurs very easily. However the enzyme cannot lyse secretory IgA, so this is a kind of protective action by the secretory component. In the gut system we have the sIgA system. This has the protective system, and IgA protease has a highly specific role in challenging the protective system.

Dr. *Shimoyama*: I think we should discuss the experimental ulcerogenecity of bacteroides. Perhaps Dr. Nakaya would like to make some comments on Dr. Kitano's paper.

Dr. *Nakaya*: If the bacteroides group is related to pathogenesis or etiology, as Dr. Hudson has suggested, then probably these are initiation agents on the one hand and maintenance agents on the other. Bacteroides may be involved in either one of these and this will be discussed later in this symposium. In the case of humans there might be some kind of genetic predisposition for initiation agents and maintenance agents. If the two are superimposed on each other, then there is the answer to the incidence of ulcerative colitis, for example. So in that sense

I think the kind of research conducted by Dr. Kitano and Dr. Kobayashi is necessary for the future.

Dr. Matsueda: We are dealing with a very controversial subject today and I have several questions. Dr. Nakaya reported that Sulphasalazine-treated IBD patients showed a decrease of bacteroides and an increase of some sorts of streptococci. We now know that metronidazole is one of the most effective drugs for Crohn's colitis and you may already know that metronidazole suppresses bacteroides and increases streptococci in the gut flora. Dr. Fukushima reported that free fatty acids seemed to be increased in active IBD patients, which suggests that patients may have increased bacteroides in the intestinal flora. My prediction is that untreated IBD patients may have increased bacteroides, especially *Bacteroides fragilis*, and decreased streptococci. However, today's results were somewhat conflicting. I would like to ask all of you why such a discrepancy exists between your research.

My second question concerns the mucosal flora and luminal flora. Dr. Hudson demonstrated the technique for culturing the mucosal flora but I feel there are a lot of problems. If you use biopsied specimens you are never able to rule out contamination of the gut flora which may bring the luminal flora into the tissue, and I do not think you can entirely wash out that kind of contamination by washing several times or even 10 times. Clearly we have to know if these are the kinds of techniques we should pursue in the future, or do we have to invent other techniques to solve these kind of problems?

The third question is for Dr. Hill. You demonstrated that IBD patients who have high risk of cancer seem to have increased bile acid concentration in the stool and increased colonization with NDC. But, as you know, almost 95% of bile acids should be absorbed in the terminal ileum, so if you see increased bile acids in the stool this may indicate some kind of disturbance of normal reabsorption or enterohepatic circulation of bile acids. This may occur because of the severity of the disease, not only because of the bacterial flora. My question is whether the increased risk of cancer is due to the severity of the disease or intestinal flora.

Dr. Mitsuoka: Your first question is a very difficult one because, as I explained earlier, it is not just a change in the flora of IBD patients. It really depends on the condition of the patients when we investigate them. It depends on the use or non-use of antibiotics and on time of use or method of use. In some cases we are looking at initial stage; in some cases we are looking at remission stage. I think it is necessary to look at the data very clearly and see what kind of data we have.

As I mentioned in my own presentation, I have got different results from other researchers. We have found an increase in *E. coli* and a decrease in anaerobes. Perhaps this is one common result, but then this seems to be the limit of agreement. We have a problem with streptococci. We have different results on streptococci. My data may differ from Dr. Hill's data; then somewhere perhaps we say they are streptococci and we send them to someone who says they are not streptococci, as Dr. Hill has just mentioned. What do we do in a case like this? If we have more such cases we may be able to find the answer. If the condition of the patient is restricted to the objectiveness of the data and if we get correlating conditions then we may be able to arrive at similar conclusions, but at present time all we can say is we cannot get identical results because we are not looking at identical conditions. As Dr. Hudson pointed out earlier, the question is how to differentiate mucosal flora from luminal flora. I think if we can get some international unity or international standard, then we will be able to carry out more international comparisons.

Dr. Hill: I agree totally with Dr. Mitsuoka that we are looking at a very complicated problem and the idea that we are all going to get identical data assumes that we are all using identical types of patients under identical conditions. Since we really have so little idea about the causes of the disease and therefore what things should be controlled, it is not surprising that we get different results. I think we have to concentrate on the areas of agreement rather than the areas of disagreement because in all of these things there are going to be lot of coincidental findings as well as relevant findings. Even in the very best possible studies there is no reason why coincidental findings should agree. It is only findings directly relevant to the disease process that we hope will agree.

As far as mucosal versus luminal flora is concerned, you may not believe it but you can wash off the luminal flora. If you count the bacteria in the washings you find very very high numbers in the first couple of washings and these drop right down, but you still have very large numbers of organisms left on the mucosa. Qualitatively you still find bacteroides, you still find clostridia, you still find streptococci, you still find coliforms and lactobacilli, but the proportions are very different from those you find in the lumen which leads us to believe that there really is a genuine mucosa-associated flora. Once again I agree totally with Dr. Mitsuoka that what we need is a nice set of defined conditions so that we know that we are comparing the same things when we talk about something. We can then define the mucosa-associated flora as that which remains on the surface after so many washings using a standard washing procedure.

The third question was whether the high fecal bile acid concentration in patients with ulcerative colitis who develop bowel cancer was due to a disturbance in the bile acids and their regulation or whether it is the result of the severity of the disease. We believe that diet is important in determining fecal loss of bile acids—98% is absorbed in the terminal ileum. This is a very efficient enterohepatic circulation system, but diet can interfere with this enterohepatic circulation and an increasing amount of dietary fat increases fecal loss, an increasing amount of dietary pectin and gelling fibers increases fecal loss, and so on. However, if you take 10 people and you put them on an identical diet and you measure fecal bile acid concentration, you will find a 4-fold range in the fecal bile acid loss. This is 10 normal healthy persons; in other words, although on average we are 98% efficient in absorbing bile acids in the terminal ileum, that masks the range of 96 to 99% still enviable from any other point of view. The gut is a marvelous system but there is this range. Some people are as low as only 96% efficient in recovering bile acids but then that gives you 4% loss compared with 99%-efficient individuals with a 1% loss and a 4-fold range. We think this is something which has to do with that person's constitution. We do not understand the terminal ileum as much as we like to think, so we do not understand why some people are 96% efficient and some are 99% efficient.

Now, when we compare ulcerative colitis patients with normal healthy control patients, the mean fecal bile acid concentration in the patients and controls is very similar, so I do not think that the severity of the disease is affecting the fecal bile acid concentration. I think what we are really doing is selecting those people who would have high fecal bile acid concentration anyway and if those people happen to develop colitis then they have a high risk. I think it is an unfortunate meeting of two unassociated factors. I do not think high fecal bile acid concentration has to do with the disease. I think it is something that is inbuilt in other characteristics of the person.

II. IMMUNOLOGY

Immunogenetic Studies on Inflammatory Bowel Disease

——HLA Antigens in Patients with Ulcerative Colitis in Japan

Norikazu Morita, Yoshiyuki Shiwaku, and Mikio Inoue

INTRODUCTION

The cause of ulcerative colitis (UC) is unknown. Evidence for the involvement of genetic factors in inflamatory bowel disease (IBD) is provided by the increased familial incidence found in both UC and Crohn's disease (CD). Also the involvement of immunological mechanisms in the causation of these diseases has been emphasized. Since HLA antigens are not only genetic markers but are probably in linkage disequilibrium with immune response or immune response-associated antigens, determination of the histocompatibility antigens in IBD could provide important information.

Most of the studies of HLA in patients with UC or CD have not been able to show an abnormal frequency of any HLA antigen. However, Delpre and his co-workers in 1980 found a significantly high frequency of HLA-Bw35 among patients with UC but not those with CD.[1)]

The aim of the present study was to investigate the possible relationship between the HLA antigens in Japanese patients with UC.

SUBJECTS AND METHODS

HLA typing was done in the 44 patients with a diagnosis of UC attending our clinic. The diagnosis was based on histopathological examination of biopsy preparation, on disease history, and on typical rectoscopic and X-ray findings.

For further analysis, the patients were divided into two groups in accordance with the time of onset of the disease: the "early onset" group, i.e., patients in whom the first symptoms occurred before the age of 30 years, and the "late onset" group, i.e., patients with symptoms occurring for the

Department of Health Care, School of Medicine, Fukuoka University, Fukuoka, Japan first time after the age of 30. One hundred and ten healthy subjects were tested for control studies.

HLA-A, -B, and -C antigens were typed by standard NIH technique. HLA-DR antigens were typed by standard microlymphocytotoxicity test recommended by the 8th International Histocompatibility Workshop in 1980.

For the evaluation of HLA association, the χ^2 test was employed.

TABLE 1. Frequencies of HLA-A, -B, and -C Antigens in Patients with Ulcerative Colitis

HLA	Ulcerative colitis ($n = 44$)	Normal controls ($n = 70$)	χ^2	Corrected p-value	Relative risk
A1	0	0		N.S.	
A2	22 (50.0)[a]	36 (51.4)		N.S.	
A3	0	0		N.S.	
Aw23	0	0		N.S.	
Aw24	31 (70.5)	42 (60.0)		N.S.	1.59
A25	0	0		N.S.	
A26	4 (9.1)	17 (24.3)	4.15	N.S.	
A11	9 (20.5)	13 (18.6)		N.S.	
A28	0	0		N.S.	
A29	1 (2.3)	0		N.S.	
Aw30	0	0		N.S.	
Aw33	6 (13.6)	8 (11.4)		N.S.	
Bw51	6 (13.6)	7 (10.0)		N.S.	
Bw52	24 (54.5)	13 (18.6)	15.95	$cp < 0.005$	5.26
B7	2 (4.5)	16 (22.9)	6.81	N.S.	
B8	0	2 (2.9)		N.S.	
B12	7 (15.9)	5 (7.1)		N.S.	
B13	4 (9.1)	2 (2.8)		N.S.	
B14	0	0		N.S.	
B15	10 (22.7)	11 (15.7)		N.S.	
B17	0	0		N.S.	
B27	0	1 (1.4)		N.S.	
B37	0	0		N.S.	
B40	7 (15.9)	32 (45.7)	10.66	$cp < 0.05$	4.45
Bw16	4 (9.1)	3 (4.3)		N.S.	
Bw21	0	0		N.S.	
Bw22	1 (2.3)	5 (7.1)		N.S.	
Bw54	3 (6.8)	9 (12.9)		N.S.	
Bw35	3 (6.8)	8 (11.4)		N.S.	
Cw1	10 (22.7)	12 (17.1)		N.S.	
Cw3	20 (45.5)	35 (50.0)		N.S.	
Cw4	3 (6.8)	9 (12.9)		N.S.	

[a]Phenotype frequencies (%). N.S.: not significant.

P-values were corrected for the number of antigens studied and then termed corrected *p*-values. Relative risk was calculated by formula.

RESULTS

In Table 1 phenotype frequencies of HLA-A, -B, and -C antigens are shown for patients and controls. In locus A, there was a decrease in the frequency of HLA-26, but this was not significant after correction for the number of antigens. In locus B, the significant differences were observed with regard to HLA-Bw52 when the patients with UC were compared with controls. Twenty-four of the 44 UC patients (54.5%) and 18.6% of the healthy individuals were positive for HLA-Bw52 ($cp < 0.005$). In Bw52 carriers, the relative risk of developing UC is 5.26. In locus C, the frequency of HLA-Cw4 in UC patients and controls was 7.7% and 12.9%, respectively, but the corrected *p*-value was not significant.

Table 2 shows the distribution of phenotype frequencies of locus DR in control individuals and the patients with UC. A highly significant increase for HLA-DR2 was observed in the patients. Twenty-eight of 40 UC patients (70%) and 32.7% of the healthy individuals were positive ($cp < 0.005$). In DR2 carriers the relative risk of developing UC is 4.8.

TABLE 2. Frequencies of HLA-DR Antigens in Patients with Ulcerative Colitis

HLA-DR	Ulcerative colitis ($n = 40$)	Normal Controls ($n = 110$)	χ^2	Corrected *p*-value	Relative risk
DR1	5 (12.5)[a]	14 (12.7)		N.S.	
DR2	28 (70.0)	36 (32.7)	15.17	$cp < 0.005$	4.80
DR3	0	0		N.S.	
DR4	11 (27.5)	52 (47.3)	3.93	N.S.	
DR5	1 (2.5)	7 (6.4)		N.S.	
DRw6	1 (2.5)	21 (19.1)	5.19	N.S.	
DR7	1 (2.5)	0		N.S.	
DRw8	6 (15.0)	13 (11.8)		N.S.	
DRw9	8 (20.0)	30 (27.3)		N.S.	

[a]Phenotype frequencies (%). N.S.: not significant.

Table 3 presents the distribution of HLA antigens in patients with UC according to age at onset of disease. Phenotype Bw52 was found in 16 of 27 patients of the early onset group. The frequency of HLA-Bw52 was higher in the early onset group, and the frequency of HLA-DR2 was also higher in the early onset group. The relative risk of developing UC before the age of 30 years is 6.38 in Bw52 carriers and 6.17 in DR2 carriers.

Table 4 shows the distribution of HLA-DR antigens in patients with

TABLE 3. Frequencies of HLA Antigens in Patients with Ulcerative Colitis by Age at Onset

	Age at Onset		Normal control
	≦ 30 y.o.	≧ 31 y.o.	
HLA-A, -B	(n = 27)	(n = 17)	(n = 70)
A2	40.7%	64.7%	51.4%
Aw24	66.7	76.5	60.0
A26	11.1	5.8	24.3
Bw51	14.8	11.8	10.0
Bw52	59.3 (RR = 6.38)	47.1 (RR = 4.03)	18.6
B7	3.7	5.9	22.9
B15	29.6	11.8	15.7
Bw16	7.4	11.8	4.2
Bw35	7.4	5.9	11.4
B40	11.1	23.5	45.7
HLA-DR	(n = 24)	(n = 16)	(n = 110)
DR1	16.6%	6.3%	12.7%
DR2	75.0 (RR = 6.17)	62.5 (RR = 3.43)	32.7
DR4	33.3	18.8	47.3
DRw6	4.2	0	19.1
DRw8	12.5	18.8	11.8
DRw9	16.7	25.0	27.3

RR: relative risk.

TABLE 4. Frequencies of HLA Antigens in Patients with Ulcerative Colitis by Extent of Involvement

	Extent of involvement		Normal control
	Proctocolitis	Proctitis	
HLA-A, -B	(n = 37)	(n = 7)	(n = 70)
A2	51.4%	42.9%	51.4%
Aw24	75.7	42.9	60.0
A26	5.4	28.6	24.3
Bw51	16.2	0	10.0
Bw52	56.8	42.9	18.6
B7	2.7	14.3	22.9
B15	21.6	28.6	15.7
Bw16	8.1	14.3	4.2
Bw35	5.4	14.3	11.4
B40	16.2	14.3	45.7
HLA-DR	(n = 33)	(n = 7)	(n = 110)
DR1	15.2%	0 %	12.7%
DR2	75.8	42.9	32.7
DR4	27.3	28.6	47.3
DRw6	3.0	0	19.1
DRw8	18.2	0	11.8
DRw9	9.1*	71.4*	27.3

*$\chi^2 = 10.40$ (with Yates' correction), $cp < 0.02$.

UC divided into proctocolitis and proctitis groups. Phenotype DRw9 was found in 3 of the 33 patients of the proctocolitis group (9.1%) and in 5 of the 7 patients in the proctitis group. The difference between the proctocolitis and proctitis groups was statistically significant for the frequency of DRw9 antigen.

The haplotype frequencies and coefficients of linkage disequilibrium of gametic association in controls and patients with UC are shown in Fig. 1. The haplotype frequency of HLA-Aw24–Bw52 in Japanese controls and in UC were 0.1070 and 0.2822, respectively. Linkage disequilibrium in controls and UC were 0.0656 and 0.1335, respectively. The haplotype frequency of HLA-Bw52–DR2 in Japanese controls and in UC were 0.0990 and 0.3059, respectively. Linkage disequilibrium in controls and in UC were 0.0750 and 0.1570, respectively. A higher haplotype frequency of HLA-Bw52–DR2 was found in patients with UC in Japan.

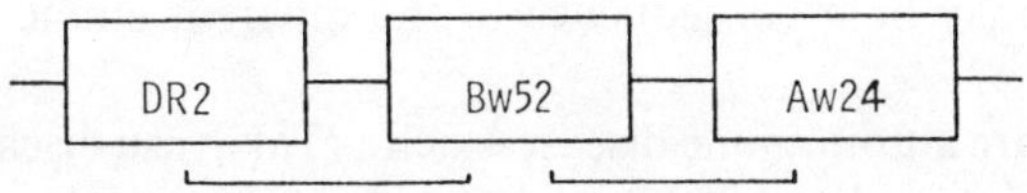

		DR2–Bw52	Bw52–Aw24
Ulcerative Colitis	HF	0.3059	0.2822
	Δ	0.1570	0.1335
	t	5.9	4.6
Control	HF	0.0990	0.1070
	Δ	0.0750	0.0656
	t	4.9	4.6

FIG. 1. Haplotype frequencies in patients with ulcerative colitis.

DISCUSSION

Previous studies of the relative frequencies of HLA antigens in patients with UC and CD have not demonstrated any clear-cut positive associations with any particular phenotypes. Recently, Delpre *et al.*[1] found a significantly high frequency of HLA-Bw35 among patients with UC. In addition, HLA-Aw24 was found with increased frequency in those with early onset of severe disease.

With regard to the HLA profile of Japanese patients with UC, Tsuchiya *et al.*[2] in 1977, Yagita *et al.* in 1977, Hiwatashi *et al.*[3] in 1979, and Tanaka *et al.*[4] in 1980 have reported an increase in HLA-B5 antigen. In the present study, we found an increase in Bw52, which is one of the split antigens of B5, and an increase in DR2, whereas Asakura *et al.*[5] reported increases in B5 and DR2. These reports in Japan are in agreement with

TABLE 5. HLA Antigens in Patients with UC in Japan

Author	HLA		
	B locus	DR locus	Haplotype
Tsuchiya *et al.*, 1977	B5↑, Bw35↓		
Yagita *et al.*, 1977	B5↑, Bw16↑		
Hiwatashi *et al.*, 1979	B5↑, B7↓		
Tanaka *et al.*, 1980	B5↑		
Shiwaku *et al.*, 1981a[6)]	Bw52↑,* B40↓		
Asakura *et al.*, 1981	B5↑, Bw22↓	DR2↑*	B5–DR2
Shiwaku *et al.*, 1981b[7)]	Bw52↑,* B40↓	DR2↑*	Aw24–Bw52–DR2
Asakura *et al.*, 1982	Bw52↑*	DR2↑*	B5–DR2

*Corrected *p*-value; significant.

regard to the increase in B5 or Bw52 and DR2 as compared with controls (Table 5).

The difference in HLA antigen between Japanese and Israeli Jewish patients may be a consequence of the different ethnic origins of the patients.

There are autoimmune diseases such as Takayasu disease in which Bw52–DR2 haplotype has been found to be significantly increased in Japanese patients. The abnormal immune responses seen in patients with UC as well as other HLA-associated diseases indicate that these patients have genes that permit the development of abnormal, even autoimmune responses. But further examination to demonstrate these points is warranted.

Figure 2 shows our hypothesis for the pathogenesis of UC. In the present study, we can demonstrate indirectly that immune responsiveness

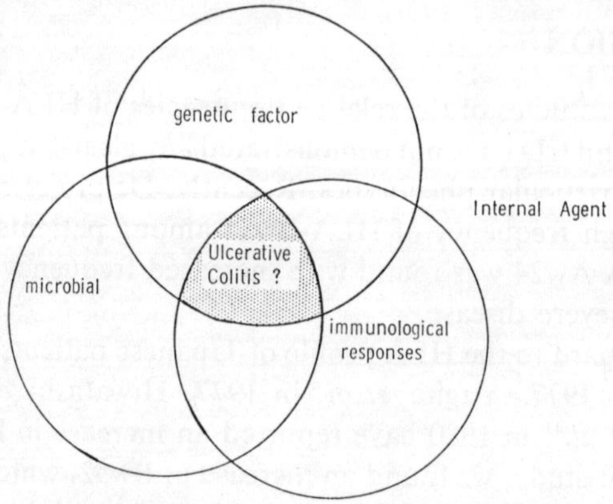

FIG. 2. Postulated pathogenesis of ulcerative colitis.

related to HLA-Bw52–DR2 haplotype plays an important role in the pathogenesis of UC in Japan.

SUMMARY

1) Japanese patients wtih UC show an association with HLA-Bw52 and DR2.
2) The relative risk to develop UC before the age of 30 years is 6.38 in Bw52 carriers and 6.17 in DR2 carriers.
3) DRw9 is higher in patients with proctitis.
4) The haplotype frequency of HLA-Aw24–Bw52–DR2 is significantly higher in patients with UC in Japan.
5) HLA-Aw24–Bw52–DR2 haplotype in Japanese patients with UC may play an important role in the pathogenesis of UC.

Acknowledgment

This study was supported by a Grant on Co-operative Research from the Ministry of Health and Welfare.

REFERENCES

1. Delpre, G., Kadish, U., Gazit, E., *et al.*: HLA antigens in ulcerative colitis and Crohn's disease in Israel. *Gastroenterology*, **78**: 1452–1457, 1980.
2. Tsuchiya, M., Yoshida, T., Asakura, H., *et al.*: HLA antigens and ulcerative colitis in Japan. *Digestion*, **15**: 286–294, 1977.
3. Hiwatashi, N., Kikuchi, T., Masamune, O., *et al.*: HLA antigens in inflammatory bowel disease. *Tohoku J. exp. Med.*, **131**: 381–385, 1980.
4. Tanaka, M., Ido, K., Sakai, H., *et al.*: HLA in ulcerative colitis. *Jap. J. Gastroenterology*, **77**: 894–897, 1980.
5. Asakura, H., Tsuchiya, M., Aiso, S., *et al.*: Association of the human lymphocyte-DR 2 antigen with Japanese ulcerative colitis. *Gastroenterology*, **82**: 413–418, 1982.
6. Shiwaku, Y., Morita, N., Sakaguchi, T., *et al.*: Histocompatibility antigens in patients with ulcerative colitis. *Igaku no ayumi*, **117**: 871–873, 1981 (in Japanese).
7. Immunogenetic Studies on Ulcerative Colitis. *Digestive Organ and Immunology* (Tokyo), **7**: 21–24, 1981 (in Japanese).

The Immunological Role of Gut Bacteria in the Patqogenesis of Inflammatory Bowel Disease

Kenzo Kobayashi, Atsuo Kitano, and Shiro Kuwajima

SUMMARY

Titers of anti-ECA (enterobacterial common antigen) antibody were high in a few cases of IBD, but there were high titers in many cases of liver disease. Differences in lymphocyte transformation response to ECA and *B. fragilis* between IBD patients and normal individuals were significant. The response of isolated lymphocytes from the intestinal mucosa to various mitogens was generally weaker. Intestinal mucosal lymphocytes of guinea pigs sensitized with ECA showed a positive response (30%) to this antigen. ECA had activity to induce delayed-type hypersensitivity (DTH) against ovalbumin in guinea pigs. Crude phospholipids of homologus intestine could enhance DTH to ECA in guinea pigs. ECA-induced cytotoxicity of lymphocytes on L cells was revealed in 24% of patients with ulcerative colitis (active stage). The inflammatory change that simulates ulcerative colitis could be produced by immunization of ECA, FIA, and phospholipid or *B. fragilis*. It was assumed from these findings that the immunological interaction between enterobacteria and gut-associated lymphoid tissues may play an important role in the etiology of IBD.

INTRODUCTION

Immunological interest has long since been drawn to the role of enterobacteria which are involved in immunological abnormalities that occur in patients with idiopathic inflammatory bowel diseases (IBD) such as ulcerative colitis and Crohn's disease. Because ulcerative colitis (UC) is known to be a disease that occurs mainly in the region where various enterobacteria inhabit, the bacteria play a significant role in the antigenicity formation to autologous colonic mucosal cells in UC.

This study was undertaken based on the possibility that various diseases

Third Department of Internal Medicine, Osaka City University Medical School, Osaka, Japan

in the intestinal mucosa are a result of complicated interrelations between the enterobacteria and the lymphatic apparatus (called gut-associated lymphoid tissues[1]) that exist abundantly in the intestinal mucosa.

EXPERIMENTS

Antibody titer in peripheral blood to enterobacterial common antigen, E. coli *014 LPS*, Bacteroides fragilis *LPS*, *and* B. vulgatus *LPS*

Enterobacterial common atigen (ECA)[2] was extracted from 85% ethanol soluble fractions of *Salmonella typhimurium* by the method of Suzuki. *E. coli* 014 LPS was obtained by phenol-water extraction according to the method of Westphal-Lüderitz.[3] The total bacillus and LPS of the obligate anaerobic bacteria, *B. fragilis* and *B. vulgatus*, were used.

The acetone dry bacillus of the strain extracted from patients with UC provided through the courtesy of Dr. T. Mitsuoka (Institute of Physical and Chemical Research) was used for preparation of the crude *B. fragilis* LPS. The hot phenol method of Westphal was employed.

Although the antibody-titer to *E. coli* 014 LPS is known to be higher in patients with IBD than in normal subjects, that to ECA is similarly higher in the former. On the contrary, the antibody to the somatic 014 antigen does not exist in patients.

In the present results, the anti-ECA antibody level was not so high in IBD, but rather, was frequently high in liver diseases (Fig. 1). However, the antibody titer to *E. coli* 014 LPS, *B. fragilis*, and *B. vulgatus* was high. The present findings stress the significance of the obvious difference in the frequency of higher antibody titer to these enterobacteria between patients with UC or Crohn's disease and normal subjects.

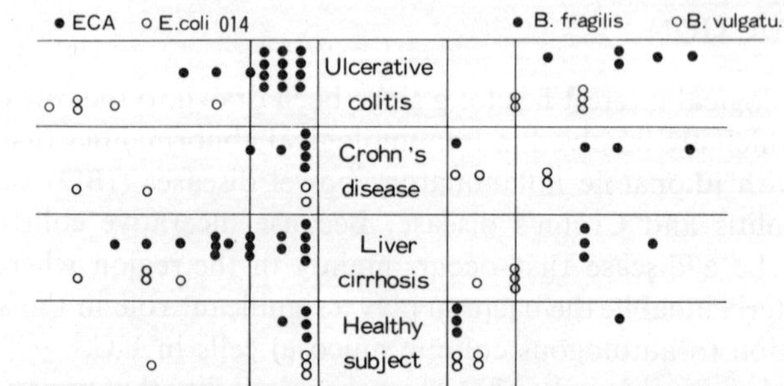

FIG. 1. Blood antibody titer to ECA, *E. coli* 014 LPS, *B. fragilis* LPS, and *B. vulgatus* LPS in patients with IBD and liver disease.

Blastoid transformation of peripheral blood lymphocytes by ECA, E. coli *014 LPS, and* B. fragilis *LPS*

The blastoid transformation reaction of lymphocytes to ECA was positive in 13 (38.2%) of 34 cases of UC and in 5 (55.6%) of 9 cases of Crohn's disease, thus significantly higher ($p < 0.01$) in patients than in normal subjects (Fig. 2). When tested with T cells, a significant increase in the positive reaction occurred in UC and Crohn's disease, as compared to testing with total lymphocytes.

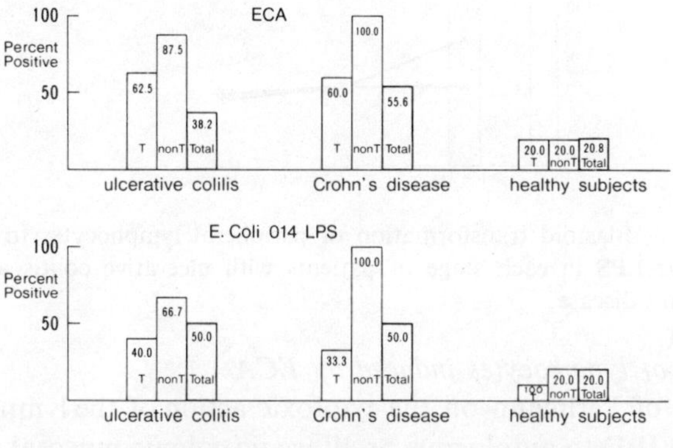

FIG. 2. Blastoid transformation of peripheral lymphocytes to ECA or *E. coli* 014 LPS in patients with ulcerative colitis and Crohn's disease.

To *E. coli* 014 LPS, on the other hand, UC and Crohn's disease patients also displayed a significantly higher ratio of positive reaction (50% equally for both) than normal subjects (20%) (Fig. 2).

In addition to the presence of antibody to ECA and *E. coli* 014 in patients with IBD, it is of interest to note that the high level of blastoid transformation by ECA and *E. coli* 014 LPS for non-T cells as well suggests the presence of immunized B cells.[4)]

On examining the production of immunized cells by the total bacillus or LPS of *B. fragilis*, when the total bacillus was used, a positive reaction was observed in active stage involving the whole colon in UC; and in Crohn's disease, in active stage with fever, abdominal pain, and hypoproteinemia. When LPS of *B. fragilis* was used as an antigen, the positive reaction appeared in two of four UC cases examined (Fig. 3). These two cases both represented the active stage. In Crohn's disease, only one out of four cases showed a positive reaction. This occurred in a female aged 18 in the active stage of Crohn's disease. Although salicylazosulfapyridine (SASP) was administered to all these patients, the three negative cases stayed in remission.

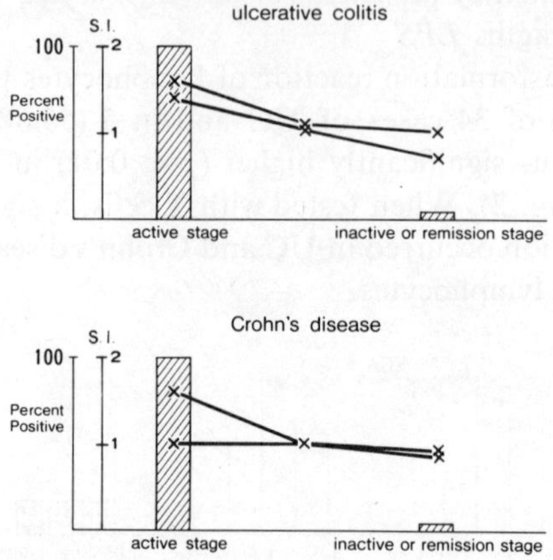

FIG. 3. Blastoid transformation of peripheral lymphocytes to *B. fragilis* LPS in each stage of patients with ulcerative colitis and Crohn's disease.

Cytotoxicity of lymphocytes induced by ECA

The study of Perlmann on the cytotoxic action of the lymphocytes of patients with IBD to autologous or allogenic colonic mucosal cells stimulated supplementary experiments by many investigators.

The normal peripheral blood lymphocytes incubated with *E. coli* 0119: B14 LPS gain cytotoxicity to colonic mucosa. This means that enterobacteria play a considerably important role in causing a cytotoxic effect to the colonic mucosa.

The presence of peripheral blood lymphocytes (T cells) sensitized by ECA or *E. coli* 014 LPS is known and these lymphocytes seem to cause cytotoxicity by inducement of killer T cells or nonspecific lymphotoxin.

We investigated ECA-induced cytotoxicity using L cells (fibroblasts) from mice successively bred by monolayer culture as target cells.[5] L-cell cytotoxicity was found in 5 (approximately 24%) of 21 human subjects with UC but in none of 20 normal controls (Fig. 4).

Common antigenicity between ECA and colonic mucosa

Three weeks after the immunization of Hartley guinea pigs with ECA, the intracutaneous reaction test was performed with a human fetal colon antigen. The results revealed a higher level of intracutaneous reaction 24 hours later in approximately 40% of the group immunized with 2 mg of ECA and in 70% of the group immunized with 20 mg of ECA than in the controls (Fig. 5). This not only confirmed the existence of common antigenicity between ECA and human fetal colon antigen, but also from the

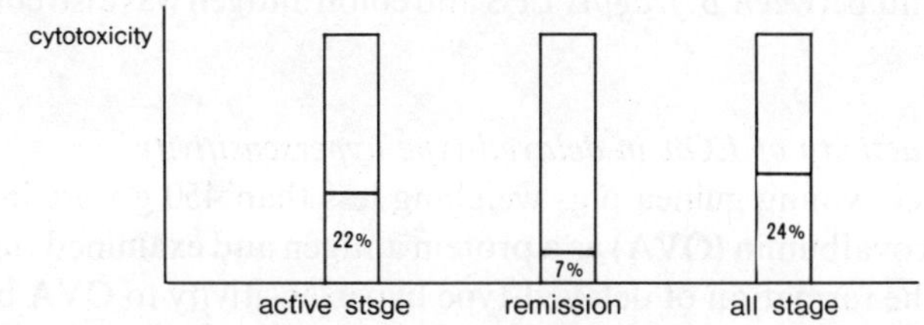

FIG. 4. ECA-induced cytotoxicity of lymphocytes on L cells in patients with ulcerative colitis.

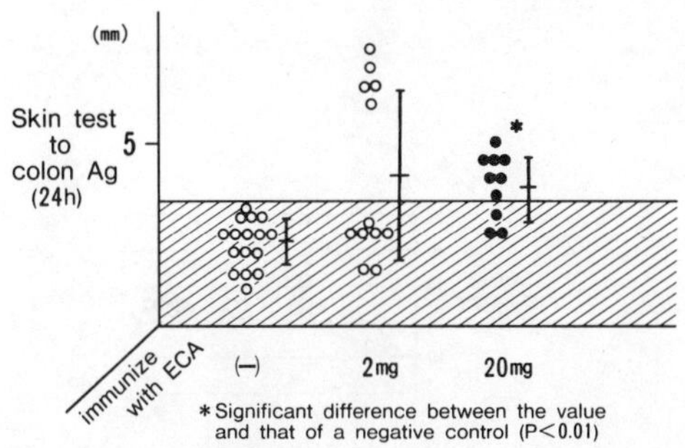

FIG. 5. Cross-reaction of colon antigen with ECA in respect of delayed-type hypersensitivity (DTH).

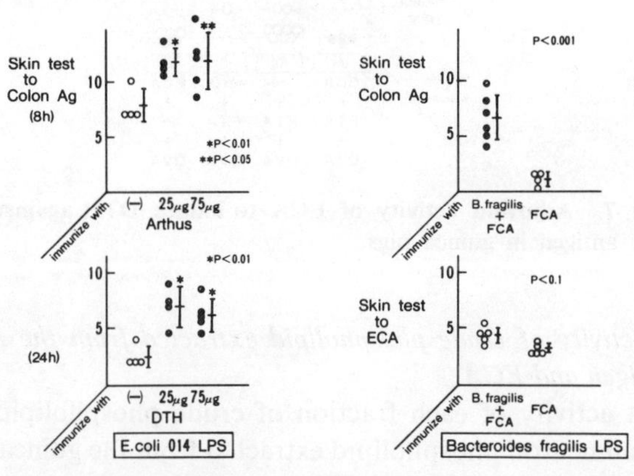

FIG. 6. Cross-reaction of colon antigen with *E. coli* 014 LPS and *B. fragilis* LPS in respect of DTH.

standpoint of cellular immunity, it evidenced that *E. coli* 014 LPS retained ECA in the form of covalent bonding.

Furthermore, common antigenicity between *E. coli* 014 LPS and colon antigen, and between *B. fragilis* LPS and colon antigen was also confirmed[6] (Fig. 6).

Adjuvant activity of ECA in delayed-type hypersensitivity

Relatively young guinea pigs weighing less than 450 g were immunized once with ovalbumin (OVA) as a protein antigen and examined three weeks later for the formation of delayed-type hypersensitivity to OVA by evaluation of the corneal reaction. Immunization without ECA produced a negative or a weak positive reaction, but immunization with ECA produced a positive reaction in 10 of 13 animals (Fig. 7). From this, it appears highly likely that ECA has the property of activating delayed-type hypersensitivity.[7]

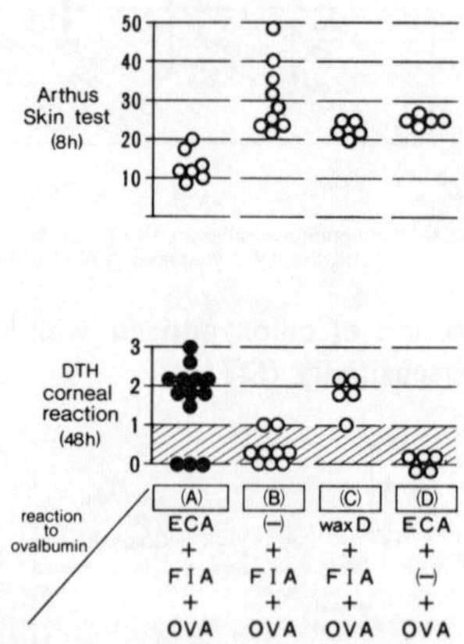

FIG. 7. Adjuvant activity of ECA to induce DTH against protein antigen in guinea pigs.

Adjuvant activity of crude phospholipid extracted from the intestine to a protein antigen and ECA

Adjuvant activity of each fraction of crude phospholipid, acid phospholipid, and neutral phospholipid extracted from the guinea pig intestine was evaluated using guinea pigs. When a protein antigen was used, strong adjuvant activity was observed in intestinal neutral phospholipid and crude phospholipid fractions (Table 1). When ECA was used, it showed a high degree of activity in inducing delayed-type hypersensitivity.[8]

The above findings seem to suggest the possibility that phospholipid contained in the intestinal tissue in UC behaves as a factor that affects the

TABLE 1. Immunoadjuvant Activities of Homologous Intestinal Phospholipids on ECA ($n = 5$)

Phospholipid	Dose (mg)	Skin test (Mean ± SD, mm)	Antibody level
MurNAC-L-Ala-D-isoglu NH_2	0.1	17.3 ± 2.2*	$< 2^2$
——	—	4.8 ± 1.5	$< 2^2$
Guinea pig intestine (crude)	0.2	11.0 ± 2.6*	$< 2^2$

*Significantly different from a negative control ($p < 0.05$).

etiology, aggravation, and protraction of the disease. The immunological interrelationship between an enterobacterial factor such as ECA and phospholipid, which is a component of the cellular membrane in the intestinal mucosa, is highly significant in analyzing the pathogenesis of IBD.

Experimental colitis induced with enterobacteria

Experimental production of the intestinal disease that simulates ulcerative colitis can be achieved by the use of a phlogogenic agent such as carrageenan or extrinsic factors such as bacteria and viruses.

Kitano, by administration of carrageenan to rabbits, has already achieved induction of the disease in the entire colon, including the rectum.[9] In his experiments, however, the disease could not be produced by oral administration of carrageenan only, but rather was achieved only in rabbits that had first been presensitized by the same agent. This suggests the importance of the role of immunological mechanisms even in an experiment performed with an extrinsic factor.

On the other hand, in human UC the peripheral blood lymphocytes are sensitized by ECA, as already described, to resultantly acquire cytotoxic action against the colonic mucosa which has common antigenicity with ECA. Sensitization with an enterobacterium and subsequent acquisition of cytotoxic action are thought to constitute a cause of IBD. In view of the above, therefore, the use of an enterobacterium as an antigenic substance for immunological preparation of an animal model is considered to be the reasonable method.

ECA (0.1 ml), FIA (0.1 ml), and phospholipid (0.2 mg) were mixed, and after ultrasonic treatment for 2–3 min, guinea pigs were immunized by injection of 0.2 ml of the mixture into the hind footpad. In order to evaluate delayed-type hypersensitivity three weeks later, reddening or induration of the skin after 48 hours of the injection was measured and expressed by the mean value of the long and short axes.

The histology of colonic mucosal tissue of the animals examined at this time revealed high concentrations of hyperplastic and irregularly arranged regenerative glands, causing a generally mild thickening of the mucous membrane and a rugged, irregular appearance of the membranous surface.

The regenerated glandular cells and surface epithelial cells were generally slightly reduced in size with a somewhat regenerative heteromorphic morphology. The interstitium was somewhat proliferated with round cells mainly composed of lymphocytes. The muscle fibers in the muscularis mucosae and lamina propria were slightly deranged.[10]

The model immunized with *B. fragilis* was also examined. After immunization with 1 mg of total bacillus or LPS of *B. fragilis* together with physiological saline and ECA, a booster injection was further administered three times at the rate of once or twice a week such that all subjects were immunized four times. The total bacillus used for immunization was prepared from the *B. fragilis* B 88221 strain (provided through the courtesy of Dr. T. Mitsuoka). The strain, after culture in a GMA semi-solid medium by a Nissui Gas Pack System, was mass cultured in 4 *l* of GMA broth, sterilized in an autoclave, and after washing, was acetone dried. *B. fragilis* crude LPS was prepared from the acetone-dried bacillus extracted from patients (provided through the courtesy of Dr. T. Mitsuoka) by the hot phenol method of Westphal. *B. fragilis* NCTC 9343 (already ultracentrifuged) provided through the courtesy of Dr. R. Nakaya, Tokyo Medical and Dental University, was further purified by treatment with RNase (3 μg/mg LPS, pH 7.5), DNase (3 μg/mg LPS, pH 5.0), and Pronase (1 μg/mg LPS, pH 7.5), according to the method of Romeo *et al.* The guinea pigs immunized with *B. fragilis* showed a skin reaction of the mean diameter of 12.1 $\pm$ 4.1 mm (mean $\pm$ SD). This reaction was significantly more conspicuous than those reactions from ECA or colon antigen, evidencing the development of delayed-type hypersensitivity to *B. fragilis*.

The histology of the colonic mucosa in the group immunized with a total bacillus of *B. fragilis* did not differ much from the histology observed in the control group or the group immunized with *E. coli* 014 LPS, except for the presence of a slight inflammatory change. However, infiltration of round cells in the lamina propria near the muscularis mucosae was observed. It appeared likely that these changes would result in tissue destruction at a later point in time. The histology of the group immunized with LPS of *B. fragilis* was characterized by an intense inflammatory change near the muscularis mucosae and a conspicuous edematous change of the mucosa mainly in this region, in spite of the preservation of the mucosal epithelium.

These findings indicate the likelihood of the involvement of an intrinsic factor, namely, an immune reaction.

Lymphocytes of guinea pigs immunized with ECA or *B. fragilis* were isolated from the colonic mucosa for investigation of blastoid transformation to immunoantigens. The results showed that the lymphocytes from the colonic mucosa of guinea pigs were sensitized by these enterobacteria (Fig. 8). Thus the formation of cellular immunity to enterobacteria in the present models is evident.

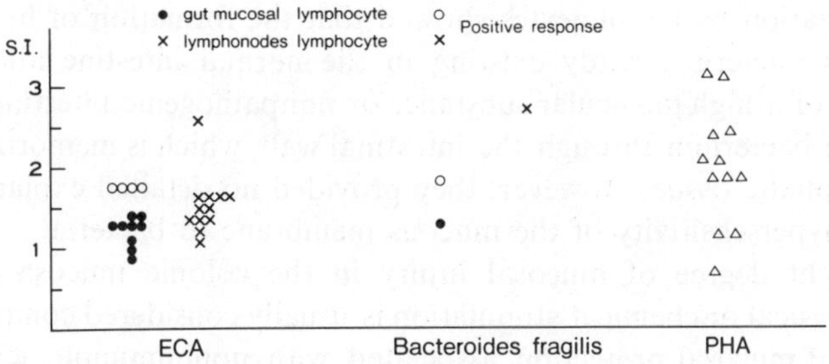

FIG. 8. Immunological responses of gut mucosal lymphocytes to enterobacterial antigen in guinea pigs sensitized with ECA or *B. fragilis* LPS.

DISCUSSION AND CONCLUSION

Serological, biochemical, and immunological analyses have so far revealed the various aspects of the role of ECA, which is believed to exist in the Gram-negative bacterium such as *E. coli* 014 and others which belong to family Enterobacteriaceae. Especially since ECA has been known to have cross-reactivity to the components of colonic mucosa, ECA in its relationship to IBD has provided extremely important subjects of study on the pathogenesis of this disease. More recently, various immunologic findings concerning anaerobic bacteria such as *B. fragilis* or *B. vulgatus*, in addition to ECA, have been published.

The existence of antibodies in the peripheral blood and colonic mucosa of patients with IBD, which react with anaerobic bacteria, has also been shown. Furthermore, common antigenicity between the *Bacteroides* genus and mouse fetal intestinal tissue has also been clarified. We confirmed, from the standpoint of cellular immunity and on the basis of delayed-type hypersensitivity, that *B. fragilis* and colonic mucosa share common antigenicity.

An antibody to ECA, *E. coli* 014, and the *Bacteroides* genus was observed in the peripheral blood of patients with IBD. Lymphocytes sensitized by these enterobacteria were also found in the peripheral blood not only of patients with ulcerative colitis but also of those with Crohn's disease. The positive reaction was frequent in the active stage of the disease but was reduced as the clinical features went into remission. This fact indicates the close association between the existence of enterobacteria-sensitized lymphocytes and the pathogenesis.

However, the mechanism by which lymphocytes are sensitized by enterobacteria still remains unknown.

The idea of Shorter *et al.* on intestinal infection of a bacterium and memorization by lymphocytes showed that the formation of hypersensitivity to bacteria already existing in the normal intestine allows easy passage of a high molecular substance or nonpathogenic intestinal Gram-negative bacterium through the intestinal wall, which is memorized from the lymphatic tissue. However, they provided no detailed explanation as to the hypersensitivity of the mucous membrane to bacteria.

A slight degree of mucosal injury in the colonic mucosa resulting from physical or chemical stimulation is usually considered common. The system of mucosal protection associated with nonimmunological mechanisms may play an important role in determining whether such slight mucosal injuries develop into disease entities or disappear. However, it would be more appropriate to attach more importance to the involvement of the local immunological mechanisms against invasion of a bacterium through the injured mucosa. Even if an inhabiting enterobacterium should invade the mucosa, disease is not necessarily the result. Thus the immunological interrelationship between the host (including the local region) and the bacteria has a great deal of significance.

We have already succeeded in producing an experimental model of ulcerative colitis using carrageenan, in which an immunological mechanism was considered to be involved. The chronic status was also obtained.

Although induction of an intestinal disease in a germ-free guinea pig by administration of *B. vulgatus* has been reported elsewhere, we were unable to obtain, by immunological procedures with bacterial antigens such as ECA and LPS, an intestinal disease comparable to the one in the previously described carrageenan model. However, the formation of delayed-type hypersensitivity to immune antigens was evident in guinea pigs immunized with *B. fragilis*. This suggests that an improvement in immunological procedures must be developed. Thus, as already described, the experimental system treated with ECA plus phospholipid, LPS, and FIA as adjuvants produced the most intense state of intestinal lesion. This, therefore, suggests that the best results may be obtained by treatment with ECA, *E. coli* 014 LPS, or *Bacteroides* genus LPS as an antigen added with various phospholipids as an adjuvant.

REFERENCES

1. Thomas, H. C. and Jewell, D. P.: Clinical Gastrointestinal Immunology. Blackwell Scientific Publications, Oxford, 1979.
2. Kunin, C. M., *et al.*: Evidence for a common hapten associated with endotoxin fraction of *E. Coli* and other Enterobacteriaceae. *Proc. Soc. Exp. Biol. Med.,* **111**: 160–166, 1962.
3. Westphal, O., *et al.*: Extraction with phenol water and further applications of the procedure. In: Methods in Carbohydrate Chemistry, Vol. 5, p. 83. Academic Press, New York, 1965.
4. Murai, M.: Isolation of intestinal lymphocytes and study of their immunological properties. *J. Osaka City Med. C.,* **29**: 417–433, 1980.
5. Yamaguchi, K., *et al.*: Immunological study on ulcerative colitis. *Jpn. J. Gastroenterol.,* **76**: 1924–1933, 1978.
6. Oka, S., *et al.*: Cross-reaction of human colon antigen with enterobacterial common antigen. *Digestive Organ and Immunology,* **6**: 105–109, 1981.
7. Kuwajima, S., *et al.*: On the activity to induce and activate delayed hypersensitivity of enterobacterial common antigen and bacterial lipopolysaccharide. *Jpn. J. Gastroenterol.,* **75**: 1642–1650, 1979.
8. Tanaka, Y., *et al.*: Immunoadjuvant activity of phospholipids extracted from animal tissues (intestine, liver and brain) to ovalbumin and enterobacterial common antigen (ECA), and their possible role in the chronic inflammatory bowel disease. *Jpn. J. Gastroenterol.,* **77**: 361–367, 1980.
9. Kitano, A., *et al.*: Study of experimental ulcerative colitis induced by carrageenan in rabbit. *Jpn. J. Gastroenterol.,* **75**: 1719–1726, 1978.
10. Kobayashi, K., *et al.*: Experimental colitis induced with colon and enterobacterial antigen. *Digestive Organ and Immunology,* **5**: 85–91, 1980.

Significance of ADCC and Autoantibodies in the Pathogenesis of Ulcerative Colitis

Hitoshi Asakura, Sadakazu Aiso,* Mamoru Watanabe,* Takeshi Yoshida,* Toshifumi Hibi,* Sumiaki Tsuru,** and Masaharu Tsuchiya**

SUMMARY

A high prevalence of anti-colon antibody and lymphocytophilic antibody in the sera from patients with ulcerative colitis was obtained by fluorescence-activated cell sorter (FACS) analysis. The anti-colon antibody had a role in antibody-dependent cell-mediated cytotoxicity against the colonic epithelial cells. On the other hand, the lymphocytophilic antibody was partially responsible for decreased suppressor cell activity which was proven by Con A-induced suppressor cell activity assay and by using monoclonal antibodies such as Anti-Leu-2a and Anti-Leu-3a. These data suggest that immunological abnormalities may have some role in the pathogenesis of ulcerative colitis.

INTRODUCTION

Ulcerative colitis is an acute and chronic inflammatory bowel disease which diffusely involves the colonic mucosa. Many patients follow a chronic course with frequent exacerbations.

There is a great deal of evidence implicating immunological mechanisms in the etiology of ulcerative colitis. Autoimmune diseases result primarily from disorders of immunoregulation, and the immune apparatus itself (such as the thymus) may become altered so that an abnormal response is elicited to antigens normally expressed on cells of tissues. Such types of autoimmunity may result from a failure of T cells to regulate lymphocyte function, either via a loss of tolerance of helper T cells to autoantigens or a loss of suppressor T cell function.

Two kinds of autoantibodies, circulating anti-colon antibodies and lymphocytophilic and/or lymphocytotoxic antibodies, have been reported

*Department of Internal Medicine, School of Medicine, Keio University, Tokyo, Japan
**Department of Bacteriology, National Defense Medical College, Tokorozawa, Saitama, Japan

in patients with ulcerative colitis.[1,2] However, these anti-colon antibodies have not been cytotoxic for colonic epithelial cells.[3] Nevertheless, these antibodies are thought to play some role in the pathogenesis of ulcerative colitis.

In order to elucidate the role of anti-colon antibody and lymphocytophilic antibody in the pathogenesis of ulcerative colitis, we investigated the nature of these antibodies in the sera of patients with this disease utilizing antibody-dependent cell-mediated cytotoxicity (ADCC) assay and fluorescence-activated cell sorter (FACS) analysis.

MATERIALS AND METHODS

Patient sera. Sera were obtained from 41 adult patients (19 of them males) with clinical, radiological, endoscopic, and biopsy findings typical of ulcerative colitis. Nineteen patients were treated with Salicylazosulphapyridine, 8 with corticosteroids, 12 with both, and 2 with neither treatment. Eleven of the 41 patients were in active stage and the others were in inactive stage. Control sera were obtained from 9 healthy laboratory workers and hospital staff. The sex and age distributions of the healthy control group were comparable to those of the ulcerative colitis group. Sera were stored at −80° C without preservatives and were centrifuged at 105,000 *g* for 90 min before use.

Lymphocyte preparation. Heparinized blood was obtained from apparently healthy individuals and patients with ulcerative colitis. Peripheral blood lymphocytes were purified on a Ficoll-Hypaque density gradient ($\rho = 1.076$) by centrifugation. After being washed in phosphate-buffered saline (PBS) at pH 7.4, the lymphocytes from healthy controls were used for the ADCC assay. For the staining, the cells were then purified further by passage through a nylon wool column to delete B cells.[4] Contamination of surface immunoglobulin (Ig)-bearing cells (B cells) as detected by staining with fluorescein-conjugated rabbit anti-human Ig was less than 5%.

Preparation of epithelial cell suspensions. Fresh specimens of colon were obtained from Wistar rats weighing 200 to 250 g. The mucosa was separated, washed several times with Hanks' balanced salt solution (BSS), and finely minced with iris scissors. The tissue was subjected to trypsinization (0.25% trypsin, GIBCO, Grand Island, NY) for approximately one hour. The suspension was filtered through a 400-μ nylon mesh to remove large pieces of tissue, washed three times in Hanks' BSS, and then resuspended in RPMI 1640 medium (Flow Labo, Rockville, MD) in a final concentration of 1×10^6 cells/ml. The percentage of viability estimated by trypan blue exclusion was more than 85% in each instance.

Indirect epithelial cell immunofluorescence for anti-colon antibodies

The 1×10^6 epithelial cells were incubated with 0.1 ml of undiluted human serum at room temperature for 30 min, and then washed three times with Hanks' BSS. The washed cells were incubated with 0.1 ml of FITC-conjugated anti-human Ig(G + A + M), anti-human IgG, anti-human IgM, or anti-human IgA of rabbit $(Fab')_2$ fragments (Cappel Labo, Cochraville, PA) at room temperature for 30 min. After having been washed three times with Hanks' BSS, the cells were resuspended at a concentration of 1×10^6 cells/ml in RPMI medium, and then filtrated through a 400-μ nylon mesh. The cell suspensions were analyzed by FACS-II (Becton-Dickinson, Mountain View, CA).[5]

ADCC assay

Target epithelial cells (1×10^5) were suspended in 1 ml of medium containing 100 μCi $Na_2{}^{51}CrO_4$ (Daiichi Radioisotope, Tokyo) and incubated for 45 min at 37° C. These labeled cells were washed three times with medium and resuspended at a concentration of 1×10^5 cells/ml. One tenth of one milliliter of the cells was dispensed into microtest plate wells and incubated with 0.05 ml of the sera for 30 min at 37° C. After 0.05 ml of normal lymphocyte suspension (2×10^6 cells/ml) was added to the wells, the plates were incubated for 8 hr at 37° C in a humidified atmosphere of 5% CO_2 and 95% air. The final ratio of effector to target cells was 10 : 1. All cultures were performed in triplicate. ^{51}Cr released from the labeled target cells was collected with a Titertek supernatant collection system (Flow Laboratories, McLean, VA) and was measured with a gamma-counter (Aloka, ARC 251). Maximum possible ^{51}Cr release was determined by three freeze-thaw cycles. The results were expressed in % cytotoxicity as follows:

$$\%\ \text{cytotoxicity} = \frac{\text{c.p.m. of experimental release} - \text{c.p.m. of spontaneous release}}{\text{c.p.m. of maximum release} - \text{c.p.m. of spontaneous release}}$$

Indirect lymphocyte immunofluorescence for lymphocytophilic antibodies

For the FACS analysis of peripheral blood lymphocytes from healthy controls and patients with ulcerative colitis, 0.1 ml of T cell-enriched preparations (1×10^6 cells/ml) was reacted with 0.1 ml of the sera from normal controls and patients with ulcerative colitis for 30 min at room temperature. After being washed in PBS, the lymphocytes were incubated with 0.1 ml of fluorescein isothiocyanate (FITC)-conjugated anti-human Ig(G + A + M), anti-human IgG, anti-human IgA, or anti-human IgM

$(Fab')_2$ fragments from rabbit for 30 min at room temperature. The F/P ratio was between 2 and 3. FITC-conjugated serum was centrifuged at 100,000 *g* for 90 min immediately before use. Cells were resuspended at 1×10^6 cells/ml and analyzed by FACS-II.

Analysis of T-lymphocyte subsets by using monoclonal antibodies

Monoclonal antibodies. Two monoclonal antibodies detecting human T cell surface antigens, termed Anti-Leu-2a and Anti-Leu-3a (Becton Dickinson Monoclonal Antibody Center, Sunnyvale, CA), were used in the present study. The preparation of specificity of these monoclonal antibodies has been amply documented.[6] Functionally, Anti-Leu-2a defines the human suppressor/cytotoxic population, while Anti-Leu-3a defines the human inducer/helper subsets. Both antibodies were fluorescein-conjugated.

Analysis of lymphocyte populations of UC patients with monoclonal antibodies. The mononuclear cell suspension (2×10^6) was incubated with 10 μl of fluorescein-conjugated Anti-Leu-2a or Anti-Leu-3a at 15° C for 20 min and washed twice. Then cells were analyzed on a fluorescence-activated cell sorter.

Con A-induced suppressor cell activity

Peripheral blood lymphocytes were separated from heparinized peripheral blood obtained from patients with ulcerative colitis and from healthy individuals by centrifugation on a Ficoll-Isopaque gradient. B and T cells were separated by rosetting with neuraminidase-treated sheep erythrocytes. Cells were suspended in RPMI 1640 supplemented with 10% fetal calf serum. Next, 3×10^6 lymphocytes in 3 ml of culture medium were incubated with 10 μg/ml of Con A in culture dishes for 48 hr at 37° C. After the incubation period, cells were harvested, washed three times with Eagle's MEM containing 5% FCS, resuspended in culture medium, and added to a PWM-stimulated PBL culture. Then 2×10^5 PBL together with 1×10^5 Con A-stimulated cells or non-stimulated cells suspended in 200 μl of culture medium were placed in a Micro Test II culture plate and cultured with 2.5 μl/ml of PWM in 5% CO_2 in air at 37° C for 7 days. On the 4th day of culture, the culture plate was centrifuged at 1,500 rpm for 5 min, and the culture medium was replaced with a fresh one without PWM. At the termination of the cultures, the culture supernatant was harvested and the amounts of IgG in culture supernatants were determined by radioimmunoassay.[7]

Human lymphocyte antigen typing

HLA typing was performed by the standard NIH technique[8] using the anti-HLA-A, -B, -C, and -DR antisera provided by Professor Terasaki. DR typing was performed on a B lymphocyte-rich suspension.[9] B-lymphocyte preparations were made from peripheral blood lymphocytes by passage through a nylon wool column. B-cell typing was performed by prolonged incubation lymphocytotoxicity testing (1 hr with antiserum at 37°C, and 1.5 hr with rabbit serum complement at room temperature). Specimens were stained with 5% solution of eosin and fixed with 25% solution of neutralized formaldehyde.

RESULTS

Anti-colon antibodies

The average of relative cell numbers with fluorescence intensity higher than the background was 9.1 ± 5.1% in healthy control sera and 33.8 ± 23.3% in sera from patients with ulcerative colitis. In the sera from the patients, the fluorescence profile of the stained cells was characterized by a large peak of cells which had a low-to-intermediate degree of fluorescence intensity. Circulating anti-colon antibodies were found in 16 of 29 (55%) patients with ulcerative colitis when the sera staining more than 19.1% of cells (above mean + 2SD in healthy controls) were regarded as positive. All of the positive sera contained IgG class anti-colon antibodies. This was proven by tests for different immunoglobulin classes.

ADCC assay

Significantly higher levels of cytotoxicity against rat colon epithelial cells were observed using the sera from 9 patients with active ulcerative colitis (% cytotoxicity = 32.5 ± 6.4) in comparison to the sera from 13 healthy controls (% cytotoxicity = 23.4 ± 3.6). Higher levels of cytotoxicity were found in 2 of 9 sera from patients with inactive ulcerative colitis.

Lymphocytophilic antibodies

The fluorescence histograms of negative control cells, which were stained with FITC-conjugated anti-human Ig serum but without intermediate sera, appeared as a narrow peak with fluorescence intensity lower than 40. Therefore, cells with fluorescence intensity of more than 40 were defined as positive cells. The percentage of fluorescence-positive cells was 20.2 ± 5.0 in 6 sera of healthy controls and 41.8 ± 26.4 in 21 sera of ulcerative colitis. The immunoglobulin class of the antibody binding to the lymphocytes was IgG. Staining of more than 30% of the normal lymphocytes was obtained with sera of 13 of 21 patients with ulcerative colitis.

T-lymphocyte subsets

Normal lymphocytes from healthy controls consist of 24.6 ± 3.6% (mean ± SD) of T cells reactive with Anti-Leu-2a and 39.9 ± 5.1% of T cells reactive with Anti-Leu-3a. The lymphocyte populations reactive with Anti-Leu-2a were 8.2 ± 3.6% in patients with active ulcerative colitis and 26.2 ± 10.7% in patients with inactive ulcerative colitis. There was a marked decrease in the Anti-Leu-2a-reactive T cells of patients with active ulcerative colitis. However, no significant difference was seen in the percentage of Anti-Leu-3a-reactive T cells among any of the patients or the controls.

Con A-induced suppressor cell activity

The percent suppression of Con A-induced suppressor cell activity was 20.6 ± 17.9 in four patients with ulcerative colitis, while it was 67.6 ± 11.8 in five control individuals. This result showed that decreased suppressor cell activity was found in patients with ulcerative colitis.

HLA-DR antigen

The distributions of phenotype frequencies of locus DR in control individuals and patients with ulcerative colitis is shown in Table 1. The antigen of markedly high frequency in patients with ulcerative colitis was HLA-DR2 ($\chi^2 = 16.4$, $p < 0.001$, corrected $p < 0.01$). The phenotype frequencies of patients with ulcerative colitis were assessed in relation to

TABLE 1. HLA Phenotype Frequencies in Patients with Ulcerative Colitis and in Controls (Locus DR)

Locus DR	Controls ($n = 51$) No. of cases	Phenotype frequency (%)	Ulcerative colitis ($n = 47$) No. of cases	Phenotype frequency (%)	χ^2	p-value	Corrected p-value
DR1	7	13.7	2	4.2		ns	ns
DR2	16	31.4	34	72.3	16.4	$p < 0.001$	$cp < 0.01$
DR3	0	0	1	2.1		ns	ns
DR4	25	49.0	14	29.8		ns	ns
DR5	4	7.8	1	2.1		ns	ns
DRw6	4	7.8	5	10.6		ns	ns
DR7	0	0	0	0		ns	ns
DRw8	4	7.8	5	10.6		ns	ns
DRw9	10	19.6	16	34.0		ns	ns
DRw10	1	2.0	0	0		ns	ns
8wDRw6y	14	27.5	10	21.2		ns	ns
8wDRw17	1	2.0	2	4.2		ns	ns
Blank	15	29.4	4	8.5			

ns: not significant.

TABLE 2. HLA Phenotype Frequencies in Patients with Ulcerative Colitis and in Controls in Relation to Clinical Pattern

	n	Aw24	Bw52	DR2	DRw9
Control	51	56.9%	31.4%	31.4%	19.6%
Ulcerative colitis					
Total	47	68.1	57.4**	72.3^{++}	34.0
Male	24	58.3	50.0	75.0^{++}	25.0
Female	23	78.2	65.2**	69.5^{+}	43.4*
Age $\leqq$ 30	30	70.0	63.3**	70.0^{++}	23.3
Age > 30	17	64.7	47.0	76.4^{+}	52.9**
Proctitis	6	50.0	16.6	66.6	50.0
Left-sided colitis	13	46.1*	61.5*	69.2*	30.7**
Total colitis	28	82.1*	64.3**	75.0^{++}	32.1
Relapsing-remitting	30	66.6**	56.6*	70.0^{++}	30.0
Chronic continuous	13	69.2*	61.5*	69.2*	30.7**
Single attack	4	75.0*	50.0*	100.0**	75.0*

*0.05 > p > 0.01, **0.01 > p > 0.001, ***0.001 > p.
$^{+}$0.05 > corrected p > 0.01, $^{++}$0.01 > corrected p.

the various clinical patterns, such as sex, age of onset, affected region, and clinical course (Table 2).

The highest frequencies of HLA-Bw52 were observed in female patients and in left-sided colitis and total colitis compared with controls, but the frequency of HLA-Bw52 was somehow higher in patients with early onset of the disease. A high frequency of HLA-DR2 was consistent regardless of sex, early or late onset, region affected, and the clinical course.

DISCUSSION

Many studies have shown that lymphocytes from patients with ulcerative colitis were sensitized to some antigens such as colonic mucosa and enterobacterial common antigen. In the leucocyte migration inhibition test, migration in patients with ulcerative colitis has shown significant inhibition in the presence of human fetal colon[10)] and the lipopolysaccharide antigen from *E. coli* 014.[11)]

Our study revealed that lymphocytes from patients with active ulcerative colitis had proliferative response to LPS from *E. coli* 014 and no response to LPS from other bacteria.[12)] The lymphocytes of controls and patients with inactive ulcerative colitis had no such proliferative response to any LPS we studied. A human fetal colon extract and the LPS from *E. coli* 014 are known to share antigenic determinants with the enterobacterial common antigen.[13)] The similarity of the colon antigen to *E. coli* 014 may raise the possibility that autoimmunization to colon in ulcerative colitis could be induced through stimulation with cross-reacting bacterial antigens. The presence of the anti-colon antibody in the sera of patients with ulcerative colitis has been revealed by various methods.[1,14] The anti-colon antibody has been reported to react with antigen in the sterile human colon as well as in rat colon or feces. But this anti-colon antibody has not been shown to be cytotoxic for colonic epithelial cells in ulcerative colitis.[3] In the present study, we demonstrated a cytotoxic effect of patients' sera on rat colon cells in collaboration with peripheral lymphocytes from healthy controls. Das, Dubin, and Nagai[15] have isolated anti-colon antibodies bound to the colonic tissue of patients with ulcerative colitis. These findings suggest that antibody-dependent cell-mediated cytotoxicity has a role in the sustained inflammation in the colon of such patients.

Lymphocytophilic or lymphocytotoxic antibody has been demonstrated in the sera of patients with ulcerative colitis by Korsmeyer *et al.*[2] They have reported that this type of antibody is detected in the sera of almost 50% of the patients studied according to Terasaki's microcytotoxicity assay. By using FACS analysis, we observed a higher prevalence of this antibody in patients with ulcerative colitis than that previously reported.[16] However, the precise clinical significance of this antibody still remains unknown. Decreased suppressor T-cell activity in inflammatory bowel disease has been demonstrated by Hodgson, Wands, and Isserbacher[17] and by this study. In addition, a severe decrease in Anti-Leu-2a-reactive T cells, suppressor subset, in patients with active ulcerative colitis was demonstrated in this study. Lymphocytophilic antibody may be partially responsible for decreased suppressor T-cell activity.[18] Such depression of suppressor activity may result in the production of anti-colon antibody.

The presence of anti-colon antibodies and lymphocytophilic antibodies in sera of patients with ulcerative colitis may suggest that immune responsiveness coded on HLA antigens, especially HLA-Bw52–DR2 haplotype in Japanese ulcerative colitis, plays an important role in the pathogenesis of ulcerative colitis.[19]

REFERENCES

1. Broberger, O. and Perlmann, P.: Autoantibodies in human ulcerative colitis. *J. exp. Med.*, **110**: 657, 1959.
2. Korsmeyer, S., Strickland, R. G., Wilson, I. D., and Williams, R. C.: Serum lymphocytotoxic and lymphocytophilic antibody activity in inflammatory bowel disease. *Gastroenterology*, **67**: 578, 1974.
3. Broberger, O. and Perlmann, P.: *In vitro* studies of ulcerative colitis. I. Reactions of patients' serum with human fetal colon cells in tissue culture. *J. exp. Med.*, **117**: 705, 1963.

4. Julius, M. H., Simpson, E., and Herzenberg, L. A.: A rapid method for the isolation of functional thymus-derived murine lymphocytes. *Eur. J. Immunol.,* **3**: 645, 1973.
5. Bonner, W. A., Hullet, H. R., Sweet, R. G., and Herzenberg, L. A.: Fluorescence-activated cell sorting. *Rev. Sci. Instrum.,* **43**: 404, 1972.
6. Ledbetter, J. A., Evans, R. L., Lipinski, M., Cunningham-Randness, C., Good, R. A., and Herzenberg, L. A.: Evolutionary conservation of surface molecules that distinguish T lymphocyte helper/inducer and cytotoxic/suppressor subpopulations in mouse and man. *J. exp. Med.,* **153**: 310, 1981.
7. Kuritani, T., Hirano, T., Kishimoto, T., and Yamamura, Y.: *In vitro* immune response of human peripheral lymphocytes. II. Properties and functions of concanavalin A-induced suppressor T cells. *Microbiol. Immunol.,* **23**: 185, 1979.
8. Mittal, K. K., Mickey, M. R., Singal, D. P., *et al.:* Serotyping for homotransplantation. XVIII. Refinement of microdroplet lymphocyte cytotoxicity test. *Transplantation,* **6**: 913, 1968.
9. Terasaki, P. I., Bernoco, D., Park, M. S., *et al.*: Microdroplet testing for HLA-A, -B, -C and -D antigens. *Am. Soc. Clin. Pathol.,* **69**: 103, 1978.
10. Bendixen, G.: Cellular hypersensitivity to components of intestinal mucosa in ulcerative colitis and Crohn's disease. *Gut,* **10**: 631, 1969.
11. Hinz, C. G., Jr., Perlmann, P., and Hammarstöm, S.: Reactivity *in vitro* of lymphocytes from patients with ulcerative colitis. *J. Lab. Clin. Med.,* **70**: 752, 1967.
12. Aiso, S., Asakura, H., Tanaka, T., and Tsuchiya, M.: Lymphocyte response to colonic antigen. Its role in the pathogenesis of ulcerative colitis. *Biochem. exp. Biol.,* **16**: 287, 1980.
13. Kunin, C. M.: Separation, characterization and biological significance of a common antigen in Enterobacteriaceae. *J. exp. Med.,* **118**: 565, 1963.
14. Marcussen, H.: Fluorescent anti-colon and *E. coli* antibodies in ulcerative colitis. *Scand. J. Gastroent.,* **14**: 277, 1978.
15. Das, K. M., Dubin, R., and Nagai, T.: Isolation and characterization of colonic tissue-bound antibodies from patients with idiopathic ulcerative colitis. *Proc. Natl. Acad. Sci. U.S.,* **75**: 4528, 1978.
16. Hibi, T., Aiso, S., Yoshida, T., Watanabe, M., Asakura, H., Tsuru, S., and Tsuchiya, M.: Anti-colon antibody and lymphocytophilic antibody in ulcerative colitis. *Clin. exp. Immunol.,* **49**: 75, 1982.
17. Hodgson, H. J. F., Wands, J. R., and Isserbacher, K. J.: Decreased suppressor cell activity in inflammatory bowel disease. *Clin. exp. Immunol.,* **32**: 451, 1978.
18. Aiso, S., Watanabe, M., Hibi, T., Yoshida, T., Tsuchiya, M., and Tsuru, S.: Characterization of immunoregulatory T cells and lymphocytophilic antibodies in ulcerative colitis: Analysis with monoclonal antibodies. *J. Clin. Lab. Immunol.,* **9**: 109, 1982.
19. Asakura, H., Tsuchiya, M., Aiso, S., Watanabe, M., Kobayashi, K., Hibi,

T., Ando, K., Takata, H., and Sekiguchi, S.: Association of the human lymphocyte-DR2 antigen with Japanese ulcerative colitis. *Gastroenterology*, **82**: 413, 1982.

Immune Complexes in Ulcerative Colitis and Crohn's Disease

Derek P. Jewell

The histological appearances of ulcerative colitis show the characteristic features of inflammation resulting from antigen–antibody reactions. These include edema, vascular congestion with diapedesis of red cells, and an infiltration of polymorphonuclear cells, eosinophils, and plasma cells. These features are similar to those of an Arthus reaction induced experimentally in animals. A possible role for antigen–antibody complexes in the pathogenesis of the disease is also suggested by the occurrence of an acute arthropathy, erythema nodosum, and uveitis in these patients. It is difficult to prove that antigen–antibody reactions are a major effector mechanism in the pathogenesis of colonic inflammation especially as the antigen involved has not been identified. Evidence to support the hypothesis is of four kinds: immunological events within the mucosa, the presence of circulating immune complexes, increased complement activation and metabolism, and experimental studies of an immune complex-mediated colitis in rabbits.

MUCOSAL IMMUNOLOGY

In the normal intestine, the predominant immunoglobulin synthesized within the lamina propria is IgA. In patients with either ulcerative colitis or Crohn's disease there is an increase in plasma cells producing all the major classes of immunoglobulin, but the greatest proportional increase is in IgG.[1,2] Even when patients with ulcerative colitis are in complete remission, the IgG-containing cells are still present in greater numbers than in normal colon.[3,4] Direct evidence for increased immunoglobulin production in the mucosa has come from studies in which rectal biopsies have been cultured in the presence of ^{14}C-leucine.[5] Studies using isolated mononuclear cells from the inflamed colon have shown a decreased spon-

Gastroenterology Unit, Radcliffe Infirmary, Oxford, England, UK

taneous antibody production.[6] This is a surprising observation and requires confirmation.

Some of this locally synthesized immunoglobulin has specificity for colonic bacteria and antibody to bacteroides can be shown in the absence of circulating antibody.[7] Therefore, it is likely that antigen–antibody reactions occur in the mucosa but the evidence for this is largely indirect and refers mainly to patients with ulcerative colitis. Free IgG and the complement components C3 and C1q have been found on the epithelial basement membrane of rectal tissue obtained from patients with active disease.[8–10] However, the specificity of these findings is still doubtful.

CIRCULATING IMMUNE COMPLEXES

Many different tests have been used to detect immune complexes in the sera of patients with ulcerative colitis or Crohn's disease. Those tests which have been used most are listed in Table 1. The interpretation of the results in the absence of a known antigen is difficult, and it has been claimed that the results of these tests are an *in vitro* artifact due to the aggregation of IgG.[19] Nevertheless, similar results have been obtained using these tests which depend on differing properties of immune complexes, control sera have been handled in a similar way, and the results have never shown any correlation with IgG.

TABLE 1. Tests Used to Detect Circulating Immune Complexes in Patients with Ulcerative Colitis or Crohn's Disease

Test	Reference
C1q binding and anti-complementary activity	11–14
Conglutinin binding	15
Inhibition of rheumatoid factor or C1q binding	13, 16
Raji cell	17
Inhibition of antibody-dependent cellular cytotoxicity	18

In general, about 30–60% of patients will show circulating complexes in the serum and, in some studies, their presence shows a positive correlation with disease activity.[12,13,18] Anti-complementary activity has been shown to correlate with the presence of extra-intestinal manifestations.[12] Hodgson *et al.*[12] also showed that circulating immune complexes were rarely found in patients whose Crohn's disease was confined to the small intestine. They suggested that this might be due to the smaller load of luminal antigen in the ileum compared with the colon and postulated that this might explain the low incidence of extra-intestinal manifestations associated with ileal Crohn's disease. Circulating complexes usually disappear following surgical resection[16] (Jewell, unpublished observations).

So far, little is known of the nature of these complexes. From gel filtration studies, they are small with a molecular weight less than 10^6 and mostly contain IgG although IgA- and IgM-containing complexes may also be present.[14,18] Whether they are true immune complexes or represent immunoglobulin aggregates will remain unknown until specific antigens can be identified within the complex.

COMPLEMENT

Measurement of serum concentrations of complement components is not helpful. Concentrations of C4, C3, and Factor B and of $C\bar{1}$ INH and C3b INA, two of the modulators of the cascade, tend to rise with active disease and return to normal as the disease goes into remission.[20–24] Nevertheless, metabolic studies have shown a greatly increased catabolism and synthesis for C1q and C3.[25,26] These studies also demonstrated extravascular sequestration of C1q and C3, presumably in the inflamed intestine.

Further evidence for complement activation is the presence of activation products in serum,[13,27] although these may occur *in vitro* during the clotting process since they are rarely found in plasma.[28] Recently, about 30% of patients with Crohn's disease have been shown to have C3i in their plasma, and the presence of this activation product correlated with disease activity.[14] Finally, the increased frequency of antibodies to activated complement components (immunoconglutinins) seen in the serum of these patients is further evidence that complement activation is occurring.[23]

When total hemolytic activity of patients' sera has been measured, it is either normal or raised during active disease.[14,22] This indicates the functional integrity of the complement cascade. However, there may be some impairment of the alternative pathway since Lake *et al.*[22] have shown an impaired response to cobra venom factor. The *in vivo* significance of this observation is unclear.

EXPERIMENTAL COLITIS

Kirsner *et al.*[29] were the first to show that a colitis could be induced in rabbits sensitized to egg albumin by instilling rectal formalin prior to an intravenous challenge with the antigen. This example of the Auer phenomenon was developed by Hodgson *et al.*[30] They used nonimmunized rabbits and injected them intravenously with pre-formed immune complexes two hours after instilling the dilute formalin into the rectum. The formalin itself causes minimal damage and serves to localize the deposition of circulating complexes. An acute colitis developed over the subsequent few days which had all the histological features of human ulcerative colitis. However, it was self-limiting and the mucosa had returned to normal within six weeks. The experiment was then repeated in rabbits who had been pre-immunized with the common enterobacterial antigen of Kunin.[31] The hypothesis was that prior immunization with an antigen found in the colon might lead to local immunological responses to the gut flora and thereby induce a chronic self-perpetuating inflammation. As in the first experiment, the rabbits developed a mild acute colitis following the intravenous injection of complexes but the inflammation continued and was still present at six months. Histologically, there was active inflammation associated with change of a chronic colitis—gland atrophy and distortion, lymphocytic infiltration along with neutrophils and plasma cells.

CONCLUSIONS

The rabbit model has shown that immune complex injury in the colonic epithelium can cause an acute colitis, resembling the human disease, which can become chronic in animals sensitized to antigens of the gut flora. In patients, there is increased local synthesis of immunoglobulins, the probability of circulating immune complexes, and increased complement activation. This represents strong evidence, even if indirect, that antigen–antibody reactions within the intestinal mucosa may play a major role in the pathogenesis of the inflammation. Most of these immunological observations apply to patients with Crohn's disease as well as to those with ulcerative colitis. It is difficult on present knowledge to explain the difference in anatomical distribution and in histological appearances of the two diseases. These differences may relate to the distribution of specific antigens and to their size and nature. The experimental observations[32] that a granulomatous response can be induced in rats by the intradermal injection of large antigen–antibody complexes made at equivalence is of considerable interest in this respect.

REFERENCES

1. Baklien, K. and Brandtzaeg, P.: Comparative mapping of the local distribution of immunoglobulin-containing cells in ulcerative colitis and Crohn's disease. *Clin. Exp. Immunol.*, **22**: 197, 1975.
2. Rosekrans, P. C. M., Meijer, C. J. L. M., Van der Wol, A. M., Cornelisse, C. J., and Lindeman, J.: Immunoglobulin containing cells in inflammatory bowel disease of the colon: a morphometric and immunohistochemical study. *Gut*, **21**: 941, 1980.

3. Soltoft, J., Binder, V., and Gudmand-Hoyer, E.: Intestinal immunoglobulins in ulcerative colitis. *Scand. J. Gastroent.*, **8**: 293, 1973.
4. Lopes Pontes, E., Piris, J., Jewell, D. P., and Truelove, S. C.: Local immune responses preceding clinical relapse in ulcerative colitis: changes in Ig-containing cells, T lymphocytes and eosinophils. *Gut*, **23** A: 895, 1983.
5. McClelland, D. B. L., Shearman, D. J. C., Lai, A., Fat, R. F. M., and van Furth, *R.*: *In vitro* synthesis of immunoglobulins, secretory component, complement and lysozyme by human gastrointestinal tissues. II. Pathological tissues. *Clin. Exp. Immunol.*, **23**: 20, 1976.
6. MacDermott, R. P., Nash, G. S., Bertovich, M. J., Seiden, M. V., Bragden, M. J., and Beal, M. G.: Alterations of IgM, IgG and IgA synthesis and secretion by peripheral blood and intestinal mononuclear cells from patients with ulcerative colitis and Crohn's disease. *Gastroenterology,* **81**: 844, 1981.
7. Monteiro, E., Fossey, J., Shiner, M., Drasar, B. S., and Allison, A. C.: Antibacterial antibodies in rectal and colonic mucosa in ulcerative colitis. *Lancet,* **1**: 249, 1971.
8. Baklien, K. and Brandtzaeg, P.: Immunohistochemical localisation of complement in intestinal mucosa. *Lancet,* **11**: 1087, 1974.
9. Otto, H. F. and Gebbers, J.-O.: Immunohistochemical observations on the local immune response in ulcerative colitis. *Inn. Med.,* **2**: 69, 1978.
10. Gebbers, J.-O. and Otto, H. F.: Evidence for local immune-complexes in ulcerative colitis. *Acta Gastroenterol.* (Belg.), **41**: 329, 1978.
11. Doe, W. F., Booth, C. C., and Brown, D. L.: Evidence for complement-binding immune complexes in adult coeliac disease, Crohn's disease and ulcerative colitis. *Lancet,* **1**: 402, 1973.
12. Hodgson, H. J. F., Potter, B. J., and Jewell, D. P.: Immune complexes in ulcerative colitis and Crohn's disease. *Clin. Exp. Immunol.*, **29**: 187, 1977.
13. Nielsen, H., Binder, V., Daugharty, H., and Svehag, S. E.: Circulating immune complexes in ulcerative colitis. *Clin. Exp. Immunol.,* **31**: 72, 1978.
14. Richens, E. R., Thorp, C. M., Bland, P. W., and Hall, N. D.: Circulating immune complexes in Crohn's disease, their characterisation and interrelationship with components of the complement system. *Dig. Dis. Sci.,* **27**: 129, 1982.
15. Pallone, F., Montano, S., Ricci, R., Iavicoli, M., and Di Mario, U.: New evidence of circulating immune complexes in Crohn's disease using two sensitive methods. *J. Clin. Lab. Immunol.*, **5**: 23, 1981.
16. Fiasse, R., Lurhuma, A. Z., Cambiaso, C. L., Masson, P. L., and Dive, C.: Circulating immune complexes and disease activity in Crohn's disease. *Gut,* **19**: 611, 1978.
17. Kemler, B. J. and Alpert, E.: Inflammatory bowel disease: study of cell-mediated cytotoxicity for isolated human colonic epithelial cells. *Gut,* **21**: 353, 1980.
18. Jewell, D. P. and MacLennan, I. C. M.: Circulating immune complexes in inflammatory bowel disease. *Clin. Exp. Immunol.*, **14**: 219, 1973.
19. Soltis, R. D., Hasz, D., Morris, M. J., and Wilson, I. D.: Evidence against

the presence of circulating immune-complexes in chronic inflammatory bowel disease. *Gastroenterology*, **76**: 1380, 1979.
20. Ward, M. and Eastwood, M. A.: Serum complement components C3 and C4 in inflammatory bowel disease. *Gut*, **15**: 835, 1974.
21. Feinstein, D. A., Kaplan, S. R., and Thayer, W. R.: The alternate complement pathway in inflammatory bowel disease. *Gastroenterology*, **70**: 181, 1976.
22. Lake, A. M., Stitzel, A. E., Urmson, J. R., Walker, W. A., and Spitzer, R. E.: Complement alterations in inflammatory bowel disease. *Gastroenterology*, **76**: 1374, 1979.
23. Potter, B. J., Brown, D. J. C., Watson, A., and Jewell, D. P.: Complement inhibitors and immunoconglutinins in ulcerative colitis and Crohn's disease. *Gut*, **21**: 1030, 1980.
24. Hodgson, H. J. F., Potter, B. J., and Jewell, D. P.: Humoral immune system in inflammatory bowel disease. I. Complement levels. *Gut*, **18**: 749, 1977.
25. Hodgson, H. J. F., Potter, B. J., and Jewell, D. P.: C3 metabolism in ulcerative colitis and Crohn's disease. *Clin. Exp. Immunol.*, **28**: 490, 1977.
26. Potter, B. J., Hodgson, H. J. F., Mee, A. S., and Jewell, D. P.: C1q metabolism in ulcerative colitis and Crohn's disease. *Gut*, **20**: 1012, 1979.
27. Teisberg, P. and Gjone, E.: Humoral immune system activity in inflammatory bowel disease. *Scand. J. Gastroent.*, **10**: 545, 1975.
28. Pepys, M. B., Druguet, M., Klass, H. J., Dash, A. C., Mirjah, D. D., and Petrie, A.: Immunological studies in inflammatory bowel disease. Immunology of the Gut. In: Ciba Foundation Symposium 46, pp. 283–304. Excerpta Medica, Amsterdam, 1976.
29. Kirsner, J. B., Elchlepp, J. E., Goldgraber, M. B., Ablaza, J., and Ford, H.: Production of an experimental ulcerative 'colitis' in rabbits. *Arch. Path.*, **68**: 392, 1959.
30. Hodgson, H. J. F., Potter, B. J., Skinner, J., and Jewell, D. P.: Immune complex-mediated colitis in rabbits. *Gut*, **19**: 225, 1978.
31. Mee, A. S., McLaughlin, J. E., Hodgson, H. J. F., and Jewell, D. P.: Chronic immune colitis in rabbits. *Gut*, **20**: 1, 1979.
32. Spector, W. G. and Heesom, N.: The production of granulomata by antigen–antibody complexes. *J. Path.*, **98**: 31, 1969.

Experimental Colitis as a Model of Ulcerative Colitis

Kiyoo Kuroe, Mitsuro Chiba, and Yutaka Yoshida

SUMMARY

Experimental colitis was induced in rabbits either by immunizing them with *E. coli* 014 which possesses cross-reacting antigenicity with colonic mucosa, or by infusing intravenously the animals' own lymphocytes sensitized with *E. coli* 014 endotoxin which contains a high concentration of enterobacterial common antigen. Hemorrhagic inflammatory changes were developed in the colon of six of fifteen rabbits immunized with *E. coli* 014 and in five of eight rabbits having received infusion of their own lymphocytes sensitized *in vitro* with *E. coli* 014 endotoxin. To study the distribution of the endotoxin-sensitized lymphocytes, the lymphocytes were labeled with ^{3}H-uridine and then infused intravenously. Marked accumulation of granules was observed in inflammatory regions in the gut by micro-autoradiography. The above suggests that the lymphocytes sensitized with bacterial antigen which had cross-reacting antigenicity with the colon mucosa caused colitis. This implies that a similar mechanism might be involved in the pathogenesis of ulcerative colitis in humans.

INTRODUCTION

Recently the pathogenesis of ulcerative colitis has been studied from the standpoint of autoimmunity. In 1959 Broberger *et al.*[1] reported anti-colon antibody in the sera of patients with ulcerative colitis. It has recently been suggested that the lymphocytes sensitized with bacterial antigen cause damage to the intestinal mucosa through the cross-antigenicity of bacterial antigens and intestinal mucosa.

In this paper we describe an experimental colitis induced in rabbits by immunizing the animals with *Escherichia coli* 014 which possesses cross-reacting antigenicity with colonic mucosa and by infusing the rabbits'

First Department of Internal Medicine, Hirosaki University School of Medicine, Hirosaki, Japan

own lymphocytes sensitized with the endotoxin extracted from *E. coli* 014 *in vitro*.

MATERIALS AND METHODS

Animals

Adult rabbits of both sexes weighing over 2 kg were used.

Enterobacterial antigen

A strain of *E. coli* 014 was inoculated into 20 ml of agar liquid medium and incubated overnight at 37° C. Subsequently the inoculum was added to one liter of the same medium and incubated for further 24 hours. *E. coli* 014 grown in media were collected by centrifugation, washed five times in sterile normal saline, lyophilized, and stored at 4° C.

E. coli *014 endotoxin*

E. coli 014 endotoxin was extracted by the phenol-water method according to Westphal *et al.*,[2] and 0.4 g of the dried *E. coli* 014 were treated with a mixer and centrifuged at 3,000 rpm for 20 minutes. The resulting water phase was obtained and dialyzed in tap water for four days to remove phenol. Then, 3 volumes of cold ethanol was added. After overnight incubation at 4° C, crude extracts were collected by centrifugation and lyophilization.

Lymphocyte transformation to E. coli *014 endotoxin*

The above endotoxin was diluted to 1 : 100, 1 : 1,000, 1 : 10,000, 1 : 50,000, and 1 : 100,000. Lymphocyte transformation to each dilution was measured in seven control rabbits.

Immunofluorescent antibody method

The indirect method of Coons was used. Rabbit colon was rapidly frozen and 4-μm sections were prepared. Then sections were fixed in 99% ethanol for 10 minutes. After drying in air, they were covered for 30 minutes with the sera from the same rabbit for the colon sample and washed in phosphate-buffered saline (pH 7.1) for 30 minutes. Finally, they were stained with goat anti-rabbit γ-globulin serum conjugated with fluorescein isothiocyanate which had been absorbed with rat liver powder.

Methods of experimental colitis

1) Fifteen rabbits were injected intracutaneously with 1 mg of the dried *E. coli* 014 with Freund's complete adjuvant once a week for seven weeks, and five of them received an enema of 5 ml of 0.5% formalin once every

four days for three times. The colonic mucosa of the rabbits was observed by endoscopy during the immunization before sacrifice. Sera from the rabbits were serologically tested for the presence of antibody against *E. coli* 014 by the ring test, the tanned-cell hemagglutination test, and the immunofluorescent antibody test.

2) Twelve milliliters of heparinized venous blood was obtained from normal rabbits and lymphocytes were isolated by Conray-Ficoll method and suspended in RPMI 1640 medium containing 20% fetal calf serum. In all instances, the preparations showed a purity of lymphocytes of over 95%. All cells were checked for viability by 1% trypan blue dye exclusion. As the preliminary experiments showed that a 1 : 10,000 dilution of endotoxin was adequate to sensitize lymphocytes, 1×10^6 lymphocytes in 1 ml medium were put in a culture tube and 20 μl of 1 : 10,000 dilution of endotoxin was added. The tubes were incubated for 18 hours at 37° C in a humidified atmosphere of 5% CO_2. Then lymphocytes were washed twice in barbital buffer solution and resuspended in a mixture of 0.5 ml of normal saline and 0.5 ml of self plasma. The lymphocytes sensitized with *E. coli* 014 endotoxin were infused intraveously into the same rabbit from which the lymphocytes were obtained. The mean count of infused lymphocytes each time was 6.7×10^5 and their viability was 84.6%. This procedure was repeated twice a week for four weeks. The colonic mucosa of the rabbits was also observed by endoscopy during the infusion. Six of eight rabbits received an enema of 5 ml of 0.5% formalin as stated before. The rabbits were sacrificed 3 to 42 days after the last infusion (Fig. 1).

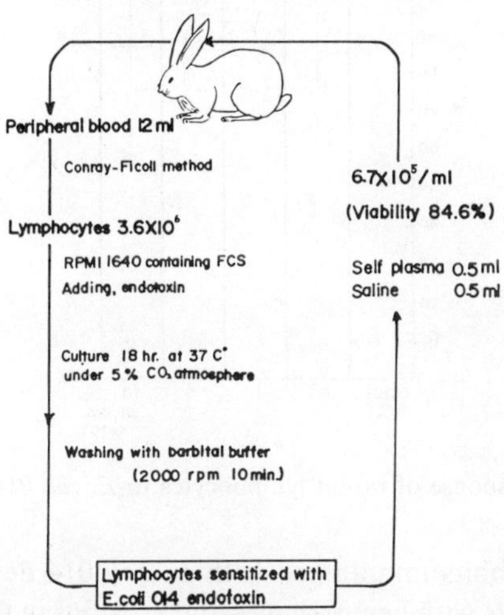

FIG. 1. Method of infusion of own lymphocytes sensitized with *E. coli* 014 endotoxin.

Autoradiograph

The lymphocytes of normal rabbits were isolated, cultured in a 1 : 10,000 dilution as stated before, and then labeled with tritium by incubating for two hours with 1 μCi of ^{3}H-uridine. After washing twice, these labeled and endotoxin-sensitized lymphocytes were infused intravenously into the same rabbits twice a week for four weeks. The rabbits were sacrificed and the colon tissue was fixed in formalin and stained with hematoxylin-eosin. These stained tissue sections were then dipped into Sakula liquid emulsion and developed with three weeks' exposure at 4° C.

RESULTS

In lymphocyte transformations to the various dilutions (1 : 100 to 1 : 100,000) of *E. coli* 014 endotoxin, the lower dilutions of endotoxin caused suppression of ^{3}H-uridine uptake. A very modest stimulation of 107 $\pm$ 18 % was obtained to a 1 : 10,000 dilution, as shown in Fig. 2. Therefore, a 1 : 10,000 dilution was used to sensitize the rabbit lymphocytes.

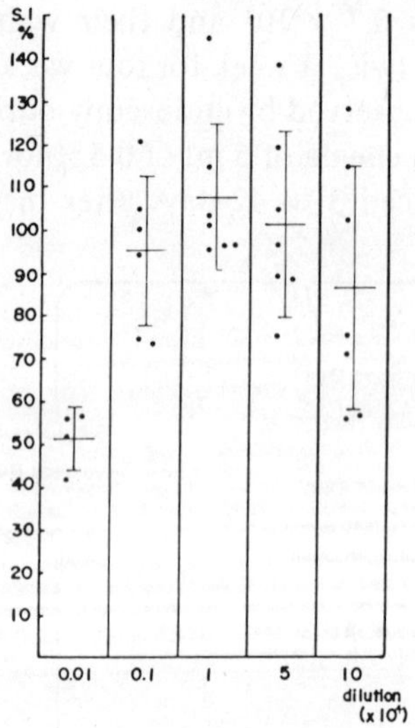

FIG. 2. Response of rabbit lymphocytes to *E. coli* 014 endotoxin.

Six of fifteen rabbits immunized with *E. coli* 014 developed diffuse inflammatory changes with hemorrhages and erosions in the colon, as shown in Figs. 3 and 4. The histologic features were hemorrhage, cellular infiltration, and denudation of the glandular epithelium (Fig. 5). In two of

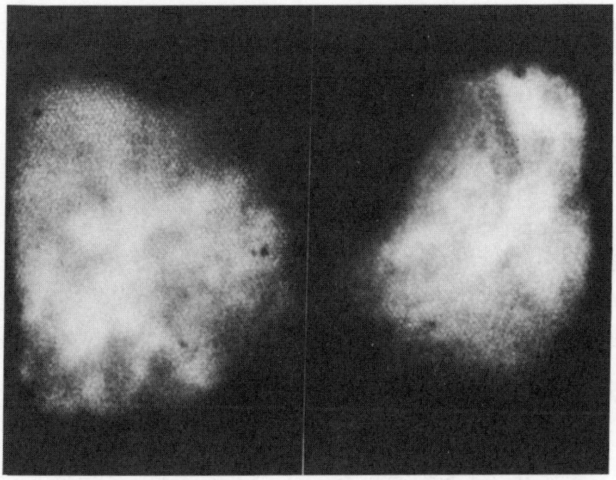

FIG. 3. Endoscopic pictures of rabbit colon revealing erosions and multiple punctate hemorrhages.

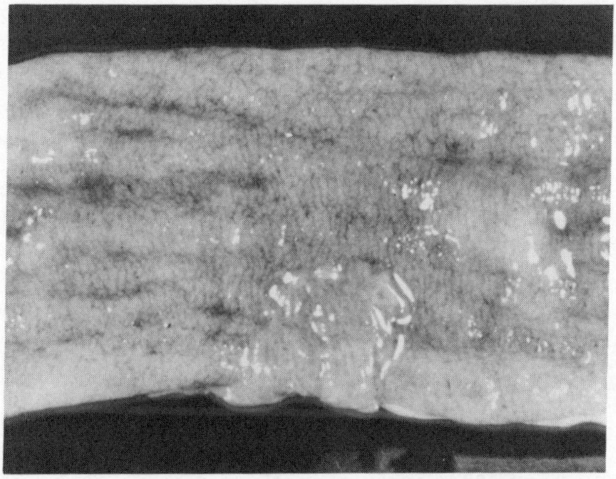

FIG. 4. Macroscopic findings of erosions and multiple tiny hemorrhages in the colon of rabbit immunized with *E. coli* 014.

these six rabbits, the inflammatory changes seen on endoscopy subsequently disappeared before exsanguination. There was no difference in the precipitin titers to *E. coli* 014 between the rabbits which developed inflammatory changes and those which did not (Table 1). The serum of rabbit No. 105 which developed colitis had an autoantibody titer of 1 : 4 to the colon by the immunofluorescent antibody method (Fig. 6). How-

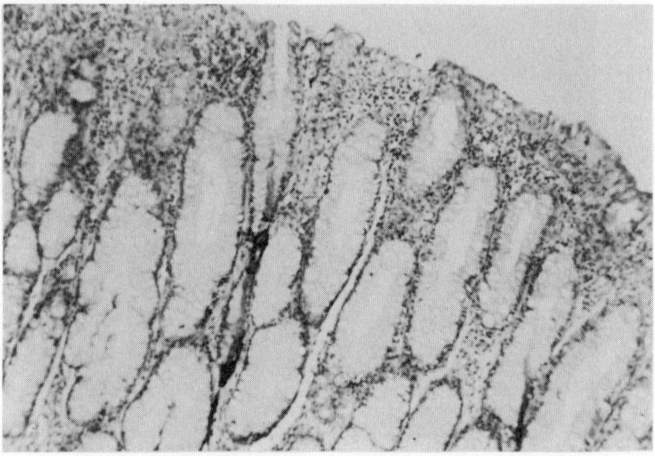

FIG. 5. Histological findings in the lesion in the rabbit colon revealing denudation of the glandular epithelium and cellular infiltrations.

TABLE 1. Antibody Titers against *E. coli* 014 in the Rabbits Immunized with *E. coli* 014 (the Ring Test)

Rabbit No.	Antibody titer	Colon response
101	1/512	None
102	1/512	Erosions, scattered small hemorrhages by endoscopy but none at autopsy
103	1/512	None
104	1/512	None
105	1/512	Erosions, tiny punctate hemorrhages at autopsy
106	1/128	None
107	1/512	None
108	1/256	Erosions, scattered small hemorrhages by endoscopy but none at autopsy
109	1/128	None
110	1/128	Erosions, scattered small hemorrhages at autopsy
111*	1/512	Erosions, small hemorrhages at autopsy
112*	1/128	None
113*	1/128	Erosions, multiple tiny hemorrhages at autopsy
114*	1/256	None
115*	1/512	None

*0.5% formalin enema after immunization.

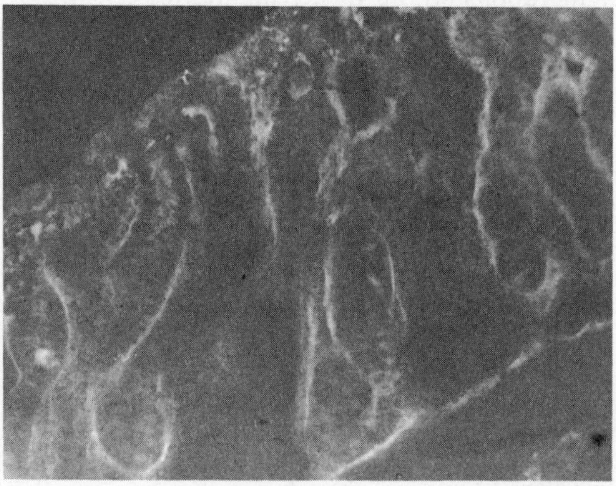

FIG. 6. Photomicrograph of cryostat sections of rabbit colon. Autoantibody is shown by staining tissue taken from the rabbit producing anti-*E. coli* 014 serum. Fluorescent staining confined to the membrane of the epithelial cell of colonic mucosa.

ever, the rabbits which did not develop colitis also had autoantibody. Five control rabbits which received enemas of formalin alone showed no colitis.

TABLE 2. Experimental Colitis in Rabbits by Infusing Their Own Lymphocytes Sensitized with *E. coli* 014 Endotoxin

Rabbit No.	Infused mean lymphocyte counts at one shot	Duration of observation after last infusion	Colon response
1	2.7×10^5	10 days	Erosions, tiny punctate hemorrhages at autopsy
2	7.1×10^5	3 days	Erosions, tiny punctate hemorrhages at autopsy
3*	2.9×10^5	21 days	Erosions, multiple scattered hemorrhages at autopsy
4*	6.9×10^5	14 days	Erosions, tiny punctate hemorrhages at autopsy
5*	6.0×10^5	31 days	Erosions, tiny punctate hemorrhages at autopsy
6*	9.2×10^5	24 days	None
7*	1.6×10^5	24 days	None
8*	9.4×10^5	42 days	None

*0.5% formalin enema after infusions.

Five of eight rabbits whose own lymphocytes sensitized with *E. coli* 014 endotoxin were infused intravenously developed changes in the colon similar to those seen in the rabbits immunized with *E. coli* 014 (Table 2). The histologic features were also similar to those seen in the rabbits immunized with *E. coli* 014. Six control rabbits in which a 1 : 150 dilution of endotoxin alone was injected intravenously developed no lesions in the colon. The frequency of colitis occurrence is summarized in Table 3.

TABLE 3. Experimental Colitis Induced by Immunological Manipulation

Method	No.	No. of developing colitis
E. coli 014 I.C.	15	6 (2)*
Lymphocytes sensitized with *E. coli* 014 endotoxin I.V.	8	5
E. coli endotoxin alone I.V.	6	0

*Colitis disappeared on postmortem examination in two rabbits.

In autoradiographs, a profuse number of labeled lymphocytes were seen in the lesions.

DISCUSSION

Until recent years, there have been few successful attempts to produce experimental ulcerative colitis in animals. Several methods, such as long-term administration of histamine or histamine releasers, local injection of collagenase, oral or intra-arterial administration of lysozymes, have been tried, but none of these experimental reactions resembles human ulcerative colitis. Immunological procedures have also been used for this purpose; however, the similarity of these types of colitis to human ulcerative colitis remains in doubt.

Recently a number of investigators have reported the possibility that normal tissue is destroyed by autoantibodies in various organ systems. A similar mechanism has been postulated in mucosal damage in inflammatory bowel disease. Bacteria normally present in the patient's gastrointestinal tract are most likely the source of the antigen which initiates a self-perpetuating sensitization. There is a possibility that bacteria may act as a hapten in sensitizing lymphocytes and then the sensitized lymphocytes may react with colon cells because of their antigenic similarity. Such a hypothesis was verified by our experiments.

We used *E. coli* 014 since an antigenic relationship between the intestinal mucosa and *E. coli* 014 has been demonstrated by several groups as well as by Kunin *et al.*[3] Six of fifteen rabbits immunized with *E. coli*

014 developed hemorrhagic inflammatory changes in the colon and autoantibody against rabbit colon was produced in the rabbits. In the immunofluorescent antibody method, staining was shown in the membranes of mucosal glands, supporting the view that the colon itself shares an antigenic determinant with *E. coli* 014. However, the autoantibody was found even in rabbits that did not develop colitis; thus other factors are thought to be necessary to develop this type of colitis.

Recent works suggest that "delayed or cellular" hypersensitivity may be more important than humoral antibodies in the pathogenesis of ulcerative colitis. The concept has been developed that ulcerative colitis may be a disease of hypersensitivity in which the immune response is directed primarily against the colon and that sensitized lymphocytes may be responsible for the initiation or perpetuation of tissue damage. Shorter *et al.*[4] induced cytotoxicity for allogeneic colon epithelial cells by prior incubation of lymphocytes from normal healthy adults with a lipopolysaccharide extract from *E. coli* 0119 : B 14. They suggested that colonic ulcerations with the resulting exposure of lymphocytes to microorganisms in the intestine may be an important factor in the induction of the cytotoxic property of the lymphocytes.

We designed an experiment based on the above hypothesis. Lymphocytes were sensitized with *E. coli* 014 endotoxin *in vitro* and then returned to the donor. By this method, five of eight rabbits developed hemorrhagic inflammatory changes in the colon. In autoradiographs a great number of ^{3}H-uridine-labeled lymphocytes sensitized with *E. coli* 014 endotoxin were seen in the lesions of rabbit colon. Therefore, the above suggests that these sensitized lymphocytes caused damage to the colonic mucosa, which possess cross-reacting antigenicity with *E. coli* 014. Similarly, the enterobacteria normally present in the intestine may sensitize the lymphocytes with resulting damage to the colonic eptihelial cells as seen in human ulcerative colitis.

Kobayashi *et al.*[5] tried to produce colitis in guinea pigs using various combinations of immunogens and adjuvants. Enterobacterial common antigen (ECA) extracted from *Salmonella typhimurium* and colonic antigen extracted from human fetus colon were used as immunogens. Phospholipid extracted from guniea pig colon, *E. coli* 014 LPS, and Freund's incomplete adjuvant were used as adjuvants. In groups immunized with ECA, colitis was produced when either phospholipid or *E. coli* 014 LPS was used as adjuvant. In addition, local mucosal lymphocytes from the guinea pigs with colitis showed transformation to ECA. From these observations, they concluded that the colitis was produced by cell-mediated immune reactions; namely, lymphocytes sensitized with ECA, which shares antigenicity with colon antigen, caused colonic damage.

Carrageenan-induced colitis has provided important information about developing ulcers in the intestine. Marcus and Watt[6,7] first reported that extracts of various red seaweeds when fed to animals in their drinking water caused ulcerative lesions of the colon in several species including guinea pigs, rabbits, rats, and mice. The extracts contained carrageenan, a sulphated polysaccharide.

Kitano *et al.*[8] also reported carrageenan-induced colitis. Rabbits were sensitized with normal saline containing 1% λ-degraded carrageenan by intramuscular injection. One week later, 5% water solution of λ-degraded carrageenan was given as drinking water for about six weeks. Endoscopically, edema was observed in the second week, and disseminated erosions and ulcers were found in various parts of the large intestine in the sixth week. Microscopic examination revealed mucosal atrophy, cryptitis, small erosions, and a marked lymphocyte and plasma cell infiltration in the ulcerative regions.

They also studied the relationship of the bacterial flora and ulcerative lesions. In guinea pigs treated with antibiotics prior to carrageenan administration, the inflammatory changes were histologically milder than those given carrageenan alone. When carrageenan was given over a long period, *Bacteroides fragilis* increased markedly in feces. The colon showed mucosal atrophy, mild lymphocyte infiltration, submucosal edema, and deformed glands. They concluded that intestinal bacteria play an important role in the production of ulcerative lesions in the intestine.

In conclusion, the studies presented here show that enterobacteria, including anaerobic bacteria, are involved in the development of experimental colitis. However, these animal models are far from the ulcerative colitis seen in humans in terms of the chronicity and nature of inflammation. Obviously, further investigations are needed to establish an animal model for ulcerative colitis.

REFERENCES

1. Brobeger, O., *et al.*: Autoantibodies in human ulcerative colitis. *J. Exp. Med.*, **110**: 657, 1959.
2. Westphal, O., *et al.*: Über die Extraktion von Bakterien mit phenol/Wasser. *Z. Naturforsch.*, **7b**: 148, 1952.
3. Kunin, C. M.: Separation, characterization and biological significance of a common antigen in Enterobacteriaceae. *J. Exp. Med.*, **118**: 565, 1963.
4. Shorter, R. G., *et al.*: Further studies of *in vitro* cytotoxicity of lymphocytes for colonic epithelial cells. *Gastroenterology*, **57**: 30, 1969.
5. Kobayashi, K., *et al.*: Experimental colitis induced by colonic antigen or enterobacterial antigen. *Digestive Organ and Immunology*, **5**: 85, 1980 (in Japanese).

6. Marcus, R. and Watt, J.: Seaweeds and ulcerative colitis in laboratory animals. *Lancet,* **II**: 489, 1969.
7. Watt, J. and Marcus, R.: Progress report. Experimental ulcerative disease of the colon in animals. *Gut*, **14**: 506, 1973.
8. Kitano, A., *et al.*: Studies of experimental ulcerative colitis induced by carrageenan in rabbits—Especially long-term treatment with carrageenan and intestinal bacteria. *Jpn. J. Gastroenterol.,* **78**: 2104, 1981 (in Japanese).

Discussion: Immunology

Derek P. Jewell and Yutaka Yoshida, Chairmen

Dr. Jewell: I'd like to ask Dr. Morita to discuss your findings in relation to the very negative findings which have come out of Europe over the last few years and also ask you whether you have any data on patients with Crohn's disease.

Dr. Morita: I think it is an ethnic difference between Europeans and Japanese. There is no data on Crohn's disease.

Dr. Jewell: Have you any family data on ulcerative colitis?

Dr. Morita: I have studied five family trees, but I have no conclusion on this point.

Dr. Muto: In your research you found that there is a difference in HLA between proctitis and proctocolitis. May I understand that proctitis and proctocolitis are different?

Dr. Morita: It is a hypothesis that ulcerative colitis might manifest as proctitis or proctocolitis by a difference in HLA. If the two are different, there might be a difference in an immune response which influences the clinical picture. I don't know how much HLA can contribute to differentiating the two conditions.

Dr. Jewell: I think it is a very interesting genetic difference. We know that only about ten percent of patients with proctitis develop extensive proctocolitis. So, clinically most patients with proctitis are a well-defined group. Immunologically most of us have been unable to find any difference between proctitis and proctocolitis although a report from Holland has shown that many patients with proctitis appeared to have an IgE response going on in the mucosa. We, in Oxford, have been unable to confirm that finding, but there is more than a suggestion that proctitis is a different disease.

Dr. Chiba: Dr. Jewell pointed out the discrepancy in the findings on HLA association in ulcerative colitis between Europe and Japan. I wonder if there is the possibility of a technical problem. Did you test microcytotoxicity in a blind way, Dr. Morita?

Dr. Morita: We did not use a blind approach. However, typing HLA is under close control by changing sera with Tokai University or in cooperation with Dr. Naito's group in our University. I think the difference in the findings on HLA is not due to a technical problem but due to an ethnic difference. As there is no ulcerative colitis in Japan associated with a certain haplotype which associates with ulcerative colitis found overseas and *vice versa*, a genetic difference between Japanese and Europeans could be concluded.

Dr. Jewell: I am sure you are right. After all we have to remember that with all these HLA types we are not necessarily measuring the genetic factor controlling a disease, but we are measuring an HLA type which is probably adjacent to the immune response gene we are actually interested in. I think the uniformity of the results you have presented from Japan is really impressive.

Dr. Jewell: I'd like to ask Dr. Kobayashi a technical question. In the patients whose mucosal lymphocytes you studied for the response to ECA, how did the response correlate with peripheral response?

Dr. Kobayashi: I used a mechanical technique. All studies on mucosal lymphocytes were obtained not from the human intestine but from the animal.

Dr. Kuroe: Recently by a similar technique, Onderdonk *et al.* reported that *Bacteroides vulgatus* was thought to be a causative agent in the development of an ulceration. You showed an overgrowth of *B. fragilis*. Did you find any specific bacterial agent?

Dr. Kobayashi: We did not use *B. vulgatus*. It would be very difficult to find that a certain bacterium causes an ulceration. Searching a species of each group of bacteria is too complicated at the present moment. Relating to your question, I think it is important what kind of immunological manipulation you use and also important is to distinguish immunological manipulations for initiation and for chronicity.

Dr. Kuroe: Relating to Dr. Jewell's question, I'd like to comment. We have studied some immunological characteristics of lamina proprial lymphocytes from the human colon. We found that suppressor cell activity decreased in ulcerative colitis as compared to that of the control colon in accordance with the findings obtained with monoclonal antibodies by the group of Keio University. This decreased suppressor activity in the gut might make a condition in which cytotoxic T cells proliferate and antibodies are easily produced.

Dr. Jewell: Dr. Asakura, you have done some experiments we would all love to do, particularly with your isolated colonic epithelial cells. Most laboratories have never been able to get the techniques to work. It's very nice to have such good data.

Dr. Kuroe: Is the cytophilic antibody you have shown the same as cytotoxic antibody seen in SLE or viral infection? What do you think about the background of cytophilic antibody production?

Dr. Asakura: I could not find the cytotoxic antibody in the patients with ulcerative colitis. Both cytophilic and cytotoxic antibodies have been found in SLE. Although the role of these antibodies is not known, it is thought to relate to a decrease of suppressor cell activity.

Dr. Kuroe: What do you speculate is the cause of the decreased suppressor cell activity? Is that a phenomenon following an infection?

Dr. Asakura: We haven't presented our study about the thymus today because of a lack of time. But we have data suggesting HLA and thymus influence the changes seen in the peripheral blood.

Dr. Jewell: In patients who had lymphocytophilic antibody, how many patients had received blood tranfusions?

Dr. Asakura: We excluded the patients who had had blood transfusions.

Dr. Jewell: In your ADCC, was that an autologous system, namely the patient's serum on the patient's epithelial cells?

Dr. Asakura: We used colonic epithelial cells not from the human colon but from the normal rat colon.

Dr. Morita: What do you think about the DR2 and the antibody?

Dr. Asakura: There was no close relation between the frequency of DR2 antigen and anti-colon antibody in the serum. It is the subject of future study how DR2 antigen relates to other antibodies and other immunological mechanisms.

Dr. Morita: Dr. Jewell, is the immune complex an initiator?

Dr. Jewell: I don't know, but the immune response may well initiate the disease.

Dr. Kobayashi: I was very much impressed by the histopathological similarity of the experimentally induced colitis by Dr. Jewell and by ourselves. The microscopic figures are unique in which edema and cell infiltration are seen in the lamina propria whereas an intact epithelial layer is restored. This suggests that an immunological process is operating and some intrinsic factor is operating. Do you agree with my interpretation?

Dr. Jewell: First a number of experimental models have been produced for colitis. I found your model very interesting because of its close histological similarity to ours. You sensitized lymphocytes to produce an inflammation which again looks very similar. So it may be that the colon can only respond in one way that is producing this sort of picture. On the second point, as I understand, one of the differences one uses to dissociate an infective colitis from ulcerative colitis is that much of the inflammation of infective colitis actually occurs superficially in the lamina propria, whereas ulcerative colitis tends to be rather deeper. We were, therefore, rather pleased we produced a model which showed an inflammation deep in the lamina propria rather than a superficial one.

Dr. *Kobayashi*: Was the histological picture in your animal model produced with a bacterial antigen or immunized with a combination of a bacterial antigen and an immune complex?

Dr. *Jewell*: It is just with an enterobacterial antigen.

Dr. *Chiba:* We understand SLE as a typical model for an immune complex disease. In an active phase of SLE it is usual that a complement level is markedly decreased. But you have shown a high level of complement in active IBD. Would you comment on this point?

Dr. *Jewell*: One has to think about two points, synthesis and catabolism. In SLE catabolism outstrips the ability of synthesis and you get a fall in the serum level. In IBD, monocytes and macrophages which increase in the peripheral blood and inflamed tissue may release complement and compensate for complement consumption. When you have less C3 catabolism, then synthesis rate increases and compensates. Why do we get an increase level in IBD? It is more difficult to understand. But most of the complement components and certainly C1q and C3 which we have looked at are actually synthesized within monocytes and macrophages, and we know there is an increase in the number of monocytes in the peripheral blood and an increased number of macrophages in the inflamed mucosa. So I think the raised level is due to a stimulated population of monocytes and macrophages. Nevertheless, there is still an underlying increase in metabolism due to these immunological events.

Dr. *Aiso*: I have two questions for Dr. Kuroe: 1) How is the distribution of lesions in your experimental colitis with sensitized lymphocytes with endotoxin and what is the relation between the lesion and the accumulation of sensitized lymphocytes observed by autoradiography? 2) Do you think a superficial epithelial lesion and a submucosal inflammation are induced by different mechanisms?

Dr. *Kuroe*: The lesions were about 10 to 20 cm in length in the distal part of the rectum. The accumulation of the sensitized lymphocytes was roughly in parallel with the degree of inflammation. We could speculate that the sensitized lymphocytes infused caused some immunological reaction resulting in mucosal damage. And then antigens entered from the lumen through the damaged mucosa, causing further damage in deeper areas.

Dr. *Kobayashi*: In an animal model, I think we had better separate on two objectives: 1) to plan a model similar to human disease by immunological and nonimmunological methods, 2) to clarify the immunological role of intestinal bacteria. Dr. Kuroe's and our experiments showed clearly that the intestinal bacteria can induce an inflammation in the gut.

Dr. *Kuroe*: You are right. It is a subject of study for the future as to how we can get a chronic inflammation in experimental colitis similar to clinical colitis.

Dr. *Morita*: Do you have an animal model which you observed for a long duration? Was there any histologic finding suggesting disease other than ulcerative colitis?

Dr. *Kuroe*: We found one rabbit in which the lesion was also seen in the small intestine. As we could demonstrate antibody against an antigen of lymphocytes infused in both the small and large intestine, I think the pathological differences seen in the small and large intestine may be the result of different reactions.

Dr. *Jewell*: In your immunofluorescence slide showing the anti-colon antibody, the staining was mainly directed towards a membrane antigen. Did you see a staining of goblet cells in your animals?

Dr. *Kuroe*: No, I didn't.

Dr. *Jewell*: One of the major fields of research at the moment we have not really discussed has been the whole field of immunoregulation. We heard from Dr. Asakura that suppressor cell activity and, indeed, the number of suppressor cells may be depressed in patients with ulcerative colitis. Dr. Kuroe in discussion mentioned his studies on isolated mucosal lymphocytes, again suggesting a depressed suppressor cell activity. This is the field which is rapidly developing and very controversial. Our own studies differ from both of these findings. We have been unable to demonstrate any abnormality in a number of suppressor or helper cells in patients with ulcerative colitis. A number of groups in the United States have found other results. So this again is a field where there is considerable confusion. Much more work needs to be done.

In terms of isolated lymphocyte studies, this has been one of the major developments and is an exciting field in IBD immunology. But again we are in a field of discrepant results. I think, however, it is disappointing that so far lymphocytes isolated from IBD patients do not behave terribly abnormally; some studies find decreased suppression, some normal, and some increased suppressor cell activity. Overall no great abnormality has been found. I'd like to inject a word of caution about the process of separation. One point is that a study in our laboratory shows the isolation procedure itself is able to alter the proportions of suppressor to helper cells. Another finding I'd like to mention is the fact that natural killer (NK) cells are infrequently found in the intestine. Everybody working in the field has found that NK cell activity is poor in the isolated population of the cells. If one correlates activity with the phenotype, the reason for depressed activity is the fact that there are very few NK cells within the intestine. That raises a very interesting question. For the first time, we have a population of lymphocytes whose recirculation pattern differs from other populations of lymphocytes. It certainly means we have to completely reappraise all the studies of NK cell activity in IBD.

Dr. Kuwajima: I feel that an immunoregulatory mechanism being established in SLE such as a defect of suppressor T cell and a deficiency of T–B cell cooperation should be taken into consideration in the future in planning an animal model or in assessing the immunological function of lymphocytes *in vitro*.

Dr. Jewell: I don't think we should get too fixated on SLE. Diseases differ from one to another. But I think the point of looking at antigen-specific suppressor cells is a very valuable one. I am sure this is going to be a next step.

Dr. Chiba: As I did characterization studies on colonic mucosal lymphocytes, I'd like to comment on a pitfall of a technique employed in my experiment. Even though I reported that a chemical (EDTA) and an enzymatic (collagenase) treatment of peripheral blood lymphocytes did not modify the ability of mediating cytotoxicities, I did not employ the exact method which was employed for the isolation of mucosal lymphoid cells. I incubated the peripheral blood lymphocytes with the agent without stirring. I don't know whether the function would have been modified if I had added the mechanical procedure of stirring. Because it has been recently demonstrated that a mechanical procedure releases prostaglandin from the cells which modify lymphocyte functions. I think there are many similar problems in our immunological research field. Therefore, we have to be very careful in interpreting the data.

Dr. Jewell: I am sure that methodological problems are enormous. We treated our peripheral blood lymphocytes exactly the same way with all the stirrings and so on, and then found that collagenase makes no difference. However, if you take the supernatant from the gut lymphocytes which are from collagenase digestion and you add that to peripheral lymphocytes then you alter the function very considerably. I am becoming very disillusioned at functional assays done on the isolated cells because there are too many factors one cannot control for.

Dr. Yoshida: We still have many problems in the methodology to be solved, as well as in the interpretation of the results. I am sure, however, we all agree that our immunological approach to the study of etiopathogenesis in IBD has achieved much as shown in the papers presented today. Finally, I would like to encourage all the investigators here to continue their immunological studies to answer the unanswered questions raised today.

III. PATHOLOGY

Dysplasia in Inflammatory Bowel Disease

Robert H. Riddell

Carcinoma in ulcerative colitis tends to develop insidiously. It is relatively rare and only about 1,000 cases *p.a.* occur in the U.S.A. Symptoms and strictures usually reflect advanced disease. Early asymptomatic carcinoma is frequently finely nodular or plaque-like, making detection difficult by all currently available methods. The relatively young age of patients with carcinoma in colitis (average early 40s) is particularly worrying. Fortunately, a clinical high-risk group exists (patients with extensive or total colitis for 7 years or more, particularly if the onset was before 25 years of age), which can be particularly closely watched.

The problem

At least 20% of patients in the high-risk group will develop carcinoma; some estimates approach 50% and are based on an estimated incidence of 2% annually after the first decade. How can these be anticipated assuming total proctocolectomy to be unacceptable?

Dysplasia

The variety of terminologies that have been applied to the epithelial changes associated with colitic cancers is very confusing. An international group of pathologists interested in this problem has now agreed on the term "dysplasia" which is defined as an unequivocally neoplastic transformation of large bowel epithelium. Because it is a neoplastic change there is an implication that invasive carcinomas may arise directly from this change. Dysplasia is synonymous with a variety of other terms that have been used but that are less well defined including premalignant change, precancerous change, precancer, atypia, and adenomatous change in

Department of Pathology, University of Chicago, Chicago, Illinois, U.S.A.
Present address: Department of Pathology, McMaster University Medical Centre, Hamilton, Ontario, Canada

ulcerative colitis. It is a spectrum now divided into "high-grade" (including carcinoma *in situ*) and "low-grade" dysplasia. In ulcerative colitis, this carcinoma *in situ* is invariably accompanied by carcinoma, and much lesser degrees of dysplasia frequently give rise to a carcinoma; indeed, it is a common error in both surgery and pathology to think that *in situ* carcinoma must be present to give rise to an invasive carcinoma. Dysplastic mucosa always has that potential, and frequently exerts it. Dysplasia is best regarded as essentially similar to an adenoma conceptually, morphologically, and in its tendency to give rise to carcinoma.

Macroscopic appearance of dysplasia

The following may be detectable radiologically[1]:

1) Polyps or polypoid masses: Sometimes this appearance is part of (2) or it may be part of a carcinoma. Typical filiform inflammatory polyps virtually never undergo neoplastic transformation. However, the entire spectrum of dysplasia from inflammatory polyps to carcinoma was one of the first indications of a precancerous lesion in ulcerative colitis.[2] For this reason, inflammatory polyps that appear atypical or adenomatous or have a distinct head of more than 1 cm in diameter are best excised to exclude these changes. If such polyps are found, it is also wise to take multiple biopsies around its base as they may be part of a more diffuse dysplasia. When this is not the case, management may be a little more difficult, for such "adenomas" might have occurred even in the absence of colitis, particularly in more elderly patients. In younger patients, such polyps are unusual in non-colitics and are probably best treated more aggressively (see below).

2) Slightly raised nodular or plaque-like areas which may harbor an underlying carcinoma: It is stressed that the appearances may be similar whether or not an underlying carcinoma is present and that macroscopically (and, therefore, endoscopically) it is impossible to make this distinction.[3] Further, biopsies of these lesions will reveal the dysplasia but rarely the underlying carcinoma if present. For this reason, any lesion with this appearance is best treated as a carcinoma if a biopsy shows dysplasia.

3) Villous change: While recognizable in opened specimens, this seems very difficult to detect endoscopically. It probably represents the earliest stage of (2) and each "villus" is rarely larger than 1–2 mm in any dimension.

4) There may be no detectable abnormality, the diagnosis being entirely histological.

Application of macroscopic appearance to endoscopic biopsy

From the above, it is apparent that in the absence of gross lesions the most likely site from which a dysplastic biopsy may be obtained is a nodular or plaque-like lesion. Unless the colonoscopist is aware of these lesions and deliberately seeks them out, they are easily missed. It follows that only in a scrupulously clean bowel will such lesions be most readily seen.

Villous change, if detected, is similarly a high-yield area. It should be remembered that this change may be seen occasionally in acutely inflamed bowel which is not dysplastic and not premalignant. Polyps should only be removed if atypical as outlined above; several biopsies should be taken around the base of these lesions.

In the absence of any of these changes, the yield will be to some extent dependent on the number of biopsies taken. Thus, if a single biopsy is taken from ascending, transverse, descending, or sigmoid colon and rectum, the return over many colonoscopies will be less than if a large number of biopsies had been taken.

University of Chicago protocol: A biopsy is obtained from the cecum, then an additional biopsy is taken every 10 cm on withdrawal of the scope. Each biopsy is oriented, put into a separate container, and labeled accurately as to the site of origin. Although a little more tedious than putting all biopsies into 3 or 5 "regional" containers, if problems of interpretation arise or it is chosen to follow a particular abnormality, then that site can be returned to with a reasonable degree of accuracy. This usually yields 10–12 biopsies. In addition, 3–4 rectal biopsies are also taken—this also being a relatively high-yield area.

Examination of colonoscopic washings for cytology has a very low yield and in our study has only been positive when obvious endoscopic lesions are present.

Microscopic appearance of dysplasia

In the vast majority of cases, this is essentially similar to the changes seen in a small adenomatous polyp with enlarged hyperchromatic nuclei which tend to be misplaced towards the lumen. There is frequently lack of mucin production and the cytoplasm may become intensely eosinophilic. In contrast to the small adenoma which it morphologically resembles, such changes may be widespread and even relatively low grades of dysplasia stand a much greater chance of harboring a carcinoma than a similar degree of dysplasia found in an adenoma. A pathology report describing "adenomatous" features should, therefore, be taken more seriously. At the University of Chicago, a diagnosis of dysplasia is not made unless it is thought severe enough to be able to give rise to a carcinoma directly. However, it should be appreciated that carcinomas in ulcerative colitis do *not* usually arise via the spectrum of mild to moderate to severe dysplasia to *in situ* carcinoma-invasive carcinoma. It is true that the more severe the dysplasia the more likelihood there is of an associated carcinoma being present, but milder forms of dysplasia are quite capable of giving rise directly to a carcinoma. The greatest risk is over-interpreting epithelial changes in mucosal biopsies. If acute inflammation is present, it may be difficult to make a reliable diagnosis of precancer even when dysplasia is marked, and some degree of epithelial change is commonly noted when there is acute inflammation or active regeneration. It is also possible to under-interpret the precancer lesion. This may occur when too much reliance is placed on a single feature such as the presence of a villous configuration. Another form of "under-interpretation" is failure to recognize that dysplasia and cancer in ulcerative colitis may have the same basic histologic appearance. On several occasions, lesions thought to be confined to the mucosa and termed "precancer" in a biopsy have proven on resection to be from areas with underlying invasion and hence to be associated with a true cancer.[3)]

Reporting of biopsies in inflammatory bowel disease

As a result of several meetings of interested pathologists that included multiple slide exchanges, biopsies are classified as positive, negative, or indefinite for dysplasia.[4)]

Positive biopsies are unequivocally neoplastic (and equivalent to adenomas in the non-colitic population). They may be divided subjectively into low-grade (relatively little dysplasia) and high-grade (previously including moderate or severe dysplasia and carcinoma *in situ*).

Negative biopsies include normal mucosa, active disease, and quiescent disease.

Indefinite biopsies can be subdivided into those that are probably negative (reactive), those that are probably positive (but in which there is some doubt so that the biopsy cannot be included with positive biopsies), and unknown.

Management of biopsies

a) Biopsies that are negative for dysplasia or indefinite for dysplasia, probably negative, are followed by routine colonoscopy and biopsies.

b) Biopsies that are positive for dysplasia-high-grade indicate a colectomy once the dysplasia has been confirmed by a second interested pathologist.

c) Biopsies from an endoscopic lesion that yields biopsies of dysplasia of any grade indicate a colectomy because there is about a 60% chance that the lesion will prove to be a carcinoma when resected. The diagnosis of dysplasia should again be confirmed by a second interested pathologist, and if necessary rebiopsy of the lesion.

d) Biopsies that are indefinite for dysplasia—unknown, or probably positive—indicate repeat colonoscopy at a shorter interval of time (months) to monitor changes in the biopsy or confirm that it is a stable lesion.

e) Biopsies showing low-grade dysplasia in the absence of a mass or endoscopic lesions may be treated either by colectomy in view of the relatively high risk of a carinoma already being present (about 15–30%), or followed if the patient is either unwilling to have a colectomy or there are other reasons against colectomy.

Relationship of dysplasia–carcinoma sequence and time

This is shown in Table 1.

TABLE 1. Relationship between Length of History and the Precancer–Cancer Sequence (St. Marks Hospital Series—personal observation)

Pathologist status	Average length of history	No. of pts.
Dysplasia, but no carcinoma	14.4 years	36
Unexpected Ca in resected specimen	15.5	6
Resection for suspected carcinoma	18.0	40
Inoperable carcinoma	22.5	10

Management of "adenomas" in ulcerative colitis

The major concern of such adenomas is that they may represent part of a larger area of dysplasia. If the latter is the case then it will be impossible to excise the lesion completely colonoscopically, for the dysplastic mucosa will continue into the stalk and the adjacent mucosa. When the possibility of this situation is encountered endoscopically, the polyps should be snared if possible and multiple biopsies taken of the adjacent mucosa, particularly in patients who are in the adenoma-bearing age range. If the adjacent mucosa proves to be dysplastic as well as the polyp, then polypectomy will not remove the entire lesion, and colectomy is recommended. However, there is theoretically no reason why colitic patients in an adenoma-bearing age group (for the sake of argument over 45 years old) should not be as susceptible to (or more susceptible to) adenoma formation as the non-colitic population. The management of such lesions is currently controversial. At one extreme, if such a lesion occurs in a 30-year-old male with a 16-year history of colitis, it can be argued that he has demonstrated the potential of his large bowel to form neoplastic lesions and is therefore in a very-high-risk category for the subsequent development of carcinoma. In addition it would seem likely that these lesions are in some way a result of the colitic process and it is unlikely that he will continue for the next 50 years without producing more of these lesions. Logically one could argue that the wisest course of action would be excision of the large bowel to ensure as far as one can the patient's longevity irrespective of the presence or absence of dysplasia in the mucosa adjacent to the polyp.

At the other end of the spectrum might be a 68-year-old patient with a 10-year history of colitis who has two typical adenomas excised from his sigmoid colon, but no other evidence of dysplasia. Why should these not be just simple adenomas and treated as such? The possibility that these may have been potentiated by the colitic process cannot be denied, but it currently seems most reasonable to treat such patients conservatively and just follow them very carefully clinically. The lack of dysplasia in the mucosa adjacent to the polyp would support this interpretation.

The most difficult patients to manage are those intermediate between these two examples, e.g., a 42-year-old patient with an adenoma but not other evidence of dysplasia and a 12-year history of colitis. Arguably he could be treated conservatively. However, if he has two or three such lesions, the possibility that these are not simple adenomas but part of the colitic process is increased, and the chance that other undiscovered lesions are present also has to be borne in mind. Under these circumstances it is difficult to escape suggesting colectomy. In such patients a variety of other factors tend to affect this decision such as the activity of disease, the amount of time lost at work in the previous year or two, the clinician's impression of the patient's attitude towards colectomy, and, of course, the patient's willingness to undergo the operation. It is apparent from these examples that clinical judgment still has a large role to play in determining when a patient should undergo colectomy.

Dysplasia in Crohn's Disease

In view of the increased incidence of carcinoma in Crohn's disease, it has become apparent that the high-risk factors are similar to those seen in ulcerative colitis but include excluded loops of bowel, and possible fistula tracts. In view of the fact that strictures are expected in Crohn's disease, the diagnosis of carcinoma is either late, in which case the tumor is invariably fatal, or found incidentally, these being the only patients to survive.

Dysplasia has now been described in Crohn's disease,[5,6)] and although it makes good sense to suggest resection of the dysplastic mucosa, the problem is knowing exactly how much bowel to resect if the dysplasia occurs in anything other than a localized segment of large bowel. The potentially diffuse or multifocal nature of Crohn's disease within the GI tract means that, unlike ulcerative colitis, it may not be possible to resect all of the bowel at risk, neither may it be desirable to do so.

The other major problem regarding dysplasia in Crohn's disease is that it may not be possible to effect the same sort of colonoscopic follow-up that has become routine in ulcerative colitis because of the difficulties in performing colonoscopy in patients with Crohn's disease. Further, unless a partial colectomy has been carried out, the terminal ileum is difficult to observe routinely.

REFERENCES

1. Frank, P. H., Riddell, R. H., Feczko, P. J., and Levin, B.: The radiological detection of colonic dysplasia (precarcinoma) in chronic ulcerative colitis. *Gastrointestinal Radiology,* **3**: 209–219, 1978.
2. Dawson, I. M. P. and Pryse-Davis, J.: The development of carcinoma of the large intestine in ulcerative colitis. *Brit. J. Surg.,* **47**: 113, 1959.
3. Blackstone, M. O., Riddell, R. H., Rogers, B. H. G., and Levin, B.: Dysplasia-associated lesion or mass (DALM) detected by colonoscopy in long-standing ulcerative colitis: An indication for colectomy. *Gastroenterology,* **80**: 366–374, 1981.
4. Riddell, R. H., Goldman, H., Ransohoff, D. F., *et al.*: Dysplasia in inflammatory bowel disease: Standardized classification with provisional clinical applications. *Human Pathology,* **14**: 931–968, 1983.
5. Craft, C. F., Mendelsohn, G., Cooper, H. S., and Yardley, J. H.: Colonic "precancer" in Crohn's disease. *Gastroenterology,* **80**: 578–584, 1981.
6. Simpson, S., Traube, J., and Riddell, R. H.: The histological appearance of dysplasia (precarcinomatous change) in Crohn's disease of the small and large intestine. *Gastroenterology,* **81**: 492–501, 1981.

Further questions frequently requiring clarification

Q.1. Can marked inflammation in colonic biopsies obscure dysplastic changes?

A. Many of the changes found in the presence of acute inflammation, and particularly in the resolving phase after an acute attack, can show nuclear and cytoplasmic changes readily confused with a true dysplasia. Most of these, particularly regenerative changes, can usually be distinguished from dysplastic changes (Ref. 4), particularly with experience. However, in a small proportion of patients these changes overlap sufficiently to request repeat biopsies to ensure that the more exuberant changes regress, and in the presence of much inflammation it is wise to repeat the biopsies from whichever area of bowel is most affected. Labeling each biopsy accurately as to the site of origin greatly facilitates this. It should be realized, however, that severe dysplastic changes can invariably be diagnosed. An adenoma is still an adenoma even if ulcerated and heavily inflamed.

Q.2. In dysplasia, is it necessary to tell the pathologist whether the biopsy was from a grossly normal area or from an inflamed-appearing area?

A. What the endoscopist recognizes as inflamed is usually readily apparent histologically as acute inflammation $\pm$ hyperemia. Conversely, chronically inflamed mucosa, even if very heavy, usually appear normal endoscopically. On the whole, therefore, this information only confirms what is obvious histologically.

Q.3. Is dysplasia in an inflammatory polyp of any significance? If so should biopsies be taken round the base of these polyps?

A. Dysplasia cannot be ignored as it implies an intrinsic ability of the large bowel to undergo changes along a neoplastic pathway. However dysplasia in the typical filiform inflammatory polyps associated with inflammatory bowel disease is excessively rare and those polyps can usually be ignored. Atypical polyps (over 1 cm diameter at the head, those that look like adenomas, and those that are dome-shaped, broad-based, and sessile or otherwise atypical) are best biopsied or excised. Biopsies should be taken around the base of all these polyps if at all possible at the same time to anticipate the question "How should I manage this patient?" if the lesion shows dysplasia. It can be very difficult to recommend proctocolectomy if a polyp is excised that looks like a typical adenoma, for why should it not be just that? If biopsies round the base also reveal dysplastic mucosa then one is on much stronger grounds in advocating surgery as the polyp is probably part of a more diffuse dysplastic process. If the biopsies reveal that the polyp is the only displastic lesion then one is on better grounds to just follow the patient if that is considered best, particularly in an elderly patient. In young patients such a change is likely to herald further neoplastic developments. Clearly each case has to be managed on an individual basis.

Q.4. Does carcinoma ever develop without a mucosal component?

A. No. Although occasionally described in the literature, in my experience the primary can always be found if looked for. However the carcinomas occurring in UC are frequently atypical and readily avoid detection. It also goes without saying that epithelial neoplasms should always begin in the epithelium. To my knowledge there are no exceptions to this.

Q.5. Should not the carcinomas in UC always be visible to the endoscopist if he can visualize the area (e.g., a stricture)?

A. No! This seems to be a very difficult area endoscopically. Carcinomas that are plaque-like or have only small nodules can easily be missed endoscopically, possibly because the intraluminal pressure depresses them to the level of surrounding mucosa, while neoplastic strictures can appear so smooth inside that the endoscopist is surprised that his biopsies are of dysplastic (*rarely carcinomatous*) mucosa. More typical carcinomas do occur and usually present no problem.

Note: Remember: endoscopic lesion + dysplastic biopsy = carcinoma until proven otherwise.

Carcinoma in Ulcerative Colitis

Tetsuichiro Muto and Fumio Konishi

JAPANESE EXPERIENCE

The risk of developing carcinoma in longstanding ulcerative colitis has been well documented in the Western literature[1)] and the concept is widely accepted. Although ulcerative colitis has been well recognized in Japan for more than 20 years, carcinoma complicating ulcerative colitis has rarely been reported in the Japanese literature. The purpose of this paper is to analyze the Japanese experience of colonic carcinoma in ulcerative colitis based on the collected cases from the Japanese literature.

Analysis of collected cases

All reported cases of alleged carcinoma complicating ulcerative colitis were carefully reviewed and only histologically proven cases were selected. Many examples of alleged carcinoma in ulcerative colitis reported many years ago were found to be stenosing carcinoma associated with proximal obstructive colitis. So far 13 examples with definite evidence of carcinoma complicating ulcerative colitis have been collected and are shown in Table 1. There were six men and seven women. The age at carcimona detection ranged from 27 to 68, with an average age of 45.8 years. The interval between the onset of the disease and the discovery of carcinoma was over 10 years except for 3 examples. In one patient the interval was reported to be one year, but symptoms might not have been recognized by the patient because clinical symptoms in these reported cases seemed to be rather mild. All but three patients had total colitis, and those three had left-sided colitis. These data agree with the Western experience in that carcinoma complicating ulcerative colitis tends to develop in the younger age group and in patients with total colitis and a history of more than 10 years. There were 4 cases with multiple carcinomas: poorly differentiated adenocarcinoma or signet ring cell carcinoma, which are rather unusual

Department of Surgery, Faculty of Medicine, University of Tokyo, Tokyo, Japan

TABLE 1. Carcinoma in Ulcerative Colitis (Japanese Collected Series)

No.	Reported year	Age when cancer detected and sex	Time sequence after onset	Site of cancer	Type of cancer	Dysplasia
1.	1962	45f	19 yr.	Rectum	?	?
2.	1976[a]	62f	35	Rectum	Well diff.	−
3.	1977	39m	10	Multiple	Poorly diff. and undiff.	+
4.	1978	49f	12	Rectum, multiple	Well, poorly diff. and signet ring cell	+
5.	1978	53m	35	Sigmoid	Mucinous	?
6.	1980	37f	20	Cecum and descending	Well and poorly diff.	+
7.	1980[a]	37m	15	Sigmoid	Moderately diff.	?
8.	1981	29f	6	Multiple	Well, poorly diff. and signet ring cell	+
9.	1981	27m	16	Rectum	Mucinous	+
10.	1981	63m	1 ?	Rectum	Signet ring cell	+
11.	1982	53f	8	Ascending	Well diff.	+
12.	1982[a]	40f	21	Rectum	Well diff.	−
13.	1983	68m	>20	Rectum	Well diff. and mucinous	+

[a]Left-sided colitis.

types among ordinary colon carcinomas, were present in six cases. Dysplastic epithelium was detected by histologic examination of the surgically resected specimens in eight cases. These histological characteristics of carcinoma also agreed with the Western experience. None of these carcinomas was detected by surveillance examination.

Case presentations

Case 1 (No. 4 in Table 1): A 49-year-old housewife complained of diarrhea and bloody discharge. Twelve years ago she was diagnosed as total ulcerative colitis and received left hemicolectomy. Although she had been suffering from continuous mild colitis since this operation, she had not had proper treatment. On proctoscopy an annular growth was found 12 cm from the anal verge and the biopsy histology showed adenocarcinoma. Proctocolectomy was performed and the entire resected specimen was histologically examined by serial step sections (Fig. 1). The main growth invaded through the muscle coat to reach the subserosa, and was surrounded by a wide area of intramucosal and submucosal carcinoma. The histological type of the carcinoma was a mixture of well to poorly differentiated adenocarcinoma and signet ring cell carcinoma (Fig. 2). There

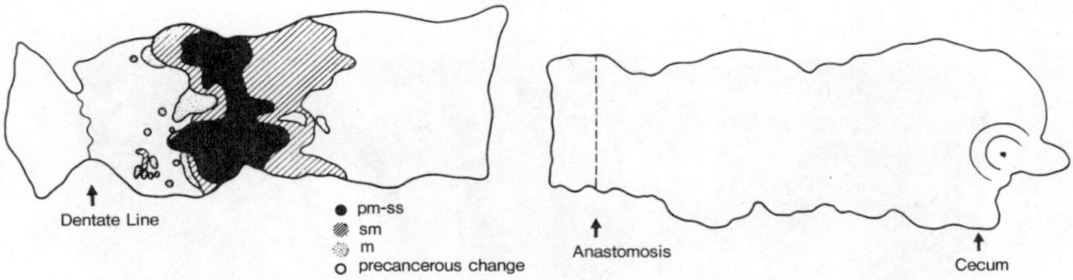

FIG. 1. Schematic illustration of the specimen according to the serial step sections of the whole colon. The main tumor invades through the muscle coat to reach the subserosa, and is surrounded by a wide area of carcinoma with submucosal invasion and carcinoma *in situ*. There are independent multiple foci of carcinoma *in situ* and a focus of invasive carcinoma only distal to the main tumor. All the remaining mucosa is covered by irregular tubules with variable degrees of dysplasia suggestive of precancerous change. No normal mucosa is found.

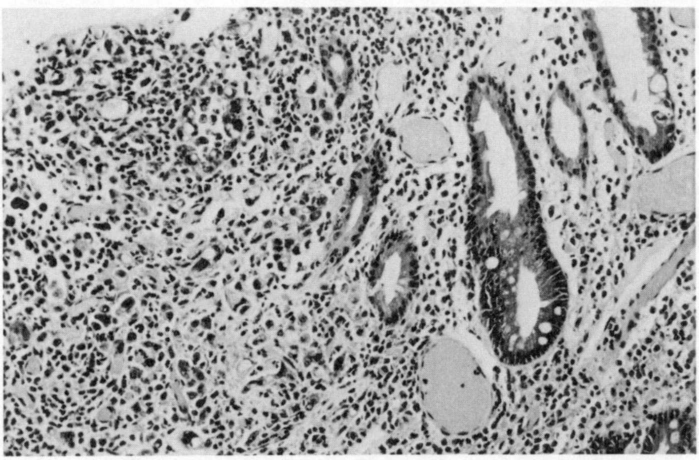

FIG. 2. Signet ring cell carcinoma (left) adjacent to the dysplastic tubules (right).

were independent multiple foci of intramucosal carcinoma and a focus of submucosal carcinoma only distal to the main growth. All the remaining mucosa was covered by irregular tubules with variable degrees of dysplasia suggestive of precancerous change, and no normal mucosa was found (Fig. 3). This is a typical example of multiple rectal carcinoma complicating longstanding ulcerative colitis.

Case 2 (No. 13 in Table 1): A 68-year-old man was found to have ob-

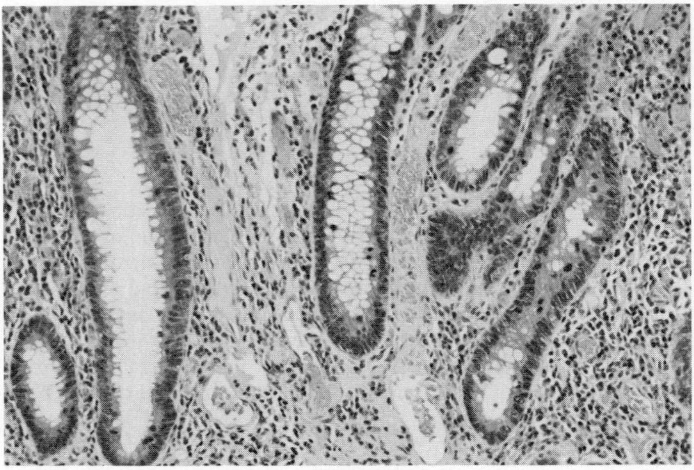

FIG. 3. Dysplastic tubules in the flat mucosa.

structive jaundice, and transcutaneous cholangiography revealed obstruction of the right intrahepatic bile duct. On digital examination a sessile mass was found in the lower rectum and was confirmed by barium enema and proctoscopy (Fig. 4). He had been having more than several bowel movements per day for more than 20 years but was never diagnosed as

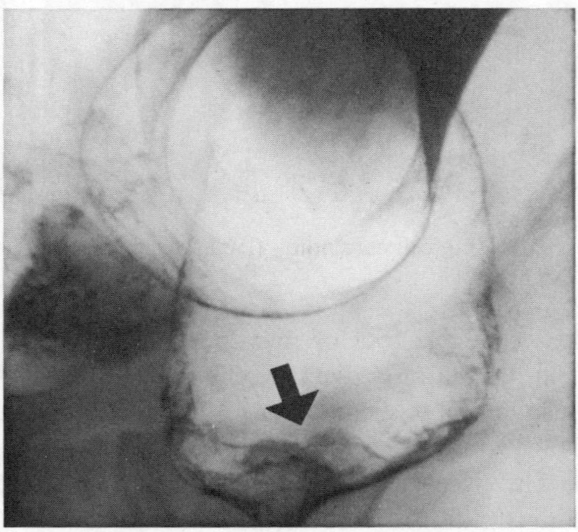

FIG. 4. Sessile growth of the lower rectum (arrow). The rectal mucosa appears normal.

ulcerative colitis. He thought his frequent bowel actions were normal and never consulted doctors. On colonoscopy his entire colon was mildly inflamed with loss of haustration, showing a typical appearance of chronic ulcerative colitis. Biopsy histology confirmed the diagnosis of mild chronic ulcerative colitis. The biopsy histology taken from the rectal mass showed severe dysplasia and submucosal invasion in part (Fig. 5). A transanal local excision was performed and the tumor was found to be mucinous carcinoma invading the submucosa (Fig. 6). The morphological characteristics of this carcinoma were quite unusual for ordinary carcinoma, and it was therefore assumed to be carcinoma complicating longstanding ulcerative colitis. He had a right hemilobectomy of the liver for the intrahepatic bile duct obstruction due to suspected malignancy and was found to have adenocarcinoma (Fig. 7). There was marked fibrosis of the Glisson's sheath and pericholangitis was also present (Fig. 8). This case seems to be a rare example of rectal carcinoma and bile duct carcinoma complicating longstanding ulcerative colitis.

Comment

It has been confirmed that colonic carcinoma complicating chronic ulcerative colitis exists in Japan, although the number of the cases reported has been quite small compared with Western countries. However, the general characteristics of carcinoma in ulcerative colitis are not so different from those in Western countries, as shown in the case presentations and in

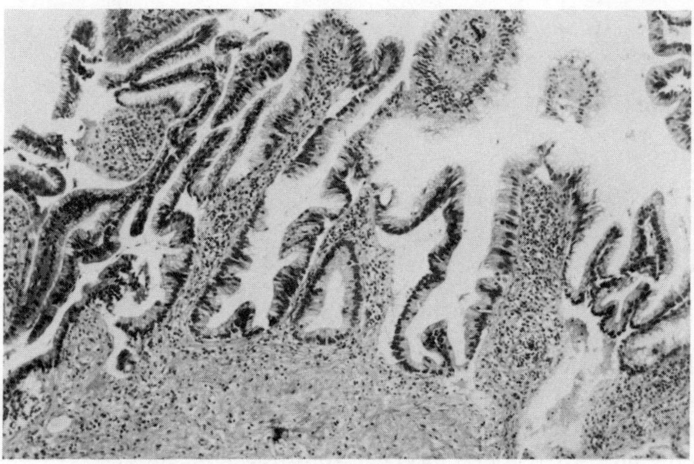

FIG. 5. Biopsy histology showing villous growth with severe dysplasia.

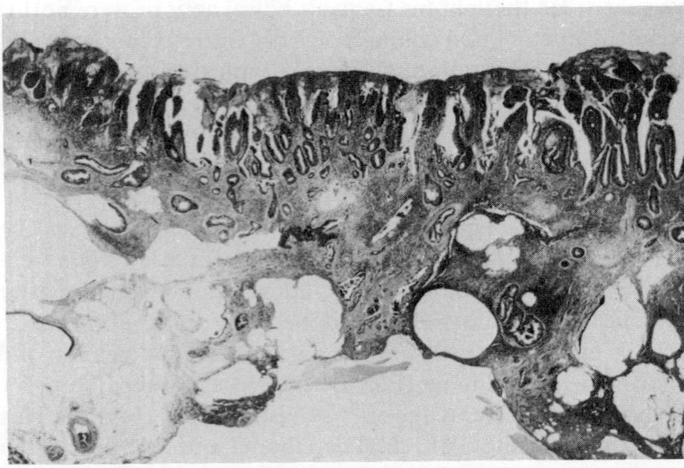

FIG. 6. Mucinous carcinoma invading the submucosa without residual adenomatous tissue.

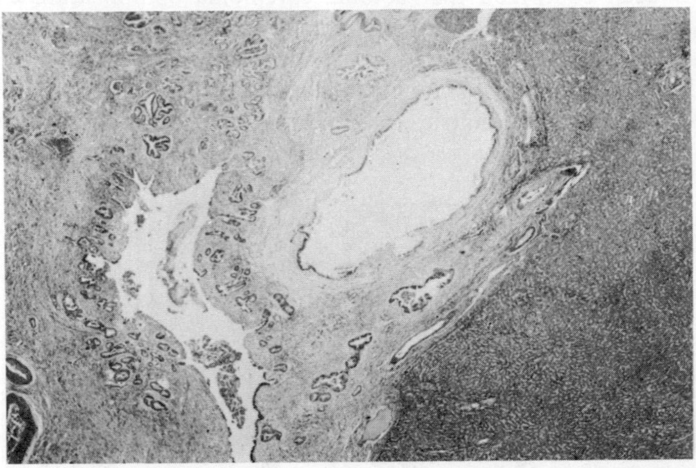

FIG. 7. Carcinoma infiltrating around the intrahepatic bile duct.

the collected series. The low frequency of carcinoma in ulcerative colitis in Japan is related to the low incidence of both ulcerative colitis and colorectal carcinoma. Another reason is that only a small number of cases of chronic ulcerative colitis has been followed long enough for carcinoma development. Since the frequency of ulcerative colitis has been increasing over the past several years and since many cases have been receiving medi-

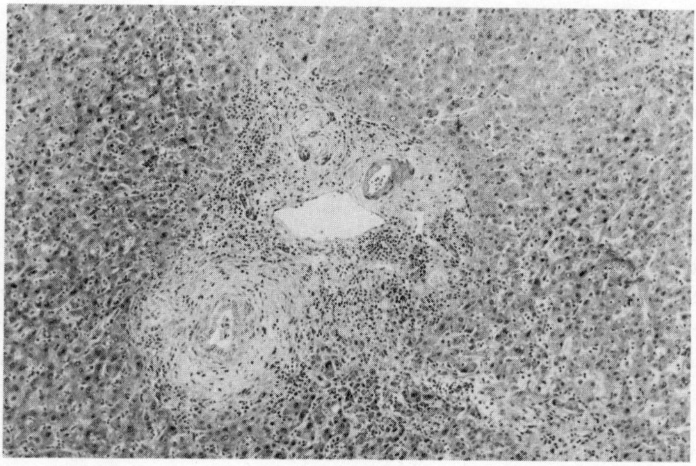

FIG. 8. Fibrosis and chronic inflammation around the Glisson's sheath of the resected liver.

cal treatment for many years with the recognition of high cancer risk in such patients, the number of carcinomas in ulcerative colitis will no doubt increase in the future in Japan. Changing environmental factors will also play a role in increasing carcinoma in ulcerative colitis as they do in ordinary colorectal carcinoma. Therefore, it is essential to study Western experience in regard to this particular problem in order to make earlier diagnosis and provide earlier treatment for better prognoses.

MUCIN STUDY OF PRECANCEROUS LESION IN ULCERATIVE COLITIS—A PRELIMINARY REPORT

Making a correct diagnosis of dysplasia in ulcerative colitis is a difficult task even for experienced pathologists. Grading of dysplasia in ulcerative colitis is also a controversial issue.[2] The criteria for grading dysplasia are based purely on histological and cytological features, and so far no method has been found to facilitate the diagnosis of dysplasia. In order to solve this problem we used special mucin staining, periodic acid-thionin Schiff/potassium hydroxyde/periodic acid-Shiff (PAT/KOH/PAS) by Culling.[3] The purpose of this section is to present recent results of this staining in dysplasia complicating ulcerative colitis together with other diseases.

Methods and Results

The detailed technique of PAT/KOH/PAS staining is described elsewhere,[3] and we followed Culling's technique. O-acetylated sialic acid at C8 is predominantly seen in the normal human colonic mucosa and stains red with this technique, whereas mucin stained blue or purple indicates the presence of O-acetylated sialic acid at C7 or C9, or C0 (unsubstituted) which is assumed to be abnormal according to Culling's paper. He claimed that all colonic carcinoma stained blue or purple with his technique.[3]

We stained 3 examples of dysplasia in ulcerative colitis, 60 examples of colonic carcinoma, 36 examples of tubular adenoma, 10 examples of villous or tubulovillous adenoma, 36 examples of the flat mucosa in adenomatosis coli, and 67 normal controls with PAT/KOH/PAS technique. The results are shown in Table 2.[4] As Culling had pointed out, almost all carcinoma and villous adenoma stained blue or purple. Although he claimed that all colonic carcinoma stained blue or purple, it was not so in our experience. It is interesting to note that all dysplastic epithelium in ulcerative colitis stained blue or purple, and in one example, blue tubules and red tubules were arranged in a mosaic pattern although both tubules appeared quite similar in hematoxilin and eosin staining. It is also interesting to note that the flat mucosa around adenomas in adenomatosis coli stained blue or purple in a high proportion (92%). These tubules appeared quite normal in ordinary hematoxilin and eosin staining, but functionally they seem to have different mucin properties from those of ordinary colonic mucosa. Adenomas on the blue surrounding mucosa always stained blue.

TABLE 2. PAT/KOH/PAS Staining Characteristics in Various Colonic Diseases

	Blue-purple	Red	Total
Carcinoma	59 (98%)	1	60
Adenoma	13 (36%)	23	36
Villous, tubulovillous adenoma	59 (90%)	1	10
Flat mucosa in adenomatosis coli	33 (92%)	3	36
Dysplasia in ulcerative colitis	3 (100%)	0	3
Normal control	26 (39%)	41	67

We also examined mucin in active and inactive ulcerative colitis with the same method used in the biopsy specimens in order to determine the effect of inflammation on the mucin staining (Table 3). It can be assumed that in active colitis the proportion of blue or purple mucin is much higher than in the inactive stage, and the mucin property seems to be influenced by mucosal inflammation, the results being similar to those of Culling.[5] Twenty-six out of 67 biopsy specimens from presumably normal colonic mucosa stained blue or purple.

TABLE 3. PAT/KOH/PAS Staining Characteristics in Ulcerative Colitis

	Blue-purple	Red	Total
Active	7	2	9
Inactive	7	10	17

Comment

Filipe *et al.*[6] have claimed that sialomucin was found predominantly in the colonic mucosa adjacent to and remote from the carcinoma, suggesting this abnormal pattern of mucin as a precancerous change. However, Isaacson *et al.* reported that this sialomucin-dominant mucosa can be found in the mucosa of colostomy orifices and of prolapsing piles, and claimed this change to be secondary and irrelevant to premalignant change. We followed this mucin staining and agree with Isaacson's opinion.[4]

PAT/KOH/PAS staining by Culling *et al.* is a more sophisticated staining of sialomucin, characterized by differing staining properties according to the site of O-acetylation at different side chains. According to their paper, normal colonic mucosa contains O-acetylated sialic acid at C8 or di- or tri-O-acetylation including C8 O-acetylation (C8 group) which stains red by this particular staining technique; and when mucin contains O-acetylation at C7 or C9 it stains blue or purple, as seen in colonic carcinoma. Although they stated that normal mucosa stained red, it was not always the case in our experience, and 39% of the biopsy specimens taken from the normal colonic mucosa stained blue or purple, which was assumed to be abnormal according to his criteria. The significance of this phenomenon is not clear. However, the presence of abnormal mucin by 90% in adenomatosis coli and by 100% in dysplastic epithelium in ulcerative colitis was striking. Although the number of cases examined is small, the difference from normal controls seems to be significant, and this staining property may well be useful as one of the markers of adenomatosis coli and dysplasia in ulcerative colitis. It can be assumed that the properties of colonic mucin in the dysplastic epithelium may have been changed prior to the morphological change, but it must be remembered that this site alteration of O-acetylation detected by PAT/KOH/PAS technique may not necessarily indicate premalignant change of the colonic mucosa due to the fact that in active colitis a high proportion of mucin stained blue or purple. It seems that the variable mucin properties of the colonic mucosa provide us with a new and interesting field of research work in which further detailed study is required to answer our questions.

SUMMARY

Histologically proven examples of colonic carcinoma complicating ulcerative colitis were collected and reviewed from the Japanese literature. There were 14 examples and the characteristics of this particular carcinoma in Japan were found to be the same as those in Western countries, although the incidence was very low.

Preliminary data on mucin study of dysplasia in longstanding ulcerative colitis were also presented. It was assumed that the site of O-acetylation of sialic acid in dysplasia of ulcerative colitis and in adenomatosis coli would be changed significantly, and this staining property could be one of the markers for making correct diagnosis.

REFERENCES

1. Riddell, R. H.: Precarcinomatous phase of ulcerative colitis. In: Current Topics in Pathology (ed. B.C. Morson), pp. 177–219. Springer-Verlag, Berlin, 1976.
2. Yardley, J. H., Bayless, T. M., and Diamond, M. P.: Cancer in ulcerative colitis. *Gastroenterology*, **76**: 221–225, 1979.
3. Culling, C. F. A. and Reid, P. E.: Specific techniques for the identification of O-acetylated sialic acids in colonic mucins. *J. Microscopy,* **119**: 415–425, 1980.
4. Muto, T., Kamiya, J., Konishi, F., Sawada, T., Sugihara, K., and Kusama, S.: Staining property of human colonic mucin by periodic acid-thionin Schiff/potassium hydroxide/periodic acid-Shiff (PAT/KOH/PAS) method. *I to Cho*, **17**: 343–348, 1982 (in Japanese).
5. Culling, C. F. A., Reid, P. E., and Dunn, W. L.: A histochemical comparison of the O-acetylated sialic acids of the epithelial mucins in ulcerative colitis, Crohn's disease, and normal controls. *J. Clin. Path.,* **32**: 1272–1277, 1979.
6. Filipe, M. I. and Branfoot, A. C.: Abnormal patterns of mucous secretion in apparently normal mucosa of large intestine with carcinoma. *Cancer,* **34**: 282–290, 1974.

Crohn's Disease in Japan
——Morphologic Features

Haruki Wakasa and Hikaru Watanabe***

Crohn's disease has been considered a rather rare disease in Japan for a long period, but in recent years the disease is becoming well recognized from clinico-pathological observations. However, in some instances, it is still difficult to differentiate it from other disorders, especially from tuberculosis.

Based on these considerations, the Japanese Research Committee for Crohn's Disease was organized under the Japanese Society of Gastroenterology. The committee has proposed criteria for Crohn's disease[1)] based on clinico-pathological considerations and has consulted on many cases from different hospitals throughout this country. During the course of the consultations, the committee has noticed some characteristic features of Crohn's disease in Japanese patients.

In the present paper, some observations on Japanese Crohn's disease obtained from consultation cases and a morphological study on granuloma by histological and ultrastructural observation will be reported.

GROSS APPEARANCE OF CROHN'S DISEASE

The Japanese Research Committee has consulted on cases of Crohn's disease and allied disorders according to the criteria proposed by the committee for the past seven years. The diagnostic criteria by different methodological steps are shown in Table 1, and diagnosis is made on a combination of these findings. In the meantime, a summary was reported in 1979 by the Japanese Research Committee for Crohn's Disease.[2)] The committee has already selected 102 cases of the disease according to the criteria.

*Department of Pathology, Fukushima Medical College, Fukushima, Japan
**Division of Gastroenterology, Sendai National Hospital, Sendai, Japan
This work was supported in part by a Grant-in-Aid for the Investigation and Research Committee for IBD from Ministry of Health and Welfare.

TABLE 1. Diagnostic Criteria for Crohn's disease (Japanese Research Committee)

	Examination	X-ray	Endoscopy	Biopsy	Surgical specimen
Discontinuity of lesion		+	+	+	+
Cobblestone appearance and/or longitudinal ulcer		+	+		+
Transmural inflammation	+ (tumor)	+ (stenosis)	+ (stenosis)		+
Granuloma				⊕	⊕
Fissures and/or fistulae	+′	+′	+′	+′	+′
Anal lesion	+′				+′

Crohn's disease: ++++′ or ++⊕.

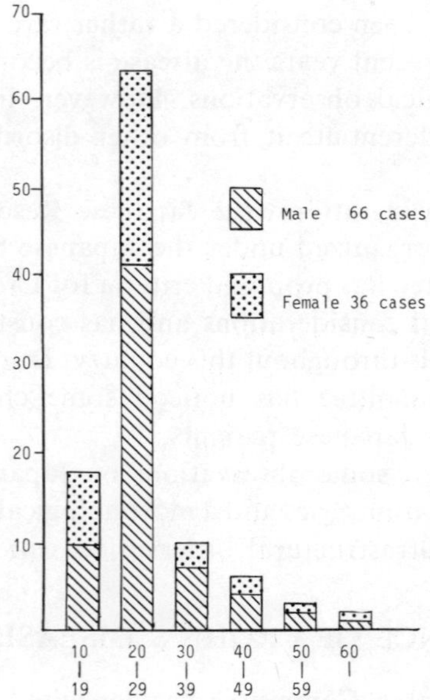

FIG. 1. Age distribution in patients with Crohn's disease. Abscissa: year range. Ordinate: number of cases.

The age and sex distributions are shown in Fig. 1. About 62% of patients were in their third decade at the time of diagnosis, followed by those in their second decade. Males outnumbered females.

With regard to lesion site, 25 patients had lesions in the small intestine only, and 29 patients had theirs in the large intestine. In 48 cases, lesions were found in both small and large intestines (Table 2). Of the 102 cases, surgical treatment was performed in 75, and the rates of surgical procedure in each lesion site were 88.0% for ileitis, 75.0% for ileocolitis, and 58.6% for colitis.

TABLE 2. Site of Lesion

Small intestine	25 cases
Small and large intestines	48
Large intestine	29
Total	102

As their most characteristic feature, 86.5% of the patients with lesions in the small intestine showed longitudinal ulcer, mainly on the side of mesenteric attachment (Table 3). It was not infrequent that longitudinal ulcers as long as 50 cm or more were observed in the terminal ileum accompanying a cobblestone-like appearance in the surrounding mucosa of the ulcer. Rarely, longitudinal ulcer in the ileum and a marked cobblestone-like appearance in the large intestinal mucosa were present together in the same case. However, in one case with a rather fresh ulcer, the mucosa, except for the ulcer, reveals a normal-looking appearance (Fig. 2). In surgical resected specimens of the small intestine of Crohn's disease, thick-

TABLE 3. Macroscopic Findings of Resected Samples

	Small intestinal lesion	Large intestinal lesion
Longitudinal ulcer	45	22
Cobblestone appearance	26	38
Thickening of intestinal wall	47	39
Stenosis	17	9
Fistulae	9	10
Aphthoid ulcer	17	8
Total	52	44

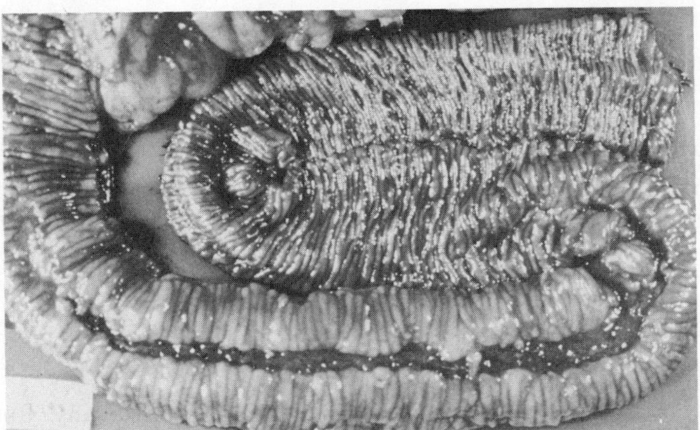

FIG. 2. Longitudinal ulcer of the small intestine.

ening of the intestinal wall of the lesion was the most prominent feature, longitudinal ulcers were the next most common, and a cobblestone-like appearance was apparent in about half of the cases.

On the other hand, in cases with large intestinal lesions, the cobblestone-like appearance and thickening of the wall were almost equally observed, and longitudinal ulcers were less frequent than in small intestinal lesions (Table 3). The marked cobblestone-like thickening is the most common morphological feature of Crohn's disease in Western countries, but such cases are less frequent in Japan.

In most of the cases, the depth of the longitudinal ulcer is usually limited to the submucosal layer, but in a few cases, muscular layers are also ruptured by the granulomatous inflammatory process. The base of the ulcer is covered with necrotic tissue or replaced by fibrous tissue (Fig. 3).

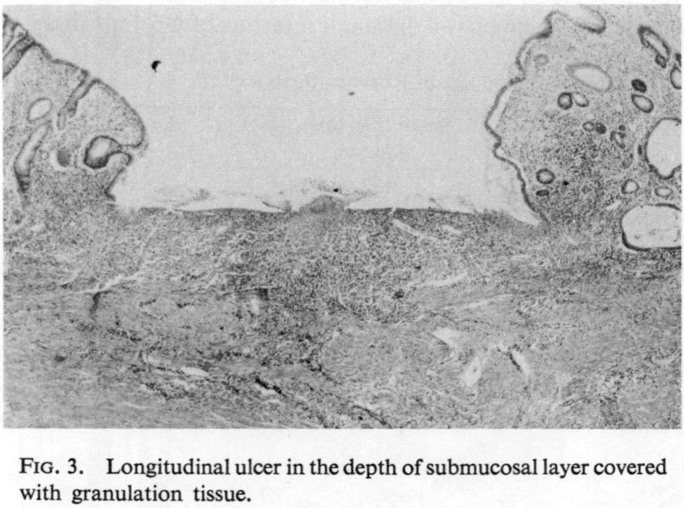

FIG. 3. Longitudinal ulcer in the depth of submucosal layer covered with granulation tissue.

In specimens with longitudinal ulcers unaccompanied by the cobblestone-like feature in the small intestine, the lesion is always limited to the area of mesenteric attachment, and granulomas are usually observed in the surrounding portion of the lesion only (Fig. 4).

EPITHELIOID CELL GRANULOMA

Morphologic features

Sarcoid-like non-caseous granuloma is characteristically found in Crohn's disease, but its occurrence differs from case to case. The occur-

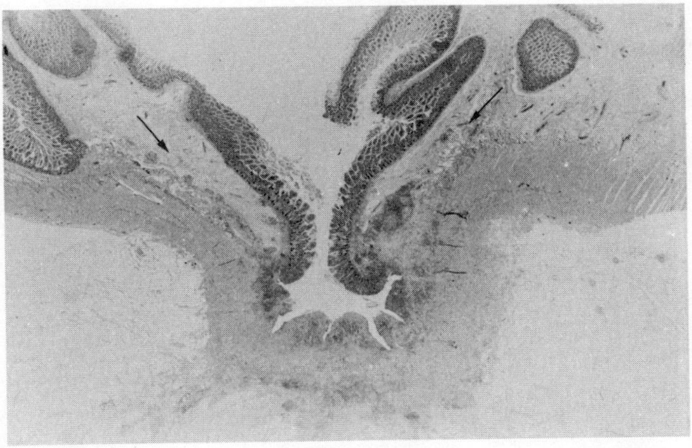

FIG. 4. Longitudinal ulcer. Granulomas in the lymphatics are found between two arrows.

rence of granuloma in biopsy materials is very helpful in making a diagnosis of Crohn's disease. In our series, granulomas were found in 90% of the small intestinal lesions and in over 80% of the large intestinal lesions (Table 4). They were present not only in the lymphatic tissue of the mucosa but in all layers of the intestine. The frequency in each layer and the size of granulomas in histologic specimens were calculated in tuberculous enterocolitis and Crohn's disease. The data were based on the results from the calculation of 159 granulomas of Crohn's disease and 247 of tuberculosis. The size of granulomas was calculated by a diameter. Granulomas in each layer of Crohn's disease were almost the same in size, and those of tuberculosis showed different sizes in different layers, probably due to a confluent tendency of tuberculous granulomas, particularly in the submucosal layer (Fig. 5).

The frequency of granulomas in each layer was not much different in

TABLE 4. Microscopic Findings of Resected Samples

	Small intestinal lesion	Large intestinal lesion
Transmural inflammation	52	45
Granuloma	47	38
Fissures	42	39
Lymphangiectasia	33	25
Total	52	46

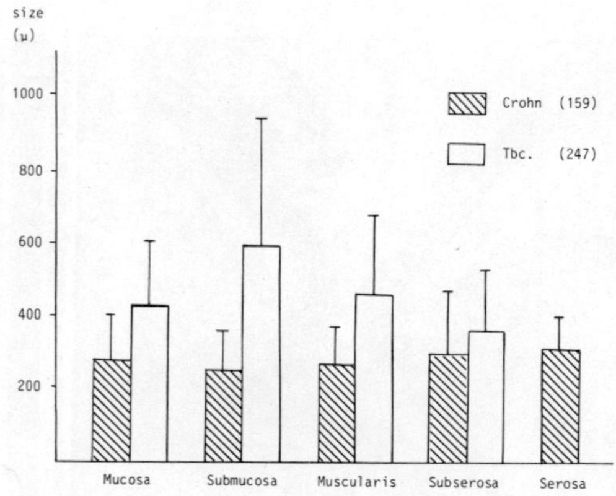

FIG. 5. Size of granulomas in each layer.

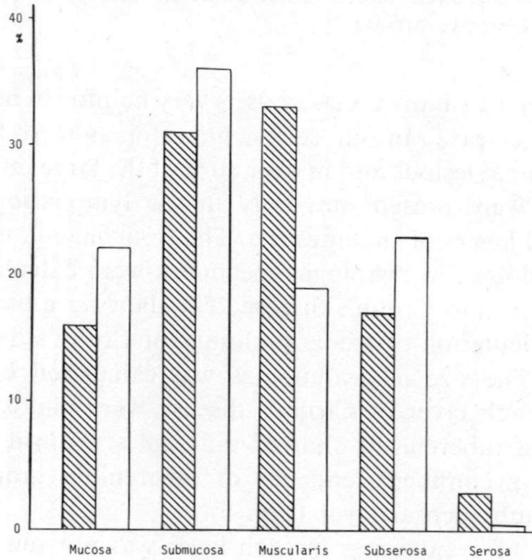

FIG. 6. Frequency of granulomas in each layer.

Crohn's disease and tuberculosis except that it was slightly higher in the muscular layers of Crohn's granuloma (Fig. 6).

Granulomas observed in mucosal and submucosal layers are composed of more numerous epithelioid cells characterized by abundant cytoplasm and oval nuclei with a diffuse chromatin pattern, and these cells show a rather compact arrangement compared with those of the muscular and subserosal layers (Fig. 7).

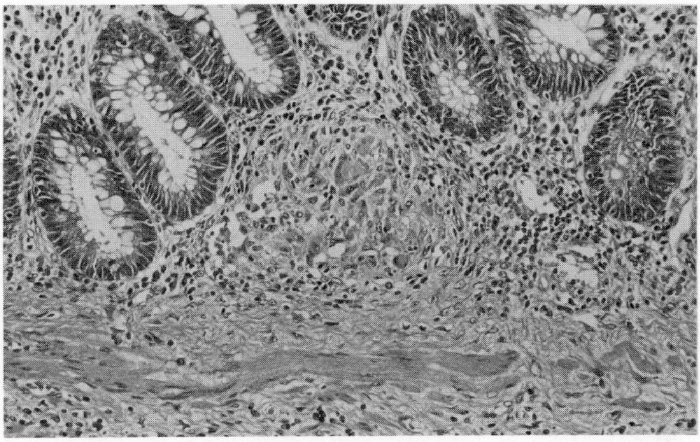

FIG. 7. Granuloma in proper mucosal layer. Epithelioid cells are compactly arranged. Langhans-type giant cell is also present.

Langhans-type giant cells are also present, but their size is not so large in comparison to those of tuberculosis, and they are surrounded by small lymphocytes as usual. Some granulomas found in muscular and subserosal layers and containing foreign body-type giant cells may not be specific for Crohn's disease, but may be formed as a result of the reaction of macrophages to necrotic tissue. Foreign body-type giant cells often phagocytize calcified material. Electronmicroscopic observation reveals that epithelioid cells have abundant cytoplasm in which electron-dense lysosomal granules are usually contained (Fig. 8).

Lysozyme staining by the PAP method shows a marked positive reaction in component cells of granuloma, revealing an intense positive reaction specifically in Langhans giant cells. The cells observed with electronmicroscopy showed parallelly arranged endoplasmic reticula, which were mainly located in the exterior portion of the cell. The cells also characteristically contain a great number of mitochondria-filling cytoplasmic space.

Relation to lymphatics

The localization of the route of granuloma formation was carefully observed in histological slides. The finding that granulomas are rarely found in the perineural lymphatic space of proper muscular layers suggests that granulomas have a close correlation to the lymphatics of the wall (Fig. 9). In the subserosal layer, numerous epithelioid cells were found in the lymphatic lumen with a close correlation to perilymphatic granulomas

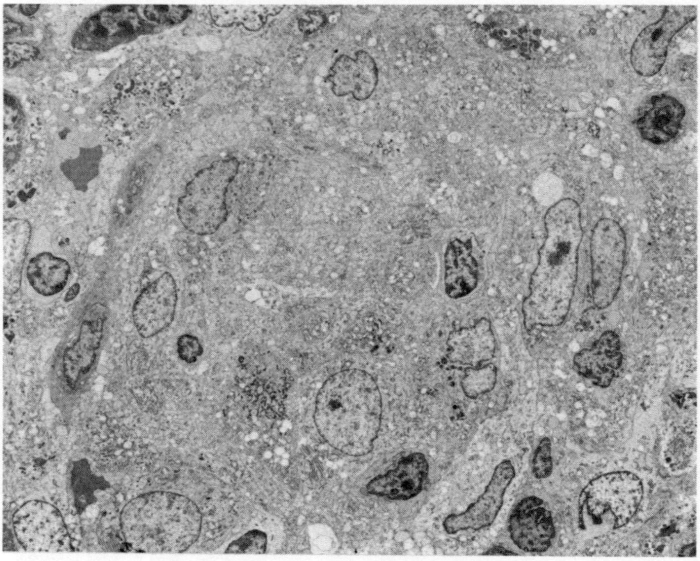

FIG. 8. Epithelioid cells have abundant cytoplasms in which electron-dense granules are present. (× 1,450)

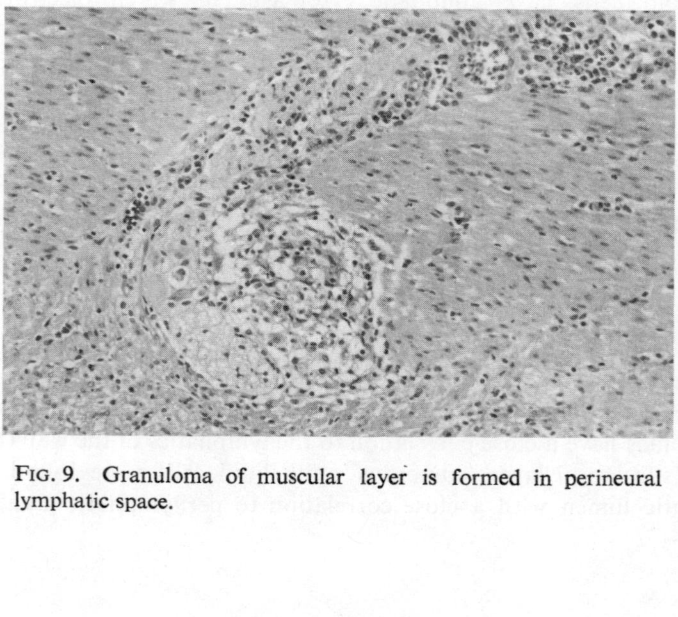

FIG. 9. Granuloma of muscular layer is formed in perineural lymphatic space.

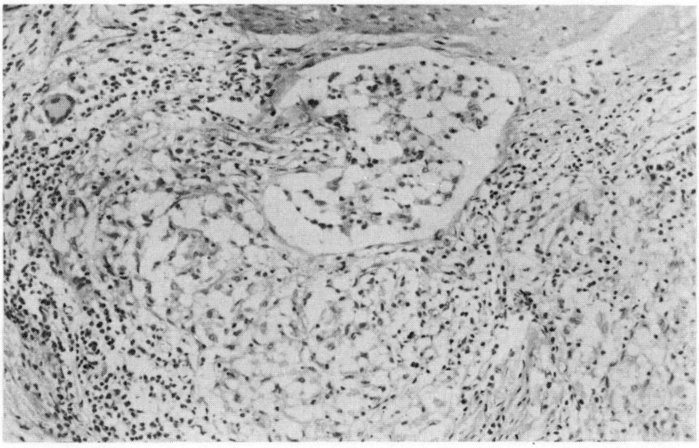

FIG. 10. Granuloma in subserosal layer. Perilymphatic and intraluminal granulomas show a close correlation.

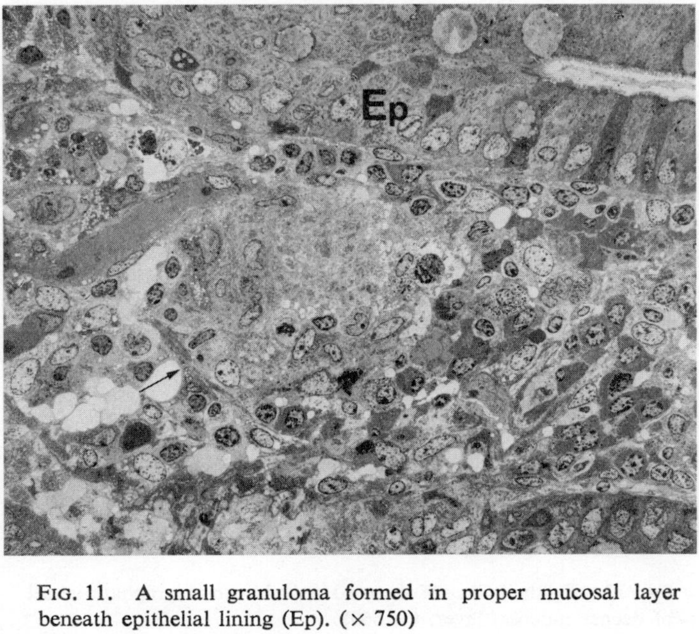

FIG. 11. A small granuloma formed in proper mucosal layer beneath epithelial lining (Ep). (× 750)

(Fig. 10). A similar phenomenon also occurs in peri-intestinal adipose tissue, showing lymphangitis or perilymphangitis, which might finally induce lymphangiectasia and edema in the mucosal and submucosal layers.

Based on these histological observations, an attempt was made to clarify the early phase of granuloma formation in a mucosal layer with ultrastructural observation. In the proper mucosal layer a small granuloma composed of a small number of epithelioid cells is found in the pericapillary area just beneath the mucosal epithelial lining (Fig. 11). This may be considered the first reaction of the histiocytic cells to an unknown agent. At this lesion, the group of a small number of epithelioid cells is surrounded by a thin wall containing endothelial-like cells, but it is still uncertain whether this space corresponds to the lymphatics. However, in slightly deeper areas of the mucosa, the close relation between granuloma and lymphatics becomes clearer. In these areas, the lymphatics are clearly surrounded by a distinct thin wall having irregularly arranged endothelial cells, and they show irregular luminal spaces where a few small lymphocytes are intermingled with large lymphoid cells or epithelioid cells (Figs. 12 and 13). In some areas, epithelioid cells are observed in a small group outside of the lymphatic wall, and therefore it is speculated that epithelioid cells may come out or enter the lumen through gaps in the thin wall.

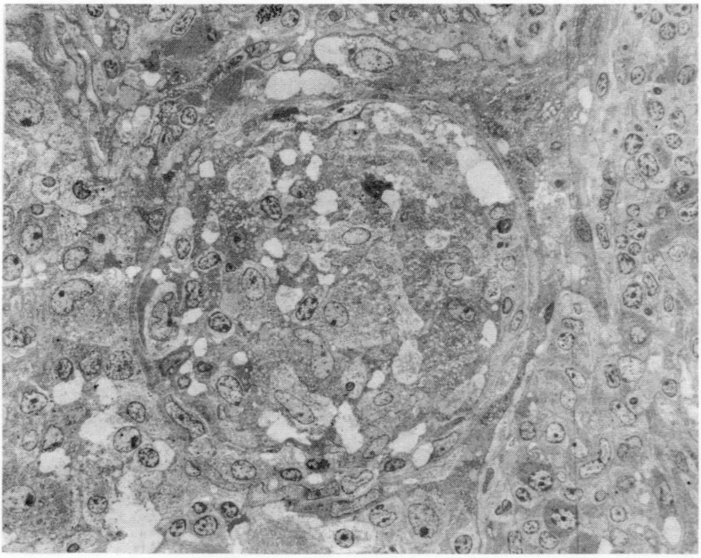

FIG. 12. Epithelioid cells observed in the lumen of lymphatic vessel of deeper mucosal layer. (× 660)

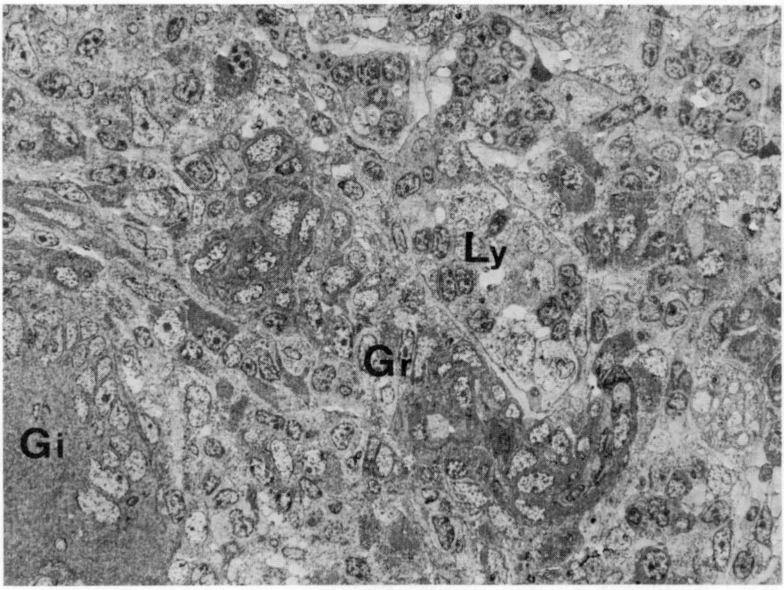

FIG. 13. Irregular-shaped lymphatic vessel containing lymphoid cells (Ly) and macrophages. Granuloma (Gr) is formed in perilymphatic tissue and a part of giant cell (Gi) is also observed. (× 600)

COMMENTS

Inflammatory bowel disease is now considered to be a disorder that has an immunological background for its etiopathogenesis.

Crohn's disease is much more common in Western countries than in Japan, and, therefore, it was rather rare in the past. However, cases have been increasing in number in recent years according to the criteria set forth by the Japanese Research Committee for Crohn's Disease organized under the Japanese Society of Gastroenterology.

Crohn's disease in Japan

The committee has proposed criteria for diagnosis of Crohn's disease and has consulted on cases all over Japan. The data reported here are based on cases collected through these consultations. These cases are considered to be Crohn's disease or allied disorders in each institution, but some of them are recognized as being tuberculous entities. Therefore, they are not based on a nationwide epidemiological population rate. In Western countries, there are two peaks in age distribution, but in our series, there was no such tendency. The difference might be due to the fact that the data of our series were calculated from the time of diagnosis, not from that of onset.

As the most promient feature of Crohn's disease, single longitudinal ulcers exceeded other features and are observed in the small intestine exclusively on the side of mesenteric attachment.

It is well recognized that aphthoid ulcer seems to be an initial morphological change in Crohn's disease. However, it is uncertain whether aphthoid ulcer progresses directly to such a longitudinal ulcer.

Cases in Western countires show the classic feature of cobblestone-like appearance and marked thickening of the wall inducing stenotic symptom.[3] Such cases are rather uncommon among Japanese cases, especially among those with small intestinal lesions. Single longitudinal ulcers might be considered a rather early change in Crohn's disease in Japanese cases.

On the other hand, in cases with large intestinal lesions, the cobblestone-like appearance is the most prominent feature, and longitudinal ulcers are usually irregular and multiple.

From our observations relating to the lymphatics, it seems that the irregularity and multiple occurrences of longitudinal ulcers observed in the colon may have a correspondence to taenia.

Based on these observations, an attempt was made to clarify the correlation between longitudinal ulcers of mesenteric attachment of the small intestine and circulatory disturbance. However, it is difficult to obtain specific evidence for the occurrence of longitudinal ulcers.

Epithelioid cell granuloma—relation to lymphatics

Epithelioid cell granulomas, which are non-caseous and rather small in size compared with those of tuberculosis, are formed in all layers of the intestine and regional lymph nodes.[4]

Among Japanese cases, the presence of epithelioid cell granuloma is highly evaluated in diagnostic determination because its frequency is higher than in Western countries. Some of the epithelioid cells contain many lysosomal granules on electronmicroscopic observation, in accordance with a marked positivity of lysozyme staining.

The finding that epithelioid cell granuloma is formed in the proper mucosal layer beneath the epithelial lining suggests an initial reaction of macrophages to an unknown agent. If the agent reaches through the epithelial barrier, macrophages will react at first to the agent and form epithelioid cell granulomas.

As described before,[5] granuloma has a close relation to intestinal lymphatics, and macrophages may move through lymphatic flow or perilymphatic space to form epithelioid cell proliferation and granuloma. Granulomas formed in or around the lymphatics of the subserosal layer

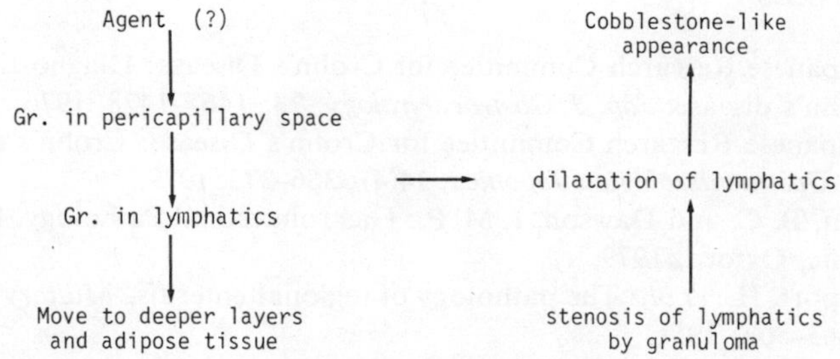

FIG. 14. Interrelation between granuloma and lymphatics.

and peri-intestinal tissue induce narrowing of the lymphatic lumen and subsequent edema in mucosal and submucosal layers, which would correspond to the cobblestone-like appearance on a gross level (Fig. 14).

Recently abnormalities in intestinal lymphatics in Crohn's disease have been indicated by Kovi,[6] who found that the lymphatics do not have gaps in the wall for tissue fluid. This might be involved in the formation of the cobblestone-like feature.

It is suggested that the lymphatics may play an important role in the pathogenesis of Crohn's disease. However, the whole pathological process based on the role of the lymphatics and granuloma formation is still obscure. Further studies including experimental work are necessary.

SUMMARY

Based on the consultation cases of the Japanese Research Committee for Crohn's Disease, the morphological features of the Japanese cases were reported with a special emphasis on longitudinal ulcers of mesenteric attachment in the small intestine.

Next, the role of granuloma and its relation to the lymphatics were discussed from histopathological and electronmicroscopical observations.

Acknowledgments

We are very grateful to the members of the Japanese Research Committee for Crohn's Disease (Chairman: Prof. S. Yamagata). We express our appreciation to Mr. T. Ito and Mr. T. Sakamoto for their technical assistance and to Mrs. M. Hangai for the preparation of the manuscript.

REFERENCES

1. The Japanese Research Committee for Crohn's Disease: Diagnostic criteria of Crohn's disease. *Jap. J. Gastroenterology,* **73**: 1467–1478, 1976.
2. The Japanese Research Committee for Crohn's Disease: Crohn's disease in Japan. *Gastroenterologica Japanica,* **14(4)**: 366–373, 1979.
3. Morson, B. C. and Dawson, I. M. P.: Gastrointestinal Pathology. Blackwell Scientific, Oxford, 1979.
4. Rappaport, H., *et al.*: The pathology of regional enteritis. *Military Surgeon,* **109**: 463–502, 1951.
5. Wakasa, H. and Yamazaki, T.: Pathology of inflammatory bowel disease. *Naika Mook*, **14**: 35–43, 1980 (in Japanese).
6. Kovi, J.: Ultrastructure of intestinal lymphatics in Crohn's disease. *Am. J. Clin. Pathol.,* **76**: 385–394, 1981.

Discussion: Pathology

Robert H. Riddell and Haruki Wakasa, Chairmen

Dr. Farmer: Please comment on the value of mucin staining in the early detection of dysplasia.

Dr. Riddell: Loss of sulfomucin seems to be an indicator of a mucosal abnormality. But the problem is that the mucin-staining technique is not specific enough to help in difficult cases.

Dr. Muto: I am not sure whether this particular technique is helpful or not. This is only a beginning according to Culling's report. I am particularly interested in the abnormal change in mucosa of adenomatosis coli. We have to wait to see what will happen in the future.

Dr. Hill: Dr. Riddell noted that in the U.S. the cumulative risk of carcinoma in colitis of 20 years' duration is 25%. In view of this and in view of the very few cases of cancer in colitis in the Japanese literature (only 5 in colitis of more than 20 years' duration), is it possible that the risk of cancer in colitis in Japan is lower than in the U.S. or the U.K.?

Dr. Muto: I don't know, because we have such limited experience that we cannot draw any final conclusion. We just started to notice the high risk of carcinoma in ulcerative colitis.

Dr. Riddell: I think it's worth putting that into perspective, because even in Western countries, carcinoma complicating inflammatory bowel disease still accounts for at best 1% of all large bowel carcinomas. These are rare tumors even in major medical centers, so we see them very infrequently. At the University of Chicago, we see at most two a year.

Dr. Farmer: What is the proximity of dysplasia to a cancer? In other words, are we more likely to find dysplasia near the lesion?

Dr. Riddell: We find dysplasia around three fourths of our carcinomas. If you find endoscopic lesions, the question is whether they are inflammatory polyps or dysplasia-associated masses. And biopsy, usually not just from the lesions, reveals dysplasia in the surrounding mucosa. It is important to distinguish between targeted biopsies, where the endoscopy sees the lesion, and other biopsies. In our experience the frequency of dysplasia is much less in patients in whom an endoscopic abnormality is not identified. We also see a degree of focality to the dysplasia.

Dr. Kino: I have a little experience with dysplasia in ulcerative colitis, and it is difficult to make a correct diagnosis from biopsy material. I would like to ask if the atypia is the same as in mild atypia in adenoma, particularly from the cytological standpoint.

Dr. Riddell: Yes. We have chosen the term dysplasia rather than atypia. Atypia is used in a variety of different circumstances; for instance, people talk about regenerative atypia or adenomatous atypia. We think that dysplasia has been less used than atypia. The important thing is that we only use the term "dysplasia" in cases of a neoplastic nature.

Dr. Muto: What staging system are you using for dysplasia in ulcerative colitis? Is it the same as the grading system for ordinary adenomas?

Dr. Riddell: It is exactly the same as what you are calling low-grade or mild dysplasia in your paper. We call it low-grade dysplasia. Moderate and severe dysplasia and carcinoma *in situ* are included with high-grade dysplasia.

Dr. Muto: I had a feeling that your severe dysplasia in ulcerative colitis is rather similar to moderate dysplasia in ordinary adenomas.

Dr. Riddell: This is because moderate dysplasia, severe dysplasia, and carcinoma *in situ* are high-grade dysplasias. You are absolutely right. When you state that you call something "moderate dysplasia" in an adenoma, we include it with high-grade dysplasia as the management is the same. We didn't need to separate it.

Dr. Muto: I suppose that a patient with a longstanding colitis may have a risk of ordinary carcinoma not related to ulcerative colitis. How could you differentiate the two types? Of 100 cases with longstanding ulcerative colitis, how many cases would be coincidental occurrence?

Dr. Riddell: I am not sure. I think a patient who is 60 and has had extensive colitis for 20 years might get carcinoma anyway. There is no doubt that we do see typical-appearing large bowel carcinoma in patients with ulcerative colitis, but I can't help thinking that the colitis may have something to do with the origination of the tumors. There is no clear answer to your question.

Dr. Muto: I have had several examples which are almost always rather ordinary-looking carcinomas which are localized and ulcerating, with a history of longstanding ulcerative colitis which is rather quiescent. There is a natural inclination to publish this as a carcinoma complicating an ulcerating colitis, but I am rather reluctant to do so.

Dr. Riddell: I think you may occasionally get a typical large bowel carcinoma incidentally in a patient with typical colitis over a long period of time. There is no one who says that carcinoma in ulcerative colitis cannot look like usual large bowel carcinoma; it is impossible to know if they were really related.

Dr. Muto: But if you find a dysplastic field surrounding the carcinoma, then you call it carcinoma in colitis.

Dr. Riddell: Yes, I agree.

Dr. Watanabe: Dr. Riddell, we have a patient who has had ulcerative colitis for the past 20 years. We conducted colostomy on the patient. In following up the carcinogenecity, we are planning to do exfoliative cytology. Do you think that this technique is valuable for the detection of carcinomas?

Dr. Riddell: We have tried cytology by a variety of different techniques. However, whatever method is used, we have a low yield. There has always been some difficulty in distinguishing regenerating lesions from neoplastic lesions. So we have now abandoned cytology as a part of routine follow-up for colitis.

Dr. Kelly: What is the incidence of high-grade dysplasia in ulcerative colitis resected from cancer?

Dr. Riddell: We are now starting a study in Chicago, because in the literature there are various figures going up to 90%. We re-examined in double-blind fashion all the colitis cases having cancer using age-matched controls. Then, it came to 73%. This is actually lower than figures in the literature. I think a part of the explanation is that large carcinomas may destroy the evidence of dysplasia that was previously present in the large bowel.

Dr. Shiratori: Dr. Riddell, you showed slides of dysplasia lying over carcinoma. I would like to know the relationship between superficial dysplasia and carcinoma.

Dr. Riddell: I think there is little doubt that there is a direct relationship between the degree of dysplasia and underlying carcinoma. It is certain that the higher the grade of dysplasia, the greater the risk. It is fairly difficult to document that. But the point that I was trying to bring out was that you don't need high-grade dysplasia for infiltrating carcinoma. Once you have dysplastic change or adenomatous change to a mild degree, it can occasionally give rise to direct infiltrating carcinomas. And I think even in Dr. Muto's adenoma study about one third of the carcinomas were described as arising from a mild dysplasia.

Dr. Shiratori: I would like to know if carcinoma occurs directly from a mild dysplastic lesion or from another portion with a more severe lesion.

Dr. Riddell: Mild dysplasia, or low-grade dysplasia, by itself can give rise to carcinoma. But your second point is also true. A biopsy is a very small piece of mucosa. Perhaps you can see low-grade dysplasia in one part of the bowel, but sometimes high-grade dysplasia is elsewhere in the bowel. Thus, this is a big sampling problem between endoscopy and biopsy. But I still maintain that you don't need high-grade dysplasia to get invasive carcinoma.

Dr. Muto: I would like to know the policy in foreign countries for patients having ulcerative colitis with mild to moderate dysplasia.

Dr. Jewell: The policy in Oxford is to examine every patient who has had the disease for 10 years by annual colonoscopy. That is a very vigorous program, and we are more and more examining even left-sided colitis on an annual basis.

Dr. Kelly: Mayo's policy is very similar. We advise yearly examination by colonoscopy and biopsy after 10 years of ulcerative colitis.

Dr. Riddell: What do we do with the patient with left-sided colitis? Is the risk raised in left-sided colitis?

Dr. Farmer: We developed a study in 1975 to find the patients at high risk for developing carcinoma from ulcerative colitis. Our policy is something different from those of Dr. Kelly and Dr. Jewell. We subdivided our patients into diagnostic colonoscopy and surveillance colonoscopy. These are people who have had ulcerative colitis of the total colon for 10 years, and that's the only reason for colonoscopy. The diagnostic colonoscopy is done to explain the adenoma by X-ray or clinical finding; and we have sorted out this surveillance group from the diagnostic group. In the patients in the surveillance group, we have found that we have a large number of patients, some 200 people, whose onset of ulcerative colitis is less than 15 years ago, and they are now 25 or 30 years old, so that complaint has become a significant factor as well. For all these reasons plus our own experiences since 1975, we recommend surveillance colonoscopy for total ulcerative colitis starting after 10 years every 2 years. When we find one of the indeterminate or other lesions required by Dr. Riddell who has called for "short-term follow-up," then we follow up those patients in a different category. We also follow the diagnostic colonoscopy patients in a different way. As far as left-sided colitis patients are concerned, the retrospective studies from both St. Marks and Mt. Sinai have determined extensive colitis primarily by single enema. With the modern techniques of double-contrast enema and colonoscopy, I think the ability to define left-sided colitis is much better. We don't know exactly what the prognosis is. I think that left-sided colitis patients have a high risk of cancer compared with the general population in the U.S.

Dr. Riddell: What do you think about the problem of Crohn's disease and carcinoma?

Dr. Farmer: As far as Crohn's disease is concerned, what you said is absolutely correct and goes along with our experience. However, you mentioned the point that large bowel cancers in ulcerative colitis constitute only 1% of the large bowel cancer seen in the U.S., and it must be 0.01% for patients with Crohn's disease.

Dr. Jegelman: Do yearly negative sequential biopsies for dysplasia in ulcerative colitis make an eventual positive biopsy more significant?

Dr. Riddell: We start to follow up after 7 years, but that's pretty arbitrary, and I usually do not start breathing easily with these patients until I have seen three series of colonoscopy biopsy that are negative, because of the chance of missing small dysplastic lesions. I think it is unlikely that the patient has dysplasia or carcinoma in the bowel that we haven't found. Subsequent biopsy really confirms your opinion. We have several patients who have developed dysplasia and are following them. Most of them seem not to want a colostomy, so we are able to follow them. Dysplasia seems to be stable and relatively unchanged. If you get changing biopsies especially to high-grade dysplasia, patients should have a colectomy at that stage.

Dr. Matsueda: Is there any relationship between the incidence of carcinoma and immunosuppressive treatments such as steroid and azathiopurine?

Dr. Farmer: Our studies on this have been retrospective. We have found no relationship of developing cancer with previous therapy, complications, type of disease, chronicity, early onset, and so on. The only thing we have found has been extent and duration, i.e., 10 years or so. In recent years, we have found that people who have quiescent disease have a higher risk of developing cancer than those whose disease is active.

Dr. Riddell: I am particularly interested in the age distribution that Dr. Wakasa showed in Crohn's disease because the peak is in the third decade and decreases with age. Certainly, in the U.S. we see a biphasic pattern. There is a definite peak in the sixth and seventh decades, and the disease we see in older people seems to be quite severe.

Dr. Wakasa: This distribution is based on consultation cases only. Doctors throughout the country refer atypical or suspicious cases for Crohn's disease.

Dr. Watanabe: These cases have been observed by the Japanese Research

Committee, and in each case we have made the diagnosis of Crohn's disease. However, age is not really the age of onset; it is the time of diagnosis. The number is limited, so if we have more cases, we may see a biphasic appearance.

Dr. Kimura: From our data obtained through a questionnaire to hospitals, there is a small peak in the sixth decade.

Dr. Riddell: Does the disease of older people tend to be severe?

Dr. Kimura: I don't know. The data are a simple collection from different hospitals.

Dr. Riddell: I was also very interested in gross examples of Crohn's disease with single longitudinal ulcers in the ileum. Could any of these be tuberculosis? Do you see tuberculosis in the large bowel?

Dr. Farmer: How do you differentiate between Crohn's disease and tuberculosis? My understanding of tuberculosis is that it is more common in the ileocecal region and that diffuse tuberculosis involving the large intestine is not a particularly common entity even in the tuberculosis seen. I wonder if in the U.S. we are missing some tuberculosis because we hardly ever see it; how do you differentiate tuberculosis from Crohn's disease?

Dr. Wakasa: In this series, we are looking at endoscopical findings and biopsy—particularly the presence of non-caseous granuloma and sometimes antitherapeutic response. We try to get all the information and then differentiate them.

Dr. Yao: We see tuberculosis quite frequently in Japan. Large intestinal lesions must be looked at to differentiate between tuberculosis and Crohn's disease. In Japan, we carry out a double-contrast barium enema because we have a very high-level technique. At first, we use endoscopy and observe many biopsies from the lesions. We do cultures from the biopsy material, whether tuberculosis or Crohn's disease. As far as the small intestine is concerned, it is rather easy to check symmetry or asymmetry by X-ray. If we still have doubts about tuberculosis, we follow the course of the cases with treatment for tuberculosis.

Dr. Riddell: In Dr. Wakasa's presentation of Crohn's disease, the distribution of the lesions was 25% in the small bowel, 25% in the large bowel, and 50% in both. Can you give some idea in tuberculosis as to how many are just small bowel or large bowel and how many are small and large bowel that involve the cecum? And how many are large bowel away from the ileocecal region?

Dr. Yao: I don't have exact accurate data. I think, however, that the ileocecal region is involved in about 90% of tuberculosis cases.

About 20% of cases are small bowel alone, about 20% large bowel alone, and others are of both small and large bowel.

Dr. Matsueda: Regarding tuberculosis from a practical point of view, we do have the problem that cultures take several months to produce results. What shall we do for treatment meanwhile? Another thing is that, as Dr. Wakasa has demonstrated, caseating necrosis could be a landmark for diagnosis. Actinomycosis may induce caseating necrosis. Is it similar?

Dr. Wakasa: Actinomycosis makes abscess with numerous granulocytic infiltrations and drusen (sulfur granules representing colonies of organisms).

Dr. Matsueda: There is some disagreement between Japanese gastroenterologists and overseas experts. I think it is necessary to develop international criteria for dealing with the disease. If only culture, inoculation, or immunofluorescence can give us definite results, it is very difficult for a gastroenterologist to deal with.

Dr. Riddell: Dr. Wakasa pointed out confluent granuloma with occasional caseous necrosis in tuberculosis. How often do you see it in Crohn's disease?

Dr. Wakasa: I don't have any confluent granuloma.

Dr. Watanabe: With regard to the differentiation between Crohn's disease and tuberculosis, I'd like to make an additional comment. In 1975, we started the Research Committee for Crohn's Disease, but at that time we had many tuberculosis cases which were mistakenly brought to the committee as Crohn's disease. After several years' experience, we are now more confident, and the majority of cases can be differentiated. I suppose we made some mistakes previously. In tuberculosis, we find small granulomas in the submucosal layer. In Crohn's disease, the mucosal gland seems to appear normal, but in tuberculosis the mucosa shows regenerative glands. We think even biopsy gives quite accurate information.

Dr. Wakasa: Yesterday Dr. Riddell commented on Crohn's disease, and I think we are using slightly narrowing criteria—in other words, stricter ones. In some cases, we are still not able to define it to be Crohn's disease, but in the future, we should continue to get more detailed information from follow-up patients and make more accurate diagnoses.

IV. INCIDENCE

Epidemiological Study on the Incidence of Idiopathic Proctocolitis in Japan
——An Enquête Study

Toshiyoshi Utsunomiya, Hisashi Shinohara, Tetsuji Kitahara, Koichi Suzuki, and Akira Yokota

Since 1973 when the Study Group for Idiopathic Proctocolitis (a disease designated by the Ministry of Health and Welfare) was formed based on the pioneering studies of Inada and Matsunaga, many new studies have been conducted. As members of this study group, we were assigned the task of conducting an epidemiological study and 10 years have now passed since we began this study on a national scale. During this 10-year period, both the overall disease concept of and diagnostic criteria for idiopathic proctocolitis have been uniformly implemented throughout the country, and thus epidemiological statistics based on our data have attained a high confidence level. In this paper we report on the results of our study concerning the incidence of idiopathic proctocolitis in Japan based on data obtained with the cooperation of various hospitals throughout Japan.

METHODS AND MATERIALS

This study was conducted by post once each year to all general hospitals in Japan.

The following information was requested in regard to new unregistered patients: name, sex, birth date, address, geographical location of occurrence, date of onset, extent of lesion(s), therapy, prognosis, etc. Follow-up information on previously registered patients included clinical course, therapy, and prognosis during each year.

Participating hospitals in this study included 85 hospitals in Hokkaido, 121 in Tohoku, 244 in the Kanto region, 199 in Chubu, 170 in Kinki, 73 in Chugoku, 58 in Shikoku, and 140 in Kyushu for a total of 1,090 hospitals.

A grand total of 5,251 patients were registered including 157 patients who were found during follow-up studies to suffer from other inflammatory bowel diseases and were then excluded; thus a total of 5,094

Division of Gastroenterology, National Okura Hospital, Tokyo, Japam patients with idiopathic proctocolitis were registered and used as subjects in this study.

The classification based on extent of lesion followed Japanese conventions. Thus lesions only in the rectum were designated as proctitis (897 cases), and lesions which had spread to the colon, both to left-sided colitis and the total colitis, were commonly termed colitis (3,952 cases). During follow-up studies on patients diagnosed as having either right-sided or segmental colitis, since these diagnoses were in many cases revised to indicate diagnoses of other inflammatory bowel diseases, we assigned them a "special type" classification (160 cases).

We also treated separately those cases in which the details of lesion extent were not noted on the Study Form (85 cases). Besides these cases, we excluded from the 4,849 cases with proctitis or colitis those in which the onset occurred before 1954 or after 1981 (31 cases and 243 cases, respectively). Thus the number of patients used in the current study included 842 cases with proctitis and 3,733 cases with colitis for a total of 4,575 cases.

RESULTS

Annual incidence rate of idiopathic proctocolitis

The annual incidence rate from 1955 over a period of years for idiopathic proctocolitis is as follows. From 1955 until 1962 there were 15 to 20 new patients per year, and the annual incidence rate was about 0.02 per 100,000 persons. (All incidence rates indicated below are based on per 100,000 of population.) In 1965 there were 75 patients (0.074), in 1970 this number increased to 246 patients (0.222), and reached its peak in 1974 with 502 patients (0.429); then in 1975 it was 402 patients (0.352), it decreased slightly in 1980 with 301 patients (0.246), and then continued at this same level.

Annual incidence rate by extent of lesion

The number of colitis patients tended to show a relatively gradual increase from 1955 to 1965. In 1965 there were 63 patients (0.064), by 1970 the number had increased to 191 patients (0.184), it reached its peak in 1974 with 386 patients (0.349), and then slowly declined after 1975 to 1980 when it became 230 patients (0.257). Thereafter the number remained at this level. Up until 1969, proctitis showed an extremely gradual increase, and in 1970 there were 39 patients (0.038). This had increased to 85 patients (0.076) by 1975, reached its peak of 96 patients (0.085) in 1976, and thereafter showed a gradual tendency to decline. Thus colitis occurs at a much higher rate than proctitis, but this may be attributable to the fact that only during the last several years has proctitis been placed in the category of idiopathic proctocolitis and positively reported here in Japan.

Annual incidence rate by sex

Among males there were 10 patients in 1955 (0.025), 34 patients in 1965 (0.07), 110 patients in 1970 (0.216), 214 patients in 1974 (0.394) when it reached its peak, 145 patients in 1977 (0.258), and 134 patients in 1980 (0.232). Among females there were 14 patients in 1955 (0.02), 39 patients in 1965 (0.07), 120 patients in 1970 (0.277), 261 patients in 1974 (0.465) when it reached its peak (similar to the males), 169 patients in 1977 (0.292), and 154 patients in 1980 (0.259) when, like the males, it remained at this same level thereafter.

Average incidence rate by geographic area

Japan was divided into six geographical regions and the mean incidence rate in each region during the last ten years was studied. It was found that in the Hokkaido–Tohoku region the rate was 0.284, in the Kanto region it was 0.353, in Chubu it was 0.26, in Kinki 0.301, in Chugoku–Shikoku 0.242, and in Kyushu 0.311. Thus the incidence rates in three regions, namely Kanto, Kinki, and Kyushu, were higher than those in the other three regions.

If we look at the different rates for colitis and proctitis, the colitis incidence rate was 0.251 in the Kanto region, 0.266 in Kinki, and 0.269 (the highest) in Kyushu. The proctitis rate was highest in the Kanto region at 0.101 and much lower in the other five regions. If we look at the incidence rate based on region, colitis tends to occur more frequently in densely populated areas, and proctitis tends to occur more frequently in northern Japan.

Age distribution at onset

Among these 4,575 patients, the mean annual incidence rate for each age group (per 5 years of age) during the last 15 years is as follows. The highest rate was 0.469 in the 20 to 24-year-old group, which was followed by the 25–29, 30–34, and 15–19 age groups. After 35, the incidence rate tended to decline with increasing age but increased slightly in the 55–59 age group showing a second peak.

Age distribution at onset by extent of lesion

The mean incidence rate of colitis by age was highest in the 20–24 age group followed by the 15–19, and 25–29 age groups. This rate tended to decline with increasing age after 30 but increased slightly in the 60–64 age group showing a second peak.

There was no special age group prone to develop proctitis, and the proctitis incidence rate remained at about the same rate from the age of 20 to 49 showing a gently rolling curve.

Age distribution at onset by sex

Among males, the mean incidence rate by age was highest in the 20–24 age group, followed by the 15–19 age group. After 25 the rate tended to decline with increasing age but reached a second peak in the 60–64 age group. Among females, the incidence rate was highest in the 20–24 age group, followed by the 25–29 age group and tended to decline with increasing age after 30 but increased slightly in both the 40–44 and 55–59 age groups showing a second and third peak. Thus the incidence rate in the 15–19 age group was relatively high among males, but there were slight aberrations in the age at onset among females; the decrease in the incidence rate with increasing age was more gradual among females than males.

Increasing tendency of colitis onset years in younger age groups

We studied the mean incidence rate for each 5-year period from 1966 to 1980 for each age group.

During the initial period from 1966 to 1970 the mean incidence rate by age showed a sharp increase among patients younger than 20, remained the same for patients ranging in age from 20 to 39, and tended to show a slight decline for patients older than 40.

During the intermediate period from 1971 to 1975, a sharp increase was observed in the 15–19 age group, reaching a peak in the 20–24 age group and declining after the age of 25 but showing a second peak in the 55–59 age group.

In the final period from 1976 to 1980, similar to the intermediate period, there was a sharp increase in the 15–19 age group, reaching a peak in the 20–24 age group, and thereafter declining but showing a second and third peak in the 40–44 and 60–64 age groups. If we compare these three curves, it is clear that the incidence rate increased in the 15–19 and 20–24 age groups during the intermediate and final periods. This tendency for colitis to occur with increasing frequency in the younger age groups becomes even more evident if we calculate the percentage of each age group during the initial, intermediate, and final periods and place them on a graph.

A comparison of the annual increase in the daily intake of animal foodstuffs and in the idiopathic proctocolitis incidence rate

We compared the daily intake of animal foodstuffs per person and the annual incidence rate of idiopathic proctocolitis during the last 25 years in Japan. It became apparent that among animal foodstuffs the intake of meat, milk, and dairy products increased parallel to the increase in the incidence rate of idiopathic proctocolitis. The daily intake of meat per person reached its peak in 1973, thereafter declined slightly, and then remained at the same level. The incidence rate of idiopathic proctocolitis reached its peak in 1974, thereafter declined slightly, and then remained at the same level. Thus the curves for both animal foodstuffs intake and incidence of idiopathic proctocolitis show very similar patterns.

CONCLUSION

We conducted a study on the incidence rate of idiopathic proctocolitis in Japan during the period from 1955 to 1980.

1) The incidence of idiopathic proctocolitis tended to increase relatively slowly during the 10-year period from 1955 to 1964, then it showed a sharp increase from 1965 to 1974, and tended to decline slightly from 1975 after reaching its peak in 1974. Thereafter it remained at the same level.

2) The annual incidence rate was found to vary between proctitis and colitis.

3) The incidence rate varies with geographical region, and it was observed that the proctitis rate tended to be higher in northern Japan whereas the colitis rate was higher in densely populated areas.

4) The incidence rate varied with age, and the age of prevalence for proctitis differed from that for colitis.

5) The age at onset of proctocolitis in females tended to be delayed by about 5 years in comparison with the age at onset in males.

6) In comparing the age distribution for each 5-year period, it was found that during the last 10 years proctocolitis tended to occur with increasing frequency in the younger age groups.

7) The per capita daily intake of such animal foodstuffs as meat, milk, and dairy products has undergone a sharp increase since 1965 and the incidence rate of idiopathic proctocolitis has shown an analogous pattern.

Based on these facts, we intend to pursue our studies by investigating the mutual correlation between the idiopathic proctocolitis incidence rate and changes in the living environment, with special emphasis on changes in food intake patterns.

Incidence of Crohn's Disease in Japan

Akira Kimura and Tsutomu Sasagawa

SUMMARY

As a result of two nationwide epidemiological studies done in 1975–1976 and 1980–1981 by post, a respective 256 and 242 cases of Crohn's disease with histological confirmation were discovered in Japan. During the past 14 years the number of cases has increased year by year, although that may be a result of improvements in the ability to detect Crohn's disease. The clinical evidence is somewhat different from that of European countries. Sixty-four percent of the cases are male; the peak of onset occurs in the third decade of life; and the prevalence among males is especially high in this decade. A tendency of the onset age to shift to younger generations was seen. We concluded that the incidence ranges between 0.25 and 0.07 per 100,000 population per annum in Japan, which is less than one-tenth that for European whites.

In 1972, Dr. Kyle mentioned in his monograph that it would be surprising if Crohn's disease did not occur in Japan with its rapidly rising standard of living and industrialization.[1] Very few others have mentioned the problems of incidence and prevalence of Crohn's disease in Japan. This paper might provide answers for some of the questions that exist.

This work was planned and undertaken by a research committee sponsored by the Ministry of Health and Welfare of Japan in 1975–1976 and 1980–1981. Sasagawa and Kimura were members of that committee and were responsible for the selection and arrangement of the data.

This is the first and only epidemiological research on Crohn's disease with histopathological confirmation in Japan. It also represents the actual situation and clinical evidence rather than the simple gathering of arbitrary diagnosed cases characteristic of former Japanese papers.

Division of Gastroenterology, Niigata Municipal Hospital, Niigata, Japan

MATERIALS AND METHODS

Before the start of actual research, we discussed and decided on the clinical criteria for the estimation of reported cases. Fundamentally our clinical criteria were based on the 1973 conception of CIOMS of WHO (Table 1).

TABLE 1. Diagnostic Criteria of Crohn's Disease Employed by the Research Committee

1) Skipped or segmental affection
2) Cobblestone appearance or longitudinal ulceration
3) Transmural inflammatory change of intestine
4) Non-caseatic epithelioid cell granuloma
5) Fissuring or fistula formation
6) Anorectal lesion (ulceration or atypical fistulation)

1) + 2) + 3) = suspected case
1) + 2) + 3) + 4) or 5) or 6) = definite case
4) + 1) + 2)
4) + 2) + 3) } = definite case
4) + 1) + 3)

Elimination of intestinal tuberculosis, ulcerative colitis, ischemic colitis, radiation colitis, intestinal Behçet's disease, simple ulcer of intestine, acute terminal ileitis, and the so-called "non-specific multiple ulcers of the small intestine" is necessary.

Given the present medical environment and general level of medicine in Japan, we had to carefully eliminate the confusion of Crohn's disease with intestinal tuberculosis and acute terminal ileitis that currently exists. Table 2

TABLE 2. Year of Diagnosed Cases (Summary of First and Second Studies)

	Male	Female	Total
–1955	19	4	23
1966	2	0	2
1967	4	4	8
1968	8	6	14
1969	10	4	14
1970	6	3	9
1971	8	12	20
1972	17	10	27
1973	18	12	30
1974	32	26	58
1975	53	22	75
1976	36	14	50
1977	32	16	48
1978	30	21	51
1979	45	24	69

shows the rate of definitely diagnosed cases among reported cases. In our study the rate is 60% in the first study and 87% in the second study (Table 3).

The outline of our study is shown in Table 3. Twice during the first year we sent out a preliminary examination sheet by post asking about the presence of Crohn's disease patients to a group of 1,379 and a group of 1,571 well-equipped and -administered hospitals throughout Japan, all of which have more than 150 beds for general use. Within six months, 556 hospitals of the 1,379 and 564 of the 1,571 hospitals had replied. The rates of reply were 40% and 36%, respectively. Totals of 615 and 501 clinically diagnosed cases were reported from the hospitals that replied.

TABLE 3. Study Outline

	First study (1975–1976)	Second study (1980–1981)
Preliminary research:		
No. of hospitals sent initial questionnaire	1,379	1,571
No. of replying hospitals	556 (40%)	564 (36%)
No. of reported cases	615	501
Final research:		
No. of closer research sheets sent to hospitals	615	501
No. of replies	424 (69%)	278 (55%)
No. of CD cases estimated as accurately diagnosed	256 (60%)	242 (87%)

The second year we tried to make a closer examination of the reported cases. Our requests included histological evidence, year diagnosed, age of onset, residence, occupation, past and family history, treatments and their effect, radiological and endoscopic findings, diagnostic value, prognosis, recovery of social activity, and so on, of every case.

Within six months, 424 of 615 and 278 of 501 of the more detailed questionnaires were returned. Finally 256 and 242 cases were identified as Crohn's disease, with histological cofirmation based on the diagnostic criteria mentioned above.

RESULTS

During the past 14 years, the number of reported cases has increased year by year. Before 1965, only 23 cases had been reported according to our research. During the next ten years, the reported cases increased gradually, and during the five years between 1975 and 1979, 232 cases were reported to our study (Fig. 1, Table 3). From our evaluation, the major part of that may depend on an improvement in Japanese doctors' ability to detect Crohn's disease.

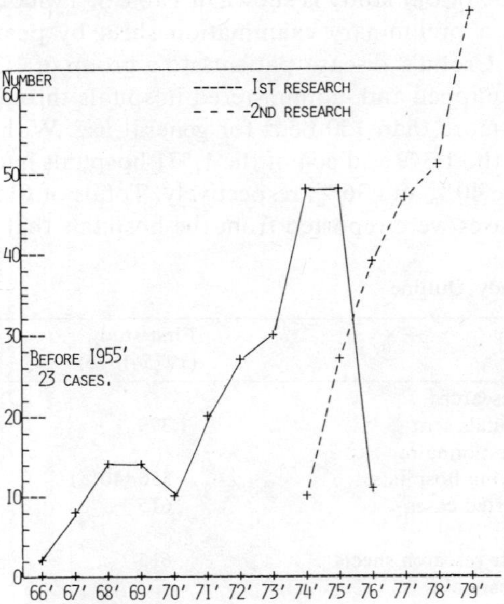

FIG. 1 Year of diagnosis in reported cases.

The decade of onset is shown in Table 4 and Fig. 2 for both males and females. Of the 498 cases, 320 (64%) are male, and in contrast to reports from Western countries, a prominent increase in males is seen in the third decade of life. We cannot find any particular reason to explain this

TABLE 4. Age of Onset

Age	First study		Second study		Total
	Male	Female	Male	Female	
0–9	3	2	1	0	6
10–19	27	17	39	22	105
20–29	71	16	43	22	152
30–39	24	17	26	7	74
40–49	14	20	16	4	54
50–59	11	7	8	8	34
60–69	7	11	3	6	27
70–	5	2	4	3	14
Unknown	5	2	16	14	37
Total	164	92	156	86	498

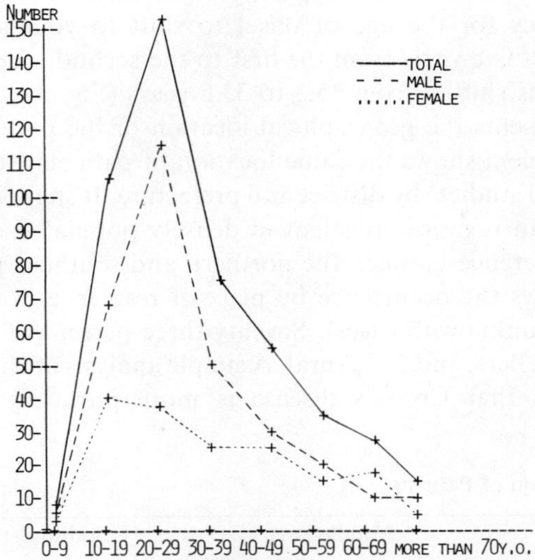

FIG. 2. Age of onset in 461 cases of Crohn's disease in Japan.

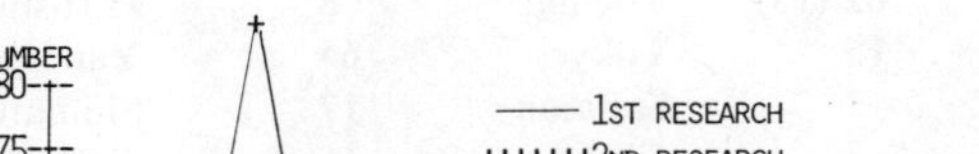

FIG. 3. Shift to a younger age of onset.

phenomenon. As noted in the reports from Western countries, there has been a tendency for the age of onset to shift to younger generations. During the past five years from the first to the second study, the average age of onset has shifted from 35.3 to 33.8 years (Fig. 3).

Figure 4 presents the geographical location of the patients of the first study, and Table 5 shows the same location of patients (summing up the first and second studies) by district and prefecture. It suggests that Crohn's disease in Japan is more prevalent in densely populated areas, and that there is no difference between the northern and southern parts.

Table 6 shows the occurrence by place of residence in the two studies (exclusive of "unknown" cases). Seventy-three percent of reported cases were urban dwellers, and 27% rural. A simple analysis of this data leads to the conclusion that Crohn's disease is more prevalent among urban

TABLE 5. Location of Patients

Northern part	No. of cases (%)	Middle part	No. of cases (%)	Southwest part	No. of cases (%)
Hokkaido district	17 (3)	Kanto district	139 (28)	Chugoku district	30 (6)
Hokkaido	17	Ibaragi	7	Okayama	5
Tohoku district	62 (13)	Tochigi	8	Hiroshima	20
Aomori	15	Tokyo	65	Yamaguchi	4
Iwate	3	Saitama	17	Shimane	0
Akita	3	Chiba	18	Tottori	1
Miyagi	17	Kanagawa	14	Shikoku district	23 (5)
Yamagata	9	Gunma	10	Kagawa	5
Fukushima	15	Hokuriku district	29 (6)	Tokushima	6
		Niigata	16	Kochi	3
		Toyama	6	Ehime	9
		Ishikawa	6	Kyushu district	64 (13)
		Fukui	1	Oita	5
		Chubu district	46 (9)	Fukuoka	28
		Nagano	4	Saga	2
		Yamanashi	1	Nagasaki	12
		Shizuoka	6	Kumamoto	9
		Aichi	23	Miyazaki	8
		Gifu	12	Kagoshima	0
		Kinki district	81 (16)	Okinawa	0 (0)
		Shiga	5	Okinawa	0
		Mie	5		
		Nara	5		
		Kyoto	8		
		Osaka	34		
		Hyogo	14		
		Wakayama	10		
Total	79 (16)	Total	295 (60)	Total	117 (24)

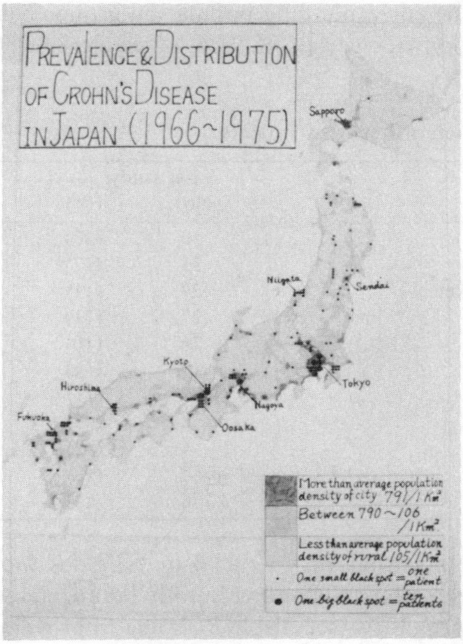

FIG. 4. Prevalence and distribution of Crohn's disease in Japan, 1966–75.

TABLE 6. Occurrence by Place of Residence

Area	First study No. (%)	Second study No. (%)	Total No. (%)
Urban	158 (72)	160 (73)	318 (73)
Urban residential area	101 (46)	117 (53)	218 (50)
Commercial area	35 (16)	28 (13)	63 (14)
Industrial area	22 (10)	15 (7)	37 (8)
Rural	61 (28)	59 (27)	120 (27)
Country town	20 (9)	24 (11)	44 (10)
Rural land	38 (17)	8 (4)	46 (11)
Mountain, seaside village	3 (1)	27 (12)	30 (7)
Unknown	37	23	60

dwellers. However, as a result of progressive industrialization following World War II, a large migration of people from rural to urban areas was seen in Japan. Thus, this analysis might be ambiguous.

Table 7 presents the incidence by occupation. Office clerks account for 20% and 17%, and students for 12% and 18%. When these groups were compared with the corresponding population groups based on data from the Japanese nationwide census of 1976, office clerks were the most often affected.

TABLE 7. Occupation of Reported Patients

Classification	First study No.	(%)	Second study No.	(%)
Office clerk	50	(20)	41	(17)
Student	31	(12)	43	(18)
Technological worker	29	(11)	26	(11)
House-keeping	27	(11)	36	(15)
Unemployed	26	(10)	25	(10)
Specialist	10	(4)	20	(8)
Light worker	27	(11)	20	(8)
Farmer	8	(3)	11	(5)
Others	4	(2)	12	(5)
Unknown	44	(17)	8	(3)
Total	256		242	

We have paid no attention to racial or religious factors because the Japanese have been ethnically and culturally homogenous for a long time.

In terms of prognosis (see Table 8), some improvement in mortality was noted between the first and second studies. Excluding "unknown" cases, crude mortality at the time of the first study was 10%, due to original Crohn's disease 5%, due to complication of Crohn's disease 2%, and due to other disease 2%. At the second study, crude mortality was 6%, due to Crohn's disease 3%, and due to complication or other disease 3%.

TABLE 8. Prognosis of Reported Patients

Criteria of prognosis	First study No. (%)	Second study No. (%)	Total No. (%)
Died	20 (10)	13 (6)	33 (8)
Due to Crohn's disease	11 (5)	7 (3)	18 (4)
Due to complication	5 (2) }	6 (3)	15 (4)
Due to other disease	4 (2) }		
Under observation	85 (42)	164 (76)	249 (60)
With medication as inpatient		9 (4) }	150 (36)
as outpatient	49 (24)	92 (43) }	
Without medication	36 (18)	63 (29)	99 (24)
Recovery	96 (48)	39 (18)	135 (32)
With minor inconvenience	65 (32)		
Complete	31 (15)		
Unknown	55	26	81

This might be evidence of recent progress in detection, diagnosis, and treatment.

DISCUSSION

Considering the present situation of hospital medical record administration in our country, estimation of the incidence of Crohn's disease is somewhat difficult. With the exception of some big hospitals which have definite divisions of gastroenterology or medical record libraries, most replies and reports depend on each doctor's individual memory. According to our analysis, mislocation of reported cases between the first and second research in 1976 is evidence of such a situation in present Japan. Nevertheless, we have attempted to establish a hypothesis (Table 9). The principle of our hypothesis is that a parallel proportion between the number of patients and the number of beds in hospitals exists, and so does the same proportional relation between the whole number of hospital beds for general use in Japan and that of hospitals corresponding to these studies.

TABLE 9. Hypothesis for Estimation

1) Almost all of Crohn's disease patients shall be admitted and diagnosed in a hospital.
2) Total number of definite CD patients who must be admitted shall correlate to the whole number of hospital beds in Japan.
3) If there is no deviation in localization and prevalence of the disease throughout Japan, the number of definite patients can be estimated from the proportion between the whole number of hospital beds in Japan and the corresponding figure in this study.
4) If the research is done at well-equipped and -administered hospitals, the prospective maximal incidence may be estimated from the original data of this study.
5) Prospective minimal incidence may be estimated from the prevalence of surgically operated patients in emergency in the above hospitals.

Regrettably, the hypothesis inevitably eliminates the mild cases who are not necessarily admitted to hospital. From the beginning of our study, we focused only on definitely diagnosed cases, so we cannot deny the omission in the results of our analysis.

On the fifth point of the hypothesis, we have to add some notes. We considered that the probability of emergency operation for Crohn's disease patients does not differ between well-equipped hospitals and those that are not well-equipped.

During 1974 and 1979, the incidence ranged between 0.25 and 0.07 per 100,000 population per annum. (The actual formula of calculation and parameters are shown in Table 10.) Even though our estimation is uncer-

TABLE 10. Formula for Estimation

Total population of Japan	108,718,000 (A)
Total number of hospital beds for general use in Japan	674,000 (B)
Number of beds in the 1,130 hospitals which responded to our studies	145,584 (C)
Estimated population covered by our studies	23,483,000 (D)
Average annual occurrence of Crohn's disease in our studies	59 (E)
Estimated average annual per 100,000 incidence among the population covered by our studies during 1974–1979	0.25 (F)

F = E/D and D = A • C/B, therefore, F = E • B/A • C

tain, we are able to say that the incidence of Crohn's disease in Japan is less than one-tenth that of European white people.

Considering the present situation of medical record administration in hospitals, statistical analysis of this data might be meaningless.

We look to further prospective studies, and if industrialization or urban living is responsible for the prevalence of Crohn's disease, Japan should be one of the best fields for such prospective epidemiological surveys.

REFERENCES

1. Kyle, J.: Crohn's Disease, pp. 8–25. William Heinemann, London, 1972.
2. Myren, J., Bouchier, I. A. D., Watkinson, G., and De Dombel, F. T.: Inflammatory bowel disease—An O.M.G.E. survey. *Scand. J. Gastroent.*, **14**: 56, 1976.
3. Mendeloff, A. I.: The epidemiology of inflammatory bowel disease. *Clinics in Gastroent.*, **9(2)**: 259, 1980.

Ulcerative Colitis and Crohn's Disease in Japanese Infants and Children

Kazuo Shiraki and Yutaka Nakasato***

SUMMARY

To know the prevalence and clinical characteristics of ulcerative colitis and Crohn's disease in Japanese infants and children, questionnaires were sent to 298 pediatric clinics throughout Japan, and 96 cases of ulcerative colitis and 31 cases of Crohn's disease were collected from the past five years. In Japanese infants and children, the incidence of ulcerative colitis was estimated as approximately 0.1 to 0.2 per 100,000 population per year, and that of Crohn's disease about 0.03 to 0.07 per 100,000 population per year.

In most patients the age at onset was more than 9 years in ulcerative colitis and more than 12 years in Crohn's disease. Growth retardation was obvious in many of the patients and was considered one of the most important complications in infants and children with inflammatory bowel disease.

INTRODUCTION

In Japan ulcerative colitis and Crohn's disease are considered rare in infants and children, and only a few cases have been reported in the literature. However, a recent survey on inflammatory bowel disease in Japanese adults suggested that the age of onset in these diseases is becoming younger. It is therefore considered necessary to know the prevalence and also the clinical characteristics of these diseases in infants and children.

METHODS AND SUBJECTS

Questionnaires were sent to 298 pediatric clinics of major hospitals throughout Japan, and a request was made for reports on all of the patients of less than 16 years old with ulcerative colitis or Crohn's disease admitted during the five years between 1976 and 1980.

*Department of Pediatrics, Tottori University School of Medicine, Yonago, Japan
**Department of Pediatrics, University of Tokyo Branch Hospital, Tokyo, Japan

RESULTS

The questionnaire was returned by 157 clinics, yielding a recovery rate of 52.7%; 96 cases of ulcerative colitis and 31 cases of Crohn's disease were collected.

Ulcerative colitis

The mean annual occurrence of ulcerative colitis in these 157 pediatric clinics was 17.3 cases, or 0.1 cases per clinic per year. We assume we were able to collect approximately one third to one half of the pediatric cases of this disease which actually occurred in Japan during the five-year period. Thus the annual occurrence of ulcerative colitis in infancy and childhood in Japan may be estimated as between 38 and 56 cases. If this estimate is correct, the annual incidence is calculated as 0.1 to 0.2 per 100,000 population in the pediatric age group. It is therefore apparent that ulcerative colitis is not a common disease in Japanese infants and children. Figure 1 shows the age distribution of the patients with ulcerative colitis during infancy and childhood. The youngest was two months old when the first symptom was noted, but most patients developed their initial symptoms after nine years of age. It appears as if the number of patients decreases after 14 years of age, but this is probably due to the fact that most patients beyond this age are not seen in pediatric clinics. There was no obvious sexual preponderance.

The geographic distribution of the pediatric patients with ulcerative colitis in Japan is shown in Fig. 2. Many patients lived in urban areas at the

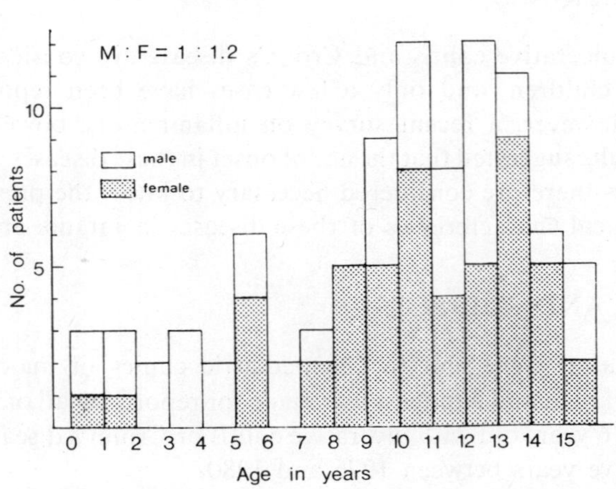

FIG. 1. Distribution of the age at onset of ulcerative colitis in infants and children in Japan (1976–1980).

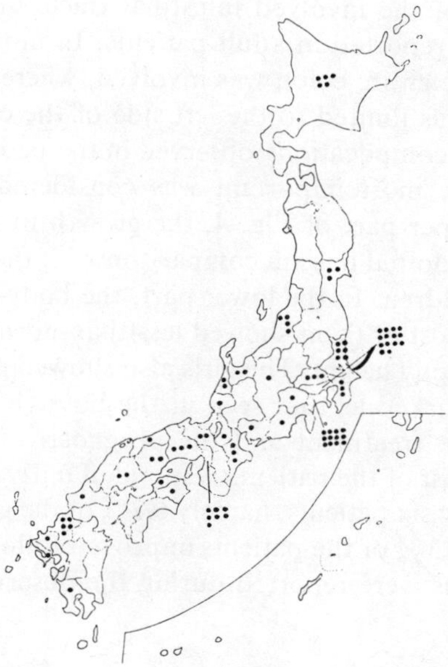

FIG. 2. Geographic distribution of patients (less than 16 years old) with ulcerative colitis in Japan.

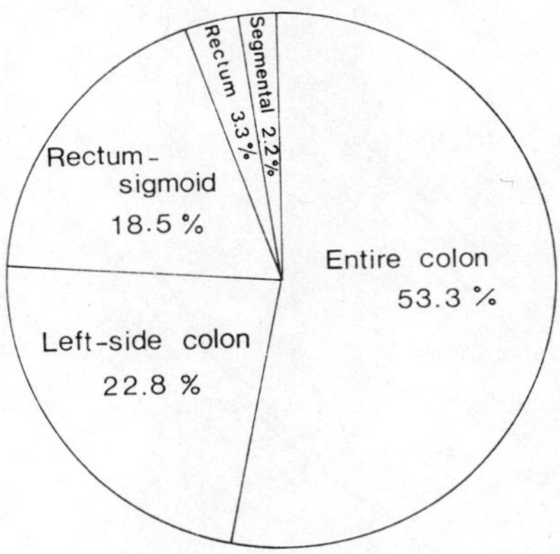

FIG. 3. Distribution of the GI tract lesions in pediatric patients with ulcerative colitis.

time of onset, but there was no significant predominance of any particular area considering the population and the number of hospitals from which the patients were reported.

The distribution of the involved intestinal tracts did not show much difference from that reported in adult patients. In more than half of the pediatric patients the entire colon was involved, whereas in 22.8% of the patients the lesion was limited to the left side of the colon (Fig. 3).

Among the many complications observed in the pediatric patients with ulcerative colitis, the most important was considered to be growth retardation. In the upper part of Fig. 4, the growth in height of the male patients is shown by dotted lines in comparison with the standard curve of normal Japanese children. In the lower part, the body-weight gain of the patients is shown. Most of them showed less-than-normal growth in body weight as well as in body height. The girls also showed growth retardation, but it was not so marked as that seen in the boys (Fig. 5).

Table 1 shows the treatment and the prognosis of the patients with ulcerative colitis. Most of the patients responded fairly well to steroid and salazopyrin, and only six patients, namely 6.7% of the group, required surgery. As a whole, 83.3% of the patients improved following various treatments, and no deaths were reported during the observation period.

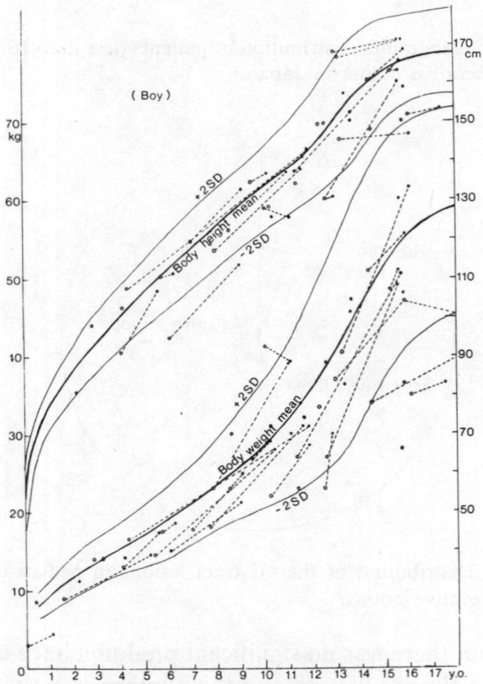

FIG. 4. Growth curves in boys suffering from ulcerative colitis.

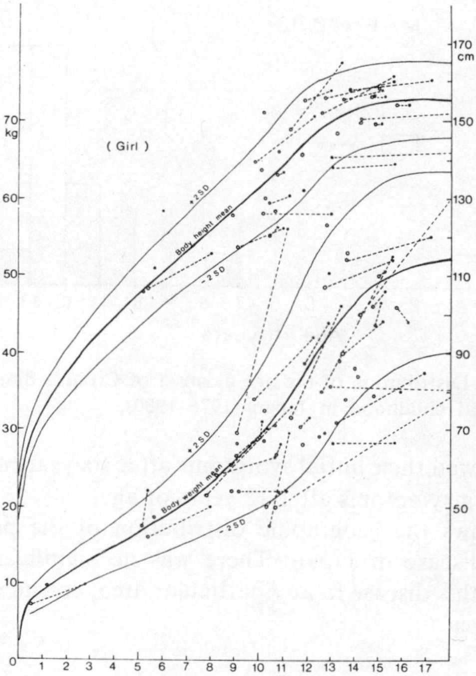

FIG. 5. Growth curves in girls suffering from ulcerative colitis.

TABLE 1. Ulcerative Colitis in Infants and Children: Treatment and Prognosis

Treatment	No. of patients	Prognosis	
		Improved	Not responded
Steroid	5	4	1
Salazopyrin	15	14	1
Steroid + salazopyrin	50	41 (82.0%)	9
Steroid + salazopyrin + surgery	6	5	1
Miscellaneous	14	11	3
Total	90	75 (83.3%)	15

Crohn's disease

The mean annual occurrence of Crohn's disease in the present series was only 5.5 cases, or 0.04 cases per clinic. It is therefore estimated that the incidence of Crohn's disease in Japanese infants and children is approximately one third that of ulcerative colitis, namely 0.03 to 0.07 per 100,000 population in the pediatric age group. Figure 6 demonstrates the distribution of the age at onset of Crohn's disease in our study. All except

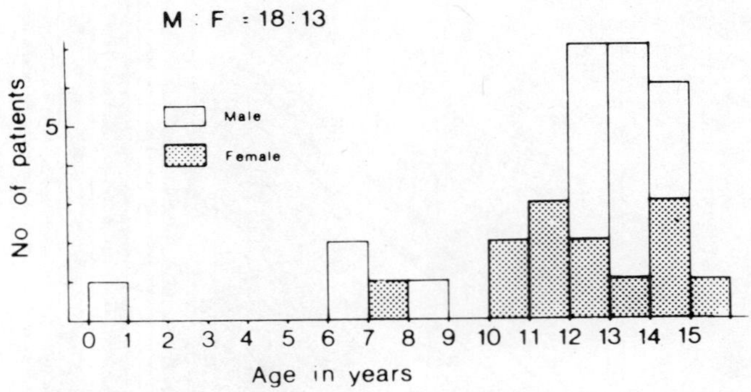

FIG. 6. Distribution of the age at onset of Crohn's disease in infancy and childhood in Japan (1976–1980).

one patient showed their initial symptoms after six years of age, with most of them showing symptoms after 12 years of age.

Figure 7 shows the geographic distribution of the pediatric patients with Crohn's disease in Japan. There was no significant accumulation of the cases of this disease in any particular area, considering the population in each area.

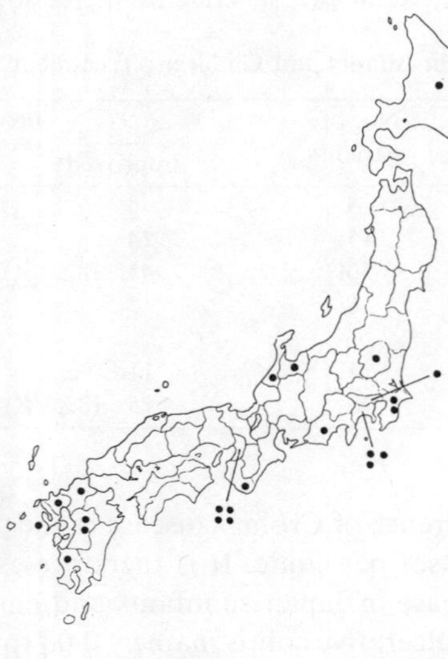

FIG. 7. Geographic distribution of patients (less than 16 years old) with Crohn's disease in Japan.

In contrast to ulcerative colitis, lesions of Crohn's disease were broadly distributed from oral cavity to anus, but in the majority of the cases the involved intestine was from the lower portion of the ileum to the transverse colon (Table 2).

TABLE 2. Crohn's Disease in Infants and Children: Multiple Lesion Site (22 Patients)

	No. of patients (%)
Oral cavity–stomach	1 (4.5)
Duodenum–middle portion of ileum	3 (13.6)
Lower portion of ileum	13 (59.1)
Cecum	8 (36.4)
Ascending colon	14 (63.6)
Transverse colon	11 (50.0)
Descending colon	8 (36.4)
Sigmoid colon	8 (36.4)
Rectum	3 (13.6)
Anus	7 (31.8)

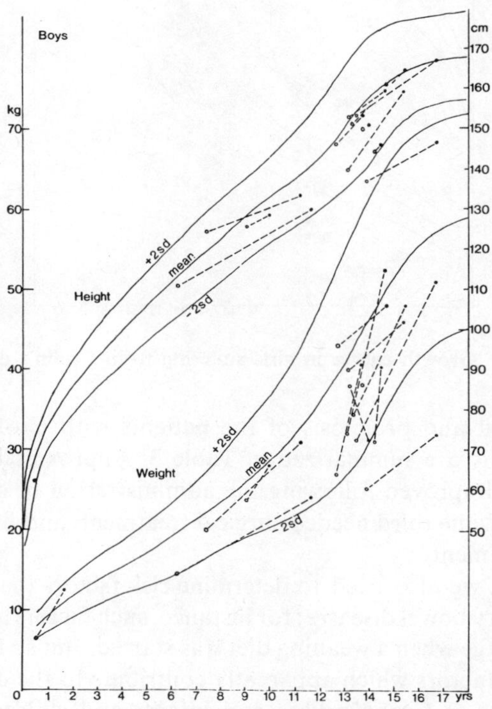

FIG. 8. Growth curves in boys suffering from Crohn's disease.

As seen in the patients with ulcerative colitis, the children with Crohn's disease also showed apparent growth retardation, and nearly all the patients showed less-than-normal growth in height, as well as in weight, after the onset of the disease, in spite of various treatments (Figs. 8 and 9).

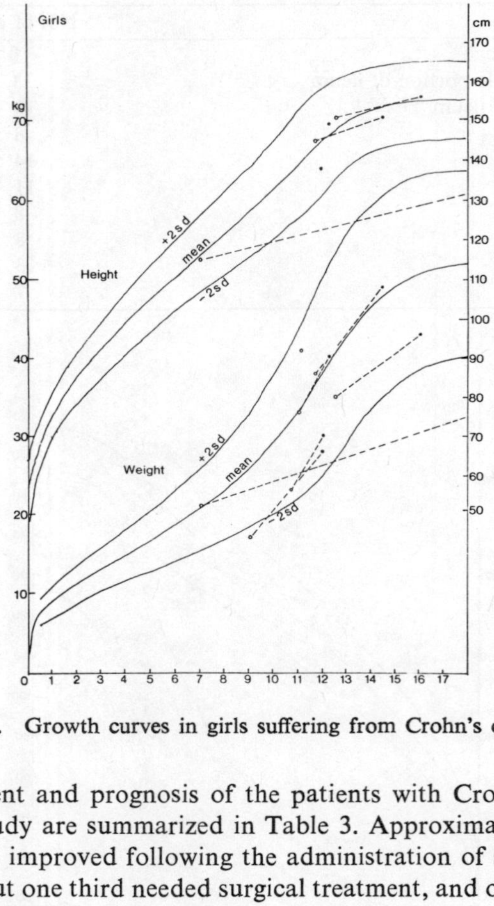

FIG. 9. Growth curves in girls suffering from Crohn's disease.

The treatment and prognosis of the patients with Crohn's disease in the present study are summarized in Table 3. Approximately two thirds of the patients improved following the administration of steroids and/or salazopyrin, but one third needed surgical treatment, and one patient died in spite of treatment.

In this study, we also tried to determine risk factors that might trigger the inflammatory bowel diseases: for instance, such factors as differences in feeding, or the age when a weaning diet was started. But so far we have not found any risk factors which apparently contribute to the development of ulcerative colitis or Crohn's disease in infants and children.

TABLE 3. Crohn's Disease in Infants and Children: Treatment and Prognosis

Treatment	No. of patients (%)	Prognosis		
		Improved (%)	Not responded	Died
Medical treatment	7 (31.8)	6 (85.7)	1	0
Medical and nutritional treatment	8 (36.4)	8 (100.0)	0	0
Medical and surgical treatment	3 (13.6)	2 (66.7)	0	1
Medical, surgical, and nutritional treatment	4 (18.2)	2 (50.0)	2	0
Total	22	18 (81.8)	3	1

Discussion: Incidence

Richard G. Farmer and Akira Yokota, Chairmen

Dr. Riddell: I was wondering if Dr. Farmer is going to compare the sort of incidences we have seen here with the incidences in U.K. and the U.S.A. so we can get an idea of the variance. I should perhaps also comment on what is apparently a very high incidence of colitis when compared to proctitis alone which does not seem to be our usual experience. The question I was going to raise is a diagnostic problem because from the discussion in this symposium I am now beginning to wonder just how accurate the figures are when comparing ulcerative colitis and Crohn's disease. It has been apparent that granulomas almost uniformly are needed at the moment to make a diagnosis of Crohn's disease and so I suspect that in the figures for ulcerative colitis there are actually quite a few patients with Crohn's disease that are buried in there. If we looked at it more carefully, we might change the diagnoses. Similarly we have heard that the Japanese have gone to great lengths to try and exclude tuberculosis in those with granulomas, and it is also possible that some patients who really have Crohn's disease may in fact still be in the tuberculous category just because anything even a little bit suspicious of tuberculosis has been put back into possible tuberculosis rather than Crohn's disease. I really wonder if in both instances we are fairly severely underestimating the amount of Crohn's disease in the population.

Dr. Farmer: Let me comment on the comparative studies in the so-called Western countries. As I mentioned, there have been attempts to define incidence in the U.S.A., U.K., and Scandinavia particularly; and various workshops like this have tried to do it for South Africa, Australia, New Zealand, and other primary Caucasian but heterogeneous population groups, usually in a relatively temperate to moderate climate. The geographical distribution is certainly impressive in that the areas I have mentioned seem to be the areas where one actually encounters the diseases.

In tropical countries, in the Middle East and in predominantly black countries, one does not see anywhere near the clinical experience with either ulcerative colitis or Crohn's disease that one sees in the predominantly Caucasian albeit heterogenous population groups that I am talking about. As I said earlier, to get somewhat accurate incidence studies is very difficult, but I will give you some numbers: for ulcerative colitis the estimates have ranged usually from approximately 3–7 per 100,000 population per year; the incidence figures for Crohn's disease in the recent past, which is to say since 1960, have ranged from approximately 2–4.7 of the incidence of new cases per 100,000 population. I would emphasize that the figures appear to be more reliable when we talk about incidence rather than prevalence. Because of the morbidity and the chronicity of the diseases, one can get a very high figure for prevalence of the diseases if one looks at certain selected populations. Problems encountered by referral centers—such as our own institution, the Mayo Clinic, the University of Chicago, Mt. Sinai in New York, the Lahey Clinic, and a few others in the U.S.A. as well as St Mark's, the Karolinska Institute in Stockholm, and a few other places where they have managed to collect large numbers of cases—have been the attraction to these centers of cases referred by physicians. It is very common to have a patient with inflammatory bowel disease referred to a specialist. In fact, a survey of gastroenterologists in the U.S.A., in terms of their hospital practice, shows that inflammatory bowel disease is the most frequent disease referred to a gastroenterologist for consultation. It exceeds liver disease, ulcer, and cancer; but certainly the most common causes for referral to a gastroenterologist are to do a procedure such as an endoscopy or because of symptoms such as an irritable bowel syndrome. Nevertheless, the most common disease referred is inflammatory bowel disease.

Several groups have noted the phenomenon of the plateauing since 1977, so the peak incidence of Crohn's disease appeared to occur between 1975 and 1977 and the incidence may even be going down slightly. Our data indicates that the number of patients referred to us has remained about the same sine 1977, following a rapid escalation beginning in 1960. What all of this means is a little hard to say, but certainly it is difficult for you to associate it with some type of causative factor such as diet, early weaning, or various psychological factors. It is made particularly difficult in the U.S.A. because of the heterogenous population, much made of the higher-than-expected Jewish incidence, and the lower-than-expected black incidence. The Jewish incidence in the U.S.A. is clearly colored by the fact that Dr.

Crohn worked at Mt. Sinai which is a predominantly Jewish hosptial in New York and that the number of patients in their large series of studies created the impression that it was a "Jewish disease." But studies, for example, from Sweden which has a small Jewish population have not shown any particular increase in Jewish preponderance. There have been attempts by the National Foundation for Ulcerative Colitis in the U.S.A. to try and get at the Jewish incidence. So far this has not been successful other than to show that, yes, there is a higher-than-expected incidence among the Jewish people, but how high, or what the relationship is to other ethnic groups is very hard to tell.

Similarly, the relationship of the urban population and the white-collar worker, as opposed to the laborer, has also been shown in multiple studies; but once again as you look at a wide spectrum of patients, you do indeed find patients from all socioeconomic groups and so on. So I think there has been a certain stereotyping that has attempted to have some causative factors implied such as a psychological factor, an environmental factor, a stress factor, or diet-related factors which may or may not be of any consequence whatsoever. What was mentioned earlier that a ubiquitous agent damaging the mucosa in a genetically predetermined, immunologically deficient person may be far more important than whether or not the patient was Jewish, whether or not they got on with their mothers, or whether or not they live in a city, suburb, or rural area. I certainly congratulate all three of these presentations in terms of trying to do the right thing in the right way, and trying to get the cooperation of the various physicians. I think getting the cooperation of the physicians is the most difficult task, and the fact that 56% responded is a cause of great concern; you then have to assume the data based on the 56%. It would certainly be nice if we could threaten or do something to them so that they will agree to fill out the forms so as to get nearly 100% response.

Dr. Yokota: As Dr. Farmer stated, there are flaws to the type of questionnaires used for our survey because not all the residents were examined, and because the results of the survey would depend upon the extent to which the physicians, who were asked to carry out the survey, cooperate.

Furthermore, because mild patients could easily be diagnosed and treated, they did not necessarily go to the trouble of returning to the hospitals which were requested to carry out the survey. For this reason, the number of reported patients did not increase; it is believed that the annual case incidence indicates either a post-peak curve or a downward trend. In other words, it may be stated that ulcerative colitis is a disease well known to physicians in Japan.

Dr. Farmer: We have found this to be the case in patients with ulcerative colitis more than in patients with Crohn's disease. The implication that was made, that most patients with Crohn's disease will require hospitalization and so hospital records tend to be more accurate, is exactly what we have found. Similarly, the experience (now I can't say incidence) at referral centers is that there has been an increasing number of patients with distal colon ulcerative colitis, usually proctitis, and also left-sided colitis. Estimates are that one third to 40% of all cases of ulcerative colitis are now of the less extensive disease. And in ulcerative colitis we can pretty much correlate the prognosis with the extent of disease. Therefore, we are indeed seeing the milder cases, and therefore, they are not coming in the hospital which could give a false low reading as far as what the relationship of the proctitis form of ulcerative colitis is to the total colon disease. For patients with Crohn's disease, it still appears that most of these patients will require hospitalization and that there has been a dramatic change in the hospital-based population for inflammatory bowel disease over the past 20 years.

Dr. Riddell made a point about the difficulty of differential diagnosis, especially if a granuloma is necessary for diagnosis. At the Cleveland Clinic and the Mayo Clinic, between 40 and 50% of patients have granulomas with Crohn's disease. We have found that we tended to overestimate the cases of ulcerative colitis and underestimate the cases of large intestine Crohn's disease. I suspect that this may be the case here with the overestimate because of the differential diagnosis with tuberculosis. Therefore I think that this problem is one that you might anticipate as well. If I were to predict what were to happen here, I would predict that over the next 10 years there would be more cases of Crohn's disease seen—probably first more cases recognized—because of either the differential diagnosis with ulcerative colitis or the differential diagnosis with tuberculosis. But then over the next 10 years, more cases of Crohn's disease would actually be identified. Why that is, whether it is a westernization or urbanization phenomenon, is very hard to say. But that would be what I would anticipate.

As I have looked over Japanese data, I am impressed that much of the incidence and prevalence-type data that you report now seems very similar to what was reported in the U.S.A. and U.K. about 20 years ago. So it would seem that one could anticipate more cases of Crohn's disease being seen in Japan in the next few years. In areas where inflammatory bowel disease is almost unheard of, such as the Middle East and Black African countries, they do see some ulcerative colitis, but it is rare to see Crohn's disease. I have seen what appear to be clinically good cases of ulcerative colitis among blacks in Africa, among Arabs in the Middle East, and among Persians in the Middle East, but I have rarely seen Crohn's disease. The cases of ulcerative colitis I have seen look very typical and do not look like a form of infectious diarrhea which would be their primary differentiation with ulcerative colitis. But the cases of suspected Crohn's disease that they see almost invariably turn out to be tuberculosis. So in areas where inflammatory bowel disease is rare, the cases that are seen do appear to be ulcerative colitis. Thus, for some reason, ulcerative colitis appears to occur first and then Crohn's disease later, perhaps reaching some type of peak or plateau and then trailing off. This may be what we are seeing in Scandinavia, U.K., and the U.S.A. at the present time.

Dr. Muto: In replying to Dr. Riddell's comment, I am a little afraid that we have misled the doctors by showing several rather indeterminate cases. I should say that almost 95% of IBD has been correctly identified and tuberculosis is almost always easily diagnosed, especially with increasing experience. So, do not take the view that we are mixing up ulcerative colitis with Crohn's disease and Crohn's disease with tuberculosis, because we have chosen very special cases which raise the problems we have seen. These are very rare examples, so please don't misunderstand. The data shown is quite correct, I think.

Dr. Farmer: I would like to ask Dr. Kimura if you have seen cases of toxic megacolon in Crohn's disease in these 461 cases. Have you had any cases of toxic megacolon, and if so, have you had trouble differentiating those from ulcerative colitis?

Dr. Kimura: According to the second study, only four cases reported the complication of toxic megacolon; it's about 2% of the total cases.

Dr. Farmer: Our experience with toxic megacolon has been that initially it was very difficult to tell the two diseases apart. Dr. Fazio and his colleagues have reported on our experience in the last 15 years with about 125 cases of toxic megacolon, and we have found that the incidence is about 50/50 for the two diseases. In the last 10 years, probably 4 out of 5 of our cases of toxic megacolon have been due to Crohn's disease. So, one of the clinical impressions we have had since about 1970 has been that Crohn's disease not only has more morbidity, but that it has more complications, more reason for hospitalization, and more difficulty with therapy. Therefore, most of the new forms in therapy such as with hyperalimentation have been directed at the Crohn's disease patient rather than the ulcerative colitis patient. Most of new therapeutic advances or attempts at therapy—for example, metronidazol, immunosuppresives, elemental diet, and home TPN—have been directed at Crohn's disease patients because of all these complications, of which toxic megacolon is yet another one.

Dr. Kelly: Dr. Utsunomiya, the thing that struck me was the decrease in the incidence of ulcerative colitis after the peak in 1974. You correlated the incidence of ulcerative colitis with perhaps the use of a Western diet in Japan, but the consumption of the Western diet seems to be steadily increasing whereas after 1974, the incidence of ulcerative colitis began to decrease. I wonder if you have any explanation for that.

Dr. Utsunomiya: The year 1974 was the year of the oil crisis, and in that year the daily amount of meat consumed in Japan decreased. Yet, whether the oil crisis had a direct impact on the consumption of meat is not known. Moreover, if we consider 1974 the borderline of economic growth in Japan, the economic growth (which was of a high level up until then) leveled off.

Compared with the average results of a 5-year survey, when a survey was carried our for the present year, the number of cases found the previous year made up only 36.2% of the number of cases reported during the current year. In the instance of cases found 2 years ago, the percentage was 22.4%, those of 3 years ago 12.7%, those of 4 years ago 6.4%, those of 5 years ago 4.5%, thus successively decreasing. The 4% of cases who were attacked by disease over 10 years ago were also included in this survey.

If we consider such points, cases attacked by disease since 1975 were supplemented after each survey was carried out, and it is believed that there was no decrease nor any marked fluctuation in the incidence curve.

Dr. Yokota: Formerly, ulcerative colitis was considered a morbid state similar to that of an extremely dramatic dysentery. However, because of changes in the concept of disease, in actual fact, there are many milder cases. We consider such cases much more difficult to collect for the questionnaires, and do not believe that the cases are decreasing in number. For instance, among questionnaires received in the mail, there were patients who were attacked by disease a long time ago. Such patients subsided, and then were re-treated in small clinics; it is assumed that when they could no longer endure the long course, they finally decided to come to our hospitals, which were carrying out the survey.

Dr. Farmer: I would like to express caution in the over-interpretation of various factors in terms of the decline or lack of decline of the incidence in the last few years. I agree entirely with this last comment and just want to mention that many different factors are now being studied. We are involved in a multicenter, international cooperative trial that Dr. Gilat in Tel Aviv is trying to do because they are attempting to look at the Jewish incidence from the Israeli point of view. There is not a particularly high incidence of inflammatory bowel disease in Israel and so they are attempting to get some data on childhood-onset inflammatory bowel disease with the appropriate controls.

I think it is very valuable to continue this type of survey, despite the limitations, but again I would certainly encourage trying to get a higher compliance rate from the positions reporting if you can.

V. MEDICAL TREATMENT

Treatment and Long-Term Course of Ulcerative Colitis

Mikio Inoue and Ichiro Yoshida

The incidence of ulcerative colitis in Japan has apparently increased in recent years. The epidemiological study carried out by the Intractable Disease Research Committee of Fukuoka Prefecture estimated the prevalence of this disease in 1980 to be 9.8 patients per 100,000 population.[1] This prevalence corresponds to about one eighth of those in Oxford in 1965[2] and in Minnesota in 1965.[3] However, up to now, because of the low incidence of ulcerative colitis, studies on the treatment and long-term course of this disease in large numbers of patients are relatively few in Japan.

In this paper, the results of treatment performed according to a standard scheme and the long-term course of this disease are described.

STUDIES ON MEDICAL TREATMENT

Therapeutic scheme and patients

In 1975, a standard scheme for medical treatment of ulcerative colitis was presented by the Japanese Ministry of Health and Welfare, Ulcerative Colitis Research Committee.[4] In this scheme, as shown in Table 1, mild and moderately severe cases are initially treated with salicylazosulfapyridine (SASP) alone, and if patients do not respond, local corticosteroids (steroid) are employed; if these fail, oral steroids are given. Severely ill patients are treated with systemic steroids. If these patients do not respond, ACTH or intra-arterial infusions of prednisolone are employed. If this treatment is not effective, immunosuppressive drugs are recommended; and if patients do not respond to these regimens, surgical treatment is considered. In fulminant attacks, the intensive intravenous regimen presented by Truelove,[5] or intra-arterial infusions of prednisolone are employed.

Department of Health Care and Administration, School of Medicine, Fukuoka University, Fukuoka, Japan

TABLE 1. Scheme for Medical Treatment of Ulcerative Colitis

I. Mild and moderately severe attacks
 1) Salazopyrin in a dose of 3 to 4 g or 0.06 g/kg a day is employed. If a patient goes into remission, maintenance dose of 2 g is continued to minimize relapses.
 2) If a patient does not respond to salazopyrin within two weeks, retention enema with 20 to 40 mg prednisolone (on going to bed, or twice a day) is used.
 3) If it is not effective, oral prednisolone 30 mg a day is administered, and if a patient does not respond, regimen for severe attacks is employed.

II. Severe attacks (except for fulminant attacks)
 1) Administration to hospital and vigorous replacement treatment is necessary.
 2) Prednisolone 40 to 60 mg daily by mouth, and during high fever and leucocytosis broad spectrum antibiotics are employed. If remission occurs, dose of prednisolone is decreased gradually, then Salazopyrin is added, and finally, a patient is put on the maintenance treatment with Salazopyrin.
 3) If a patient does not respond to oral prednisolone within two weeks, ACTH 40 to 50 u. i.v. or i.m., or intra-arterial infusion (into superior and inferior mesenteric arteries) of 30 to 40 mg prednisolone is used.
 4) If it is not effective, immunosuppressive drug (Azathioprine 1.5 to 2.0 mg/kg a day) is recommended, and if a patient fails to respond, surgery is considered.

III. Fulminant attacks
 1) Nothing is given by mouth except water; choose one of the following two regimens.
 2) Intravenous drip is maintained for a seven-day period with water, electrolytes, glucose, amino acid, vitamins, etc. Prednisolone 40 to 60 mg a day in divided doses and antibiotics are given with the intravenous drip. ACTH 40 to 50 u. and blood transfusion may be added.
 2′) Intra-arterial infusion of prednisolone is employed, together with vigorous intravenous replacement therapy.
 3) If rapid clinical remission occurs within seven days, treatment is switched to oral prednisolone as for severe attacks. If a patient fails to respond, emergency surgery is indicated.

*Japanese Ministry of Health and Welfare, Ulcerative Colitis Research Committee, 1975.

If patients fail to pass into remission within seven days, emergency surgery is indicated.

Fifty-two inpatients (25 males and 27 females) were treated according to this scheme in Fukuoka University Hospital. Diagnosis was confirmed by clinical pictures, barium enema study, colonoscopy, and pathologic examination of biopsy specimens. Among the patients, 29 were classified as mild, 18 moderately severe, and 5 severe. As to the extent of involvement of colitis, 25 had total involvement, 23 left-sided colitis, and 4 proctitis. Remission was assessed by disappearance of both clinical symptoms and active colonoscopic findings. Outpatients were excluded from this study because of difficulties in confirming the accuracy of medications.

Results of treatment

The effect of treatments and regimens required to induce remission are shown in Fig. 1. As a whole, 49 out of 52 patients went into remission by medical treatment. Among the 49 patients, 9 patients (18.4%) passed into remission with SASP alone, and 17 patients (34.7%) with the combination of SASP and local steroids. Systemic steroids were required in half of the patients; in 7 patients (14.2%) the responses to SASP and steroids were insufficient, and ACTH or immunosuppressive drugs were used to induce remission. Patients who failed to have remission by medical treatment were one death from serum hepatitis (moderately severe, total colitis), one patient discharged without remission (moderately severe, total colitis), and one patient who received colostomy (mild, left-sided colitis).

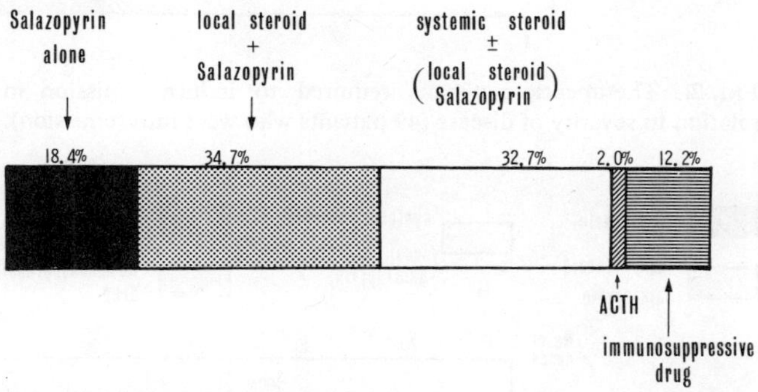

FIG. 1. Therapeutic regimens required to induce remission (49 inpatients who went into remission by medical treatment).

Of the 49 patients who went into remission, the regimens required to induce remission were analyzed. Figure 2 shows the results of the analysis in relation to the severity of disease. In mild cases, 25.0% passed into remission with SASP alone, and 46.4% by the combination of SASP and local steroids. Oral steroids were required in about 30% of the cases. On the other hand, in moderately severe cases, about 60% needed systemic steroids to have remission, and 16.7% required additional immunosuppressive drugs. In severely ill patients, two out of five cases received ACTH or immunosuppressive drugs because of poor response to oral steroids.

Figure 3 shows the regimens required to induce remission in relation to the extent of involvement of the colitis. All four proctitis patients had remission by the combination of SASP and steroid enema. In left-sided colitis, about 70% went into remission without systemic steroids. On the other hand, in total colitis, only 30% of the cases went into remission without systemic steroids. About 15% of both left-sided and total colitis

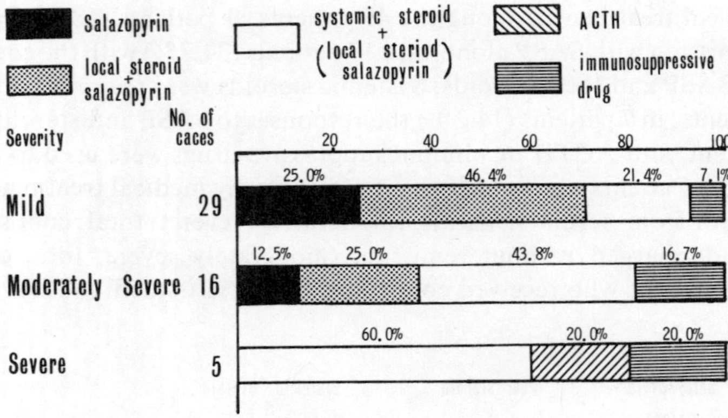

FIG. 2. Therapeutic regimens required to induce remission in relation to severity of disease (49 patients who went into remission).

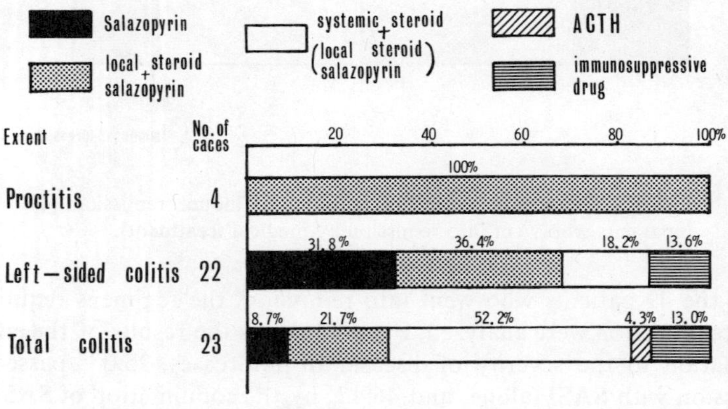

FIG. 3. Therapeutic regimens required to induce remission in relation to extent of involvement (49 patients who went into remission).

patients were SASP- and steroid-fast, and received additional immunosuppressive drugs.

To analyze the relation between the extent of involvement of colitis and the regimens required to induce remission more precisely, the required regimens were analyzed on mild and moderately severe cases in relation to the extent of involvement of colitis.

As shown in Fig. 4, among the mild cases all of the proctitis patients and 80.0% of the left-sided colitis patients went into remission by SASP

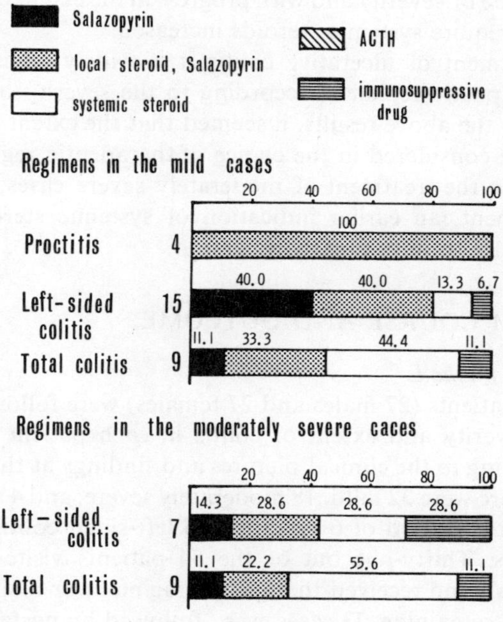

FIG. 4. Regimens required to induce remission in mild and moderately severe cases in relation to extent of involvement.

or the combination of SASP and local steroids; however, 55.5% of the total colitis patients needed systemic steroids. In the treatment of moderately severe cases, systemic steroids were also needed more often in the total colitis patients (66.7%) than in the left-sided colitis patients (57.2%).

Discussion

In the treatment of ulcerative colitis, two types of drugs have been known to be effective, corticosteroids (or corticotropin) and SASP. Recently immunosuppressive drugs have been advocated in the treatment of ulcerative colitis, especially in steroid-resistant patients. In general, SASP and steroid enema are indicated in mild or moderately severe attacks, and systemic steroid is indicated in severe attacks or moderately severe attacks with systemic upset.[6,7] However, Truelove[8] recommended oral steroids in all mild cases together with SASP and local steroids.

We observed the effects of treatment performed in accordance with the standard scheme presented by the Ulcerative Colitis Research Committee of the Japanese Ministry of Health and Welfare and assessed the propriety of this therapeutic scheme. The results obtained showed that, with increasing grade of severity and with progress in the extent of involvement, patients who require systemic steroids increased.

In the treatment of ulcerative colitis it is widely advised to employ different therapeutic regimens according to the severity of attack; however, based on the above results, it seemed that the extent of involvement should also be considered in the choice of therapeutic regimen. It is our opinion that in the treatment of moderately severe cases, or cases with total involvement, an earlier indication of systemic steroids would be rational in order to induce early remission.

LONG-TERM COURSE AND OUTCOME

Materials and methods

Fifty-four patients (27 males and 27 females) were followed for 3 to 10 years. The severity and extent of colitis in each patient were classified mainly according to the clinical pictures and findings at their first visit to this clinic. There were 32 mild, 18 moderately severe, and 4 severe patients; and they were consisted of 6 proctitis, 26 left-sided colitis, and 22 total colitis patients. Thirty-one out of the 54 patients visited our clinic at regular intervals and received therapeutic regimens or maintenance doses of SASP. The remaining 23 cases were followed by postal questionnaire or by telephone.

In the study of long-term course, the concept of patient-years of observed follow-up was used according to Watts *et al.*[9] In the patients who visited this clinic regularly, relapse and remission were assessed by clinical symptoms and colonoscopic findings; in the cases followed by questionnaire or telephone, assessment was made by clinical symptoms. Years in which colitis symptoms lasted only one or two weeks were classified as attack-years.

Results

During the follow-up period, there were three direct colitis deaths. All three patients who died from colitis during the follow-up period had total involvement, and among them two were severely ill and one was moderately severe at the time of their first visit to this clinic. Another patient (moderately severe, total colitis) died from fulminant viral hepatitis (type B), probably due to the transfusion at the time of previous attack. One patient (mild, total colitis) received proctocolectomy because of massive bleeding, and one patient (mild, left-sided colitis) received colostomy due to intractable disease.

The years in which patients died or received surgical operations, the years following surgery, and the years in which the course was unknown

(12.4% of the total patient-years) were excluded from patient-years. Thus, 290 patient-years of 54 patients in which the course was known were analyzed.

Out of 290 patient-years, 27.2% were in remission, and in 72.8% one or more attacks of colitis occurred (Fig. 5). To study the course more precisely, the concept of patient-months of observed follow-up was used according to the same principle as that of patient-years. Of 3,047 patient-months in which the course was known, 58.1% was spent in remission. These results suggest that in our patients relapses occurred frequently, but the duration of colitis symptoms was relatively short.

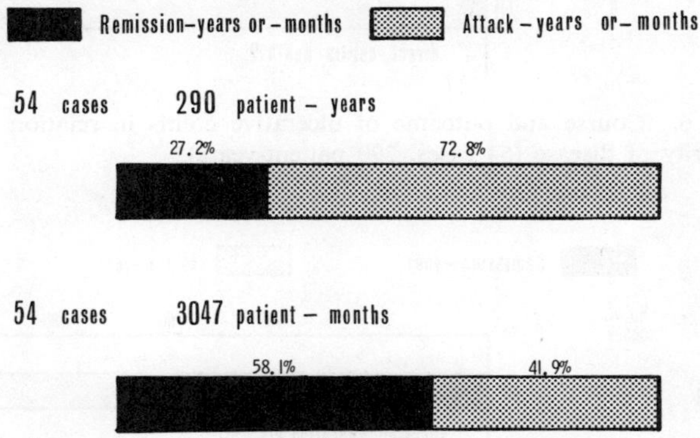

FIG. 5. Course of ulcerative colitis.

Figure 6 shows the course and outcome in relation to severity of disease at the time of the first visit. Severely ill patients showed the worst prognosis; two out of four severe cases died from colitis. The long-term course observed using the concept of patient-years suggested that with the increase in severity the proportion of remission-years decreased markedly, namely, from 32.6% in mild cases to 5.0% in severe cases. However, among mild cases, two patients received surgical operations.

In Fig. 7 the course and outcome are analyzed according to the extent of involvement. All of the three direct colitis deaths and a colitis-related death were observed in the total colitis patients, and in this group, the proportion of remission-years was the smallest (22.3%). However, the proportion of remission-years in the proctitis group (23.5%) was almost the same as that of the total colitis group. By analysis of the courses of proctitis patients, it was found that some of the proctitis patients were indifferent to treatment, so that mild symptoms continued or relapses occurred frequently, thus resulted in the low proportion of remission-years in the proctitis patients.

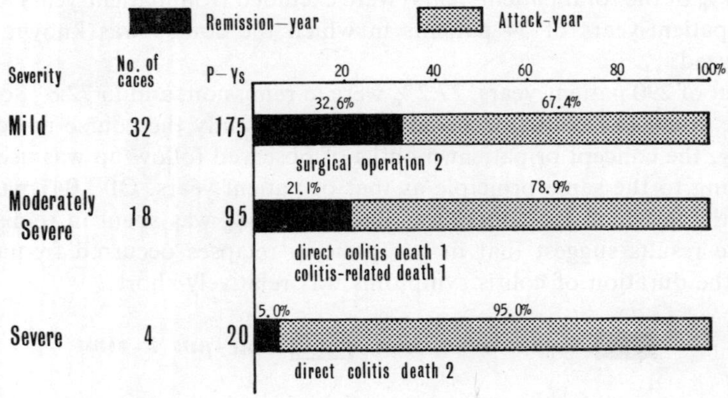

FIG. 6. Course and outcome of ulcerative colitis in relation to severity of disease (54 cases, 290 patient-years).

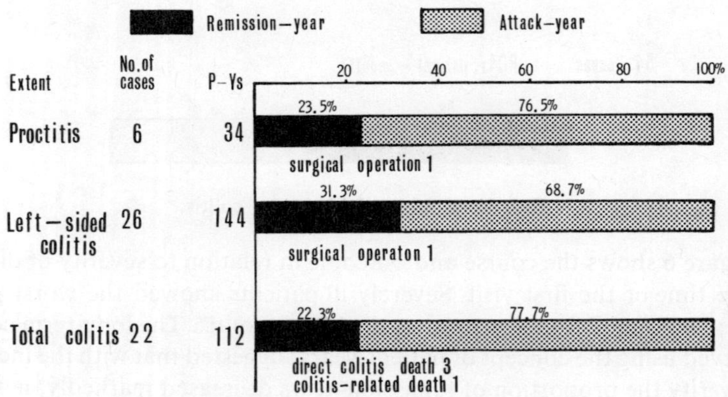

FIG. 7. Course and outcome of ulcerative colitis in relation to extent of involvement (54 cases, 290 patient-years).

Course and outcome were analyzed in relation to age at onset of colitis in Fig. 8. All of the three colitis deaths were observed in patients with early onset (below 29 years of age), and the proportion of remission-years was the smallest (17.0%) in this age group. On the other hand, patients with late onset (over 50 years old) had the most favorable course, the remission-years being 59.4%.

The relationship between the age, severity, and extent of colitis at the time of the first visit is shown in Fig. 9. In the young group (under 29 years of age) cases with severe and moderately severe attacks were most common

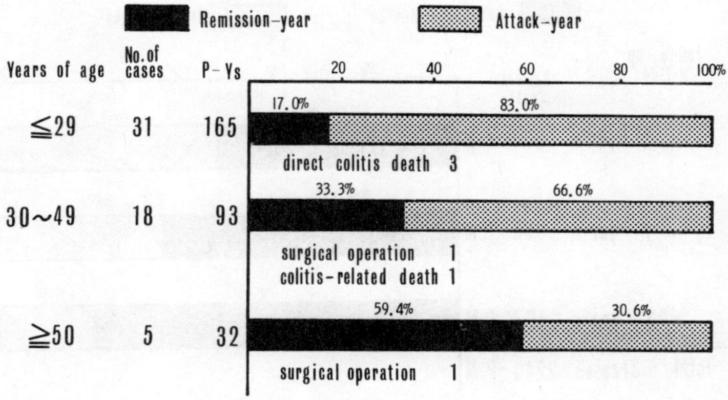

FIG. 8. Course and outcome of ulcerative colitis in relation to age at onset (54 cases, 290 patient-years).

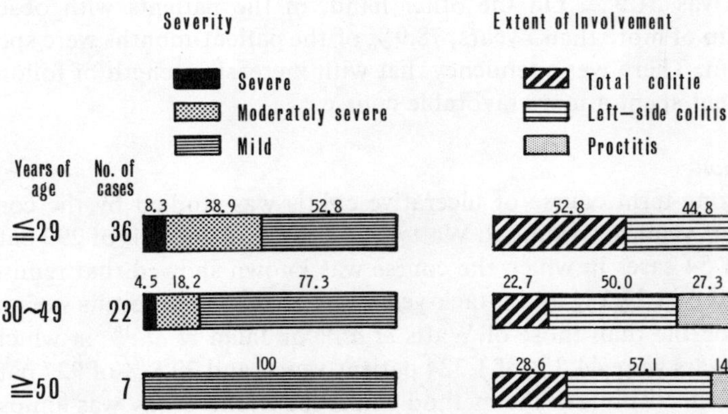

FIG. 9. Relation of severity and extent of involvement to age at first attack (65 cases).

(47.2%), and the proportion of the cases with total involvement was the largest (52.8%). On the other hand, all of the patients over 50 years of age had mild symptoms and had relatively narrow involvement. It was suggested that the above-mentioned differences in course among the various age groups were largely due to the differences in severity and extent of colitis.

In Fig. 10, the course expressed as patient-months is analyzed in relation to the length of the follow-up period after the first visit to this clinic. In the cases with follow-up of less than 4 years, the proportion of remission-

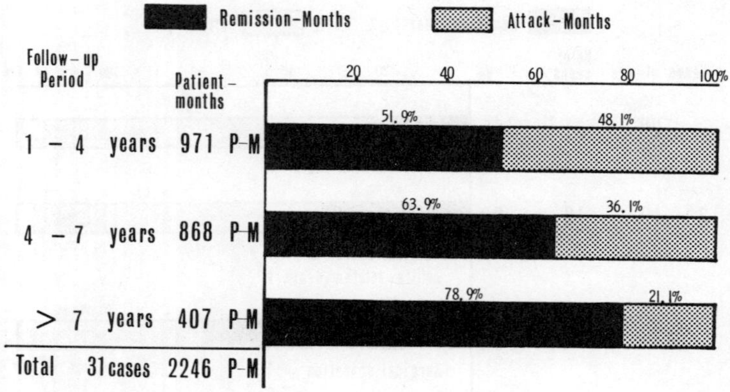

FIG. 10. Relation of follow-up period to proportion of remission- and attack-months.

months was 51.9%. On the other hand, in the patients with observed follow-up of more than 7 years, 78.9% of the patient-months were spent in remission. There was a tendency that with increasing length of follow-up, the patient spent a more favorable course.

Discussion

The long-term course of ulcerative colitis was studied by the concept of patient-years according to Watts *et al.*,[9] and an analysis of 290 patient-years of 54 cases in which the course was known showed that remission-years were in 27.2% and attack-years in 72.8%. These results were much less favorable than those of Watts *et al.*[9] or Jalan *et al.*,[10] in which the attack-years were 44.3% of 1,324 patient-years, and 39.8% of 927 patient-years, respectively. As the method employed in this study was almost the same as that of Watts and Jalan, and two thirds of our patients received maintenance doses of SASP after induction into remission, the reason for the unfavorable course of our patients was not clear. When the course was studied by the concept of patient-months, the proportion of remission-months was 58.1%, suggesting that in our patients relapses occurred frequently, but the duration of attacks was relatively short.

Investigation of the factors influencing the long-term course showed that high severity and early onset of disease had a significantly unfavorable effect on the proportion of remission-years. On the other hand, the extent of involvement had little effect on the proportion of remission-years, a view in agreement with Watts *et al.*[9] However, all three colitis deaths were in patients with total involvement (severely ill in two patients and moderately severe in one patient), and one patient who received radical surgery had total involvement. Thus, it was strongly suggested that severity, extent of involvement, and age at onset were the major factors affecting the course and prognosis of ulcerative colitis. The adverse effects of severe attack and total colonic involvement on prognosis are well established by many authors.[11–13]

In this study, early onset had a pronounced effect on the course and outcome of this disease, probably because of greater incidence of severe attacks and extensive colonic involvement in the early onset group. On the other hand, patients with late onset above 50 years of age showed the most favorable course and outcome. Contrary to these results, European observations showed that patients with late onset or elderly patients over the age of 50 or 60 had high mortality rates.[11–13] According to Watts, in the late onset group or elderly patients, the incidence of total colonic involvement was significantly lower than that in young groups; however, the incidence of severe attacks was relatively high. Edwards and Truelove[11] attributed the high mortality of elderly patients to the fact that they did not survive colitis attacks as readily as the younger patients. The favorable course and outcome of late onset patients in this study were considered to be due to the absence of severe attacks.

When the course was analyzed according to the length of follow-up period, the proportion of remission-months increased with the increase in the length of follow-up. On the contrary, Gilat *et al.*[13] reported that with increasing length of follow-up, there was an increase in the severity of disease, and Watts *et al.*[9] reported that the prognosis of colitis was not affected by the duration of symptoms from the onset of colitis.

SUMMARY

1) Fifty-two inpatients were treated according to the therapeutic scheme presented in 1975 by the Japanese Ministry of Health and Welfare, Ulcerative Colitis Research Committee. In this scheme mild and moderately severe cases are treated initially with SASP alone, then local steroids are added, and if these are not effective, oral steroids are administered. Severe cases are treated with systemic steroids.

2) Forty-nine out of 52 cases went into remission following medical treatment.

3) In terms of the therapeutic regimens required to induce remission, about 30% of mild cases and 70% of moderately severe cases needed systemic steroids. In relation to the extent of involvement, patients who required systemic steroids increased with the progress of colonic involvement; and in patients with total colonic involvement, 55% of mild

attacks and 67% of moderately severe attacks required systemic steroids. It was suggested that in the choice of therapeutic regimens, extent of colonic involvement should be taken into consideration together with severity of symptoms.

4) From the above results, it was thought that in the treatment of moderately severe cases, or cases with total involvement, an earlier indication of systemic steroids would be desirable for early remission.

5) In several patients with poor responses to steroids, immunosuppressive drugs were effective.

6) Fifty-four patients were followed for 3 to 10 years. During the follow-up period, three patients died from colitis, one patient died from serum hepatitis, and two patients received surgical operations.

7) The long-term course was observed using the concept of patient-years. In about 73% of 290 patient-years one or more attacks occurred. The proportion of attack-years in this study was significantly greater compared with that of Watts or Jalan (44.3% and 39.8%, respectively).

8) Severe disease and early onset of disease had pronounced effects on the proportion of attack-years, and patients with mild attacks and cases with late onset spent a more favorable course. The extent of colonic involvement had little influence on the proportion of attack-years; however, as to the outcome of colitis, all three patients who died from colitis, and one patient who received radical surgery, had total colonic involvement.

It was concluded that severity, extent of involvement of disease, and age at onset were the major factors influencing the course and prognosis of colitis.

9) With the increase in length of follow-up, the proportion of remission-months increased; namely, from 52% in the cases with follow-up of less than 4 years to 79% in the cases with follow-up of more than 7 years.

REFERENCES

1. Intractable Disease Research Committee of Fukuoka Prefecture: Report of Epidemiological Study on the Intractable Diseases. Fukuoka Prefecture, 1980 (in Japanese).
2. Evans, J. G. and Acheson, E. D.: An epidemiological study of ulcerative colitis and regional colitis in the Oxford area. *Gut*, **6**: 311, 1965.
3. Sadlack, R. E., Nobrega, F. T., *et al.*: Inflammatory colon disease in Rochester, Minnesota, 1935-1964. *Gastroenterology*, **62**: 935, 1972.
4. Inoue, M.: Medical treatment of ulcerative colitis. In: Proceedings of the Ulcerative Colitis and Crohn's Disease Research Committee of the Japanese Ministry of Health and Welfare, 1975 (in Japanese).
5. Truelove, S. C. and Jewell, D. P.: Intensive intravenous regimen for severe attacks of ulcerative colitis. *Lancet,* **1**: 1067, 1974.

6. Lennard-Jones, J. E.: Observations on the treatment of colitis. *Schweiz. Med. Wschr.*, **101**: 701, 1971.
7. Roth, J. L. A.: Ulcerative colitis. In: Gastroenterology (ed. H. L. Bockus) Vol. II, p. 645. Saunders, Philadelphia, 1976.
8. Truelove, S. C.: The management of ulcerative colitis. *Brit. J. Clin. Practice*, **28**: 5, 1974.
9. Watts, J. McK., de Dombal, F. T., Watkinson, G., and Goligher, J. C.: Long-term prognosis of ulcerative colitis. *Brit. Med. J.*, **1**: 1447, 1966.
10. Jalan, K. N., Prescott, R. J., Sircus, W., *et al.*: An experience of ulcerative colitis. II. Short-term outcome. III. Long-term outcome. *Gastroenterology*, **59**: 589, 598, 1970.
11. Edwards, F. C. and Truelove, S. C.: The course and prognosis of ulcerative colitis. *Gut*, **4**: 299, 1963.
12. Watts, J. McK., de Dombal, F. T., Watkinson, G., and Goligher, J. C.: Early course of ulcerative colitis. *Gut*, **7**: 16, 1966.
13. Gilat, T., Lilos, P., Benaroya, Y., *et al.*: Risk factors in ulcerative colitis. *Digestion*, **14**: 400, 1976.

Studies on Blood Coagulation in Ulcerative Colitis and Crohn's Disease

Kazuo Mori, Nobuo Hiwatashi,* and Hikaru Watanabe***

Though there have been many papers concerning the thromboembolic complications of ulcerative colitis and Crohn's disease in foreign countries,[1-5] only a few reports have appeared in Japan.[6,7] The authors reported the first case in Japan in 1978 by an autopsy of a 32-year-old male patient with ulcerative colitis complicated with pulmonary thrombosis.[8] Thereafter Kobayashi *et al.* reported one similar case in 1978.[9] Since then the authors have undertaken studies on blood coagulation in cases of ulcerative colitis and Crohn's disease and found that a large number of cases were in a hypercoagulable state.[10]

This report focuses on the differences in blood coagulability between patients in the active stage and remission of the disease. Two cases of ulcerative colitis associated with disseminated intravascular coagulation syndrome (DIC) after emergency surgery are also presented.

SUBJECTS AND METHODS

The subjects consisted of 35 patients with ulcerative colitis and 19 patients with Crohn's disease. All 54 cases were hospitalized or treated as outpatients in the Third Department of Internal Medicine, Tohoku University Hospital or in the Sendai National Hospital. Twenty-seven of the ulcerative colitis patients had total colitis, seven left-sided colitis, and one proctocolitis. The disease was in active stage in 32 and in remission in 10 at the time of examination. All 19 cases of Crohn's disease were in active stage, and 3 of them were also examined at the stage of remission.

The following methods were used in determining the blood coagulability and platelet function of these patients: bleeding time (BT) (Duke's

*Third Department of Internal Medicine, Tohoku University School of Medicine, Sendai, Japan
**Division of Gastroenterology, Sendai National Hospital, Sendai, Japan

method), whole blood clotting time (CT) (Lee-White method), clot retraction (CR) (MacFarlane's method), capillary resistance (Cap-R) (positive pressure method), kaolin partial thromboplastin time (K-PTT) (Langdell's method), one-stage prothrombin time (PT) (Quick's method), fibrinogen content (Fbg) (thrombin time method), fibrin and fibrinogen degradation product (FDP) (latex particle agglutination method), platelet count (Plt-C) (direct method), clotting factor activity (factors II through XII) (one-stage method), platelet retention rate (Plt-ret) (Salzman's method), platelet factor 3 availability (PF-3) (Weiss's method). The platelet aggregation rate (Plt-aggre) was determined by means of an aggregation meter (Chrono-log, America) using ADP (at a final concentration of 1×10^{-6} M), collagen (at a final concentration of 5 μg/ml), and Ristocetin (at a final concentration of 1.3 mg/ml) as inducers, and the highest platelet aggregation rate was taken as representative.

Using the above methods, investigations were made on the changes in coagulability in these patients, referring to the criteria of functional increase and decrease given in Table 1.

TABLE 1. Criteria of Hypo- and Hyperfunction

	Hypofunction	Hyperfunction
BT (min.)	>7.0	<1.5
CT (min.)	>15.0	<5.0
CR (%)	>70	< 40
Cap-R	> 10	
K-PTT (sec.)	> 40.0	< 30.0
PT (%)	< 70	> 100
TT (%)	< 70	> 100
HT (%)	< 70	> 120
Fbg (mg/dl)	< 150	> 300
FDP (μg/ml)		> 10
STT-30 (sec.)		> 20.0
Plt. count ($\times 10^4$/mm^3)	< 15.0	> 30.0
Clotting factor activity II–XII (%)	< 70	> 120
Plt. aggregation rate (%)	< 30	> 70
Plt. retention rate (%)	< 25	> 40
PF-3	> CT of control	< CT of control

RESULTS

Coagulation screening tests

Active stage. The tests showed that BT, CT, CR, and Cap-R of the 32 active ulcerative colitis patients were within normal range (Table 2). PT activity was also within normal range in all patients, whereas K-PTT was

TABLE 2. Coagulation Screening Test (Active)

	Ulcerative colitis		Crohn's disease	
	Hypofunction	Hyperfunction	Hypofunction	Hyperfunction
BT	2/21 (9.5%)	0/21	3/10 (30.0%)	1/10 (10.0%)
CT	0/24	0/24	0/12	0/12
CR	0/24	4/24 (16.7%)	0/13	1/13 (7.7%)
Cap-R	3/17 (17.7%)		0/ 4	
K-PTT	12/32 (37.5%)	0/32	10/19 (52.0%)	1/19 (5.3%)
PT	0/32	0/32	1/19 (5.3%)	0/19
TT	7/32 (21.9%)	0/32	9/19 (47.4%)	6/19 (31.9%)
HT	0/32	23/32 (71.9%)	0/19	15/19 (78.9%)
Fbg	2/32 (6.3%)	7/32 (21.9%)	0/19	12/19 (63.2%)
FDP		6/32 (18.8%)		4/19 (31.5%)
STT-30		14/32 (43.8%)		5/20 (25.0%)
Plt. count	1/32 (3.1%)	22/32 (68.8%)	0/19	18/19 (94.7%)

slightly prolonged in 12 of 32 cases (37.5%). Seven patients (21.9%) showed slightly decreased TT activity, while 23 cases (71.9%) had increased HT activity greater than 120%. Fibrinogen content was below 150 mg/dl in 2 cases (6.3%) but above 300 mg/dl in 7 cases (21.9%). Mild increases in FDP (to 20 μg/ml) were seen in 6 cases (18.8%). STT-30 showed increased fibrinolysis in 14 of the 32 patients (43.8%). Platelet count was increased in 22 of 32 cases (68.8%). Except for one case of disseminated intravascular coagulation syndrome (DIC), there were no cases of platelet count less than $15 \times 10^4/mm^3$, indicating a definite tendency for platelet increase in ulcerative colitis.

Similar results were obtained in 10 cases of Crohn's disease, and the notable findings were a marked increase in platelet count (18 of the 19 cases, 94.7%), HT activity (15 of the 19 cases, 78.9%) and Fbg content (12 of the 19 cases, 63.2%).

Remission. At the time of remission, the hypercoagulability was generally normalized in 10 cases of ulcerative colitis and 3 cases of Crohn's disease, but HT, Plt-C, etc., still remained in the hypercoagulable state (Table 3).

Coagulation factor activities

Active stage. As shown in Table 4, factor VIII and IX activities of 13 active ulcerative colitis patients were found to be increased in 8 cases (61.5%) and 9 cases (69.2%), respectively (mean values were 117.7% and 193.7%, respectively), while factor XI activity was decreased in 12 (93.2%) of these cases (mean value was 36.0%). Five patients with Crohn's disease showed similar results. In addition, activities of factors II, V, VII, X, and XII were also increased in some cases.

TABLE 3. Coagulation Screening Test (Remission)

	Ulcerative colitis		Crohn's disease	
	Hypofunction	Hyperfunction	Hypofunction	Hyperfunction
BT	3/6 (50.0%)	0/5	0/1	0/1
CT	0/5	0/5	0/2	0/2
CR	0/4	0/4	1/1 (100.0%)	0/1
Cap-R	1/4 (25.0%)	——	0/1	
K-PTT	1/10 (10.0%)	1/10 (10.0%)	1/3 (33.3%)	0/3
PT	0/10	0/10	0/3	0/3
TT	1/10 (10.0%)	2/10 (20.0%)	0/2	0/2
HT	0/10	9/10 (90.0%)	0/3	2/3 (66.7%)
Fbg	1/10 (10.0%)	2/10 (20.0%)	0/3	0/3
FDP	——	1/10 (10.0%)	——	2/3 (66.7%)
STT-30	——	3/10 (30.0%)	——	0/5
Plt. count	0/10	5/10 (50.0%)	0/4	3/4 (75.0%)

TABLE 4. Clotting Factor Activity (Active)

	Ulcerative colitis		Crohn's disease	
	Hypofunction	Hyperfunction	Hypofunction	Hyperfunction
II	1/13 (7.7%)	4/13 (30.8%)	0/5	2/5 (40.0%)
V	2/13 (15.4%)	1/13 (7.7%)	0/5	2/5 (40.0%)
VII	6/13 (46.2%)	1/13 (7.7%)	1/5 (20.0%)	2/5 (40.0%)
VIII	3/13 (23.1%)	8/13 (61.5%)	1/5 (20.0%)	3/5 (60.0%)
IX	3/13 (23.1%)	9/13 (69.2%)	1/5 (20.0%)	4/5 (80.0%)
X	2/13 (15.4%)	0/13	0/5	3/5 (60.0%)
XI	12/31 (92.3%)	0/13	4/5 (80.0%)	0/5
XII	3/13 (23.1%)	4/13 (30.8%)	0/5	2/5 (40.0%)

Remission. The activities of coagulation factors in three cases of ulcerative colitis indicated a tendency to hypercoagulability (Table 5). None of the Crohn's disease patients were examined at this stage.

TABLE 5. Clotting Factor Activity (Remission)

	Ulcerative colitis	
	Hypofunction	Hyperfunction
II	0/3	0/3
V	0/3	1/3 (33.3%)
VII	0/3	0/3
VIII	0/3	2/3 (66.7%)
IX	0/3	1/3 (33.3%)
X	0/3	1/3 (33.3%)
XI	1/3 (33.3%)	0/3
XII	0/3	1/3 (33.3%)

Platelet functions

Active stage. With regard to platelet function, neither major changes in BT, Cap-R, and CR nor decreases in platelet count were seen, except for one case associated with DIC syndrome (Table 6). On the contrary, 22 of the 32 active ulcerative colitis patients showed an increase in platelet count (68.8%). Only 1 of 26 ulcerative colitis patients examined showed a decrease in collagen- and Ristocetin-induced platelet aggregation; rather an increased rate in platelet aggregation in many cases and an increase in platelet retention rate in 20 of 21 patients (95.2%) were seen.

TABLE 6. Platelet Function Test (Active)

	Ulcerative colitis		Crohn's disease	
	Hypofunction	Hyperfunction	Hypofunction	Hyperfunction
BT	2/21 (9.5%)	0/21	3/10 (30.0%)	1/10 (10.0%)
CR	0/24	4/24 (16.7%)	0/13	1/13 (7.7%)
Cap-R	3/17 (17.7%)	—	0/9	—
Plt. count	1/32 (3.1%)	22/32 (68.8%)	0/19	18/19 (94.7%)
Plt. aggregation rate				
ADP (1×10^{-6} M)	0/28	16/28 (57.1%)	0/18	15/18 (83.3%)
Collagen (5 μg/ml)	1/26 (3.9%)	16/26 (61.5%)	0/16	11/16 (68.8%)
Ristocetin (1.3 mg/ml)	1/25 (4.0%)	13/25 (52.0%)	0/17	14/17 (82.3%)
Plt. retention rate	0/21	20/21 (95.2%)	1/18 (5.6%)	15/18 (83.3%)
PF-3			1/2 (50.0%)	0/2

Similar results were also obtained in Crohn's disease patients. Increased platelet count in 18 of 19 patients (94.7%), accelerated platelet aggregation rate induced by ADP, collagen, and Ristocetin, in 15 of 18 (83.3%), 11 of 16 (68.8%), and 14 of 17 (82.3%) cases, respectively, and accelerated platelet retention rate in 15 of 18 cases (83.3%) were recognized. There was no decrease in platelet count or platelet aggregation rate, but one case showed a slight decrease in platelet retention rate.

Remission. As shown in Table 7, the number of cases with hyperactivities of the platelet functions generally decreased at the stage of remission rather than at the active stage in ulcerative colitis. However, platelet count was found to be increased in 5 of 10 ulcerative colitis patients; accelerated platelet aggregation rate induced by ADP, collagen, and Ristocetin was found in 2 of 8, 3 of 7, and 2 of 7 cases, respectively; and accelerated platelet retention rate was observed in 6 of 7 cases. Decreases in ADP- and collagen-induced platelet aggregation rates were statistically significant ($p<0.01$ and $p<0.05$, respectively).

Similar results were also obtained in Crohn's disease patients.

TABLE 7. Platelet Function Test (Remission)

	Ulcerative colitis		Crohn's disease	
	Hypofunction	Hyperfunction	Hypofunction	Hyperfunction
BT	3/6 (50.0%)	0/5	0/1	0/1
CR	0/4	0/4	1/1 (100.0%)	0/1
Cap-R	4/4 (100.0%)		0/1	
Plt. count	0/10	5/10 (50.0%)	0/4	3/4 (75.0%)
Plt. aggregation rate				
ADP	1/8 (12.5%)	2/8 (25.0%)	0/3	1/3 (33.3%)
Collagen	0/7	3/7 (42.9%)	0/3	3/3 (100.0%)
Ristocetin	0/7	2/7 (28.6%)	0/1	1/1 (100.0%)
Plt. retention rate	0/7	6/7 (85.7%)	0/3	2(3 (66.7%)
PF-3				

Statistical analysis on the mean values between two groups

The mean values of the hemostatic tests were as follows: increased HT, factor VIII and IX activities; decreased factor XI activity; increased number of platelets; and accelerated platelet aggregation and retention

TABLE 8. Means and Standard Deviations of Hemostatic Test (Active)

	Ulcerative colitis		Crohn's disease	
BT (min.)	5.1 ± 1.6	(n = 21)	5.4 ± 1.7	(n = 10)
CT (min.)	6.9 ± 1.2	(n = 24)	6.6 ± 1.2	(n = 12)
CR (%)	44.7 ± 8.0	(n = 24)	46.0 ± 7.7	(n = 13)
Cap-R	normal	(n = 13)	normal	(n = 7)
K-PTT (sec.)	37.4 ± 5.3	(n = 32)	39.5 ± 6.0	(n = 19)
PT (%)	92.1 ± 8.5	(n = 32)	90.4 ± 11.2	(n = 19)
TT (%)	85.4 ± 17.7	(n = 32)	78.0 ± 21.1	(n = 19)
HT (%)	138.5 ± 39.7	(n = 32)	136.2 ± 30.9	(n = 19)
Fbg (mg/dl)	258.8 ± 70.0	(n = 32)	361.2 ± 35.6	(n = 19)
STT-30 (sec.)	21.5 ± 9.6	(n = 32)	18.7 ± 7.0	(n = 20)
FDP (μg/ml)	9.8 ± 7.8	(n = 32)	6.1 ± 2.1	(n = 19)
Clotting factor II (%)	101.0 ± 29.1	(n = 13)	123.2 ± 37.3	(n = 5)
V (%)	81.2 ± 32.4	(n = 13)	132.0 ± 38.2	(n = 5)
VII (%)	76.9 ± 26.0	(n = 13)	109.4 ± 35.9	(n = 5)
VIII (%)	177.7 ± 116.0	(n = 13)	143.0 ± 62.4	(n = 5)
IX (%)	193.7 ± 127.1	(n = 13)	153.6 ± 109.3	(n = 5)
X (%)	89.5 ± 14.5	(n = 13)	131.0 ± 28.8	(n = 5)
XI (%)	36.0 ± 17.9	(n = 13)	51.0 ± 30.7	(n = 5)
XII (%)	110.1 ± 63.1	(n = 13)	115.4 ± 55.9	(n = 5)
Plt. count (× 10^4/mm^3)	36.4 ± 12.0	(n = 32)	52.9 ± 25.6	(n = 19)
Plt. aggregation rate (%)				
ADP (1 × 10^{-6} M)	69.9 ± 12.2	(n = 28)	78.0 ± 9.0	(n = 18)
Collagen (5 μg/ml)	71.5 ± 12.2	(n = 25)	63.8 ± 11.0	(n = 16)
Ristocetin (1.3 mg/ml)	67.9 ± 20.3	(n = 25)	79.7 ± 9.9	(n = 17)
Plt. retention rate (%)	58.8 ± 16.2	(n = 21)	56.9 ± 17.5	(n = 18)

TABLE 9. Means and Standard Deviations of Hemostatic Test (Remission)

	Ulcerative colitis		Crohn's disease	
BT (min.)	6.3 ± 2.0	(n = 5)	3.5	(n = 1)
CT (min.)	6.2 ± 0.5	(n = 5)	6.5	(n = 1)
CR (%)	42.0 ± 2.8	(n = 4)	32.0	(n = 1)
Cap-R	normal		normal	
K-PTT (sec.)	35.6 ± 4.6	(n = 10)	39.0 ± 3.5	(n = 3)
PT (%)	97.7 ± 3.6	(n = 10)	99.0 ± 1.7	(n = 3)
TT (%)	90.9 ± 13.2	(n = 10)	83.0 ± 18.4	(n = 2)
HT (%)	148.6 ± 20.5	(n = 10)	94.7 ± 20.2	(n = 3)
Fbg (mg/dl)	235.9 ± 94.4	(n = 10)	212.0 ± 47.0	(n = 3)
STT-30 (sec.)	18.1 ± 4.1	(n = 10)	13.9 ± 1.2	(n = 3)
FDP (μg/ml)	7.5 ± 4.9	(n = 10)	8.3 ± 2.9	(n = 3)
Clotting factor II (%)	105.7 ± 17.2	(n = 3)		
V (%)	123.3 ± 25.2	(n = 3)		
VII (%)	87.3 ± 10.3	(n = 3)		
VIII (%)	135.7 ± 10.3	(n = 3)		
IX (%)	118.3 ± 27.5	(n = 3)		
X (%)	113.3 ± 23.1	(n = 3)		
XI (%)	65.7 ± 11.2	(n = 3)		
XII (%)	117.7 ± 41.0	(n = 3)		
Plt. count (× 10^4/mm^3)	32.0 ± 15.8	(n = 11)	35.9 ± 10.3	(n = 4)
Plt. aggregation rate (%)				
ADP (1 × 10^{-6} M)	54.7 ± 16.7	(n = 8)	69.6 ± 7.5	(n = 3)
Collagen (5 μg/ml)	60.8 ± 12.8	(n = 8)	75.9 ± 6.9	(n = 3)
Ristocetin (1.3 mg/ml)	65.6 ± 12.9	(n = 7)	80.0	(n = 1)
Plt. retention rate (%)	64.2 ± 18.1	(n = 8)	54.2 ± 24.8	(n = 3)

rates. At the stage of remission, these hyper- or hypofunctions were generally normalized in many cases, but some still showed a tendency of hyperfunction. In these hemostatic tests, increases in activities of PT and platelet aggregation rate induced by ADP and collagen and the decrease in factor XI activity were statistically significant ($p<0.05$, $p<0.01$, $p<0.05$, $p<0.05$, respectively) between the active stage and the stage of remission in ulcerative colitis patients (Tables 8 and 9).

CASE REPORTS

Case 1. 46-year-old male

Present illness. He noticed lower abdominal pain together with bloody diarrhea and fever in October 1981. He was admitted to the Department of Gastroenterology of Sendai National Hospital on November 30, 1981.

Laboratory examinations. Urinalysis was normal, but fecal occult blood reaction was strongly positive. Blood sedimentation rate was markedly decreased: 1 mm in 1 hr and 4 mm in 2 hr. Slight impairment in liver function tests, but no abnormalities in renal function tests were observed. Hemostatic tests revealed no abnormalities without an increase in platelet count; there were no accompanying signs of disseminated intravascular coagulation (DIC) syndrome at this time.

Clinical course. The patient's clinical course is illustrated in Fig. 1. After admission, elementary diet (ED), 2,400 kcal/day, was given. Administration of 0.1% prednisolone oil 30 ml/day per anus and prednisolone 40 mg/day intravenously were also given. However, he continued to have diarrhea 5–7 times a day throughout November and the diarrhea became more frequent from the middle of December. At that time, there were no major changes in the hemostatic tests, and no signs suggestive of DIC syndrome were seen.

After colectomy, a decrease in platelet count ($33.3 \times 10^4/mm^3$) and fibrinogen content (110 mg/dl) and an increase in FDP, etc., were noticed. The developement of DIC syndrome was considered. Thereafter, platelet count rapidly and continously decreased to $4.3 \times 10^4/mm^3$; prothrombin time and Thrombotest activities also decreased to 47% and 43% of normal, respectively, but in contrast, fibrinogen content increased from 110 to 425 mg/dl.

The diagnosis of DIC syndrome was confirmed and intravenous administration of fresh blood (total 11,400 ml), fibrinogen concentrate (total 11 g), and FOY (600 mg/day, anticoagulant, Ono Chemicals, Japan) was begun. Platelet count gradually normalized two weeks later and intravenous administration of FOY was discontinued. Six days later, however, he developed hematemesis and tarry stool, and finally died of renal failure.

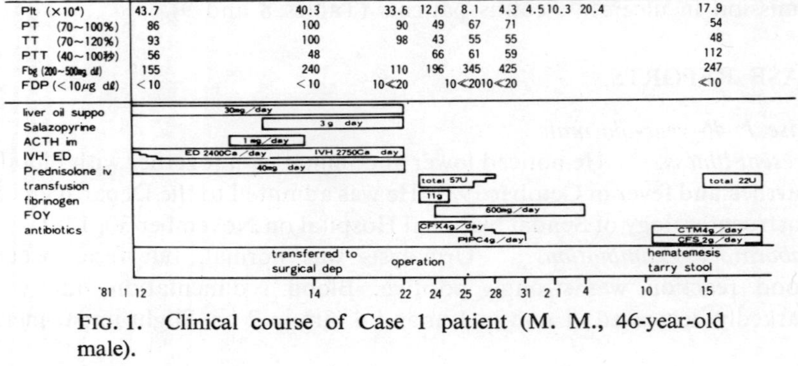

FIG. 1. Clinical course of Case 1 patient (M. M., 46-year-old male).

Case 2. 27-year-old male

Present illness. He had bloody diarrhea with lower abdominal pain and was diagnosed as ulcerative colitis at the age of 15. He had received rectal resection at that time. At the age of 17, he relapsed but improved with medication. In May 1981, he again developed bloody diarrhea with toxic megacolon. He was admitted to the Department of Gastroenterology of Sendai National Hosptial on May 19, 1981.

Laboratory examinations. Urinalysis was normal, but fecal occult blood reaction was positive. His increased blood sedimentation rate was 63 mm in 1 hr and 96 mm in 2 hr. There was slight impairment of liver function, but no abnormalities of serum protein or electrolytes were seen. Hemostatic tests revealed no abnormalities, and no signs of accompanying DIC syndrome were found at that time.

Clinical course. The patient's clinical course is illustrated in Fig. 2. Immediately after admission, administration of 0.1% prednisolone oil directly into the bowel, ACTH 1 mg/day intramuscularly, and prednisolone 40 mg/day intravenously were instituted. Nevertheless, he continued to have diarrhea 2–6 times/day and gradually became febrile. Two weeks after admission, his platelet count decreased to $15.5 \times 10^4/mm^3$ and sigmoidectomy was performed. After operation, the fibrinogen content decreased to 102 mg/dl. Prothrombin time and Thrombotest activities also

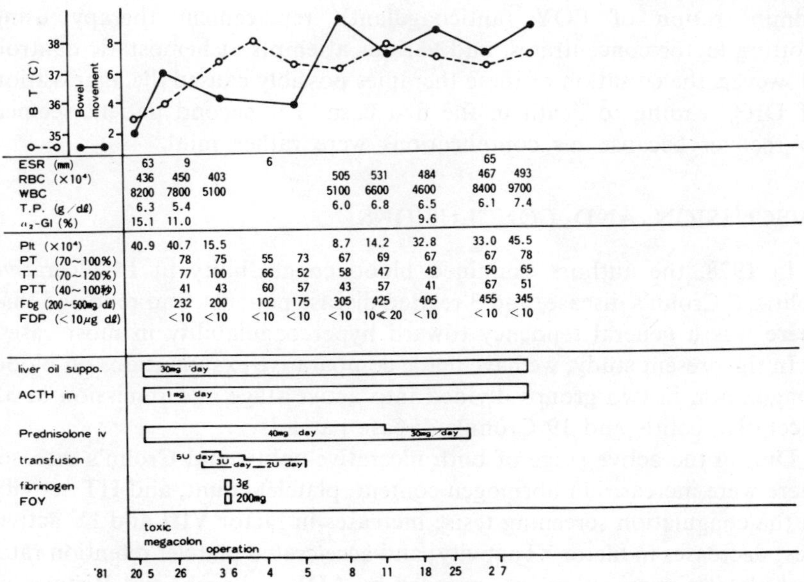

FIG. 2. Clinical course of Case 2 patient (C. H., 27-year-old male).

decreased to 55% and 66% of normal, respectively, and there was a tendency toward prolongation of partial thromboplastin time.

Blood transfusion was instituted from three days before operation and 3 g of fibrinogen concentrate and 200 mg of FOY were given intravenously after operation. Platelet count gradually rose to $8.9 \times 10^4/mm^3$ on the fifth day and $14.2 \times 10^4/mm^3$ on the eighth day after operation. Fibrinogen content increased from a minimum of 102 mg/dl to normal, and abnormalities of prothrombin time and partial thromboplastin time were also normalized.

Of marked interest is that the blood sedimentation rate was increased (63 mm in 1 hr) immediately after admission, whereas it returned to normal (6–9 mm in 1 hr) after operation. At that time, the patient's general condition was serious, with accompanying DIC syndrome.

DIC syndrome in IBD patients

Our findings on investigations of blood coagulation in ulcerative colitis, including the above-mentioned case reports, indicate that hypercoagulability in ulcerative colitis patients is thought to indicate a pre-DIC state, and patients often develop DIC syndrome from surgical operation or other factors.

It is apparent that these two cases developed DIC syndrome after abdominal operation. Improvements in clinical features and blood coagulation abnormalities were achieved in these two cases by intravenous administration of FOY (anticoagulant), replacement therapy using clotting factor concentrates, and various attempts at hemostatic control. However, the cessation of these therapies possibly caused the aggravation of DIC, leading to death in the first case. The second patient seemed to recover because his complications were rather mild.

DISCUSSION AND CONCLUSIONS

In 1978, the authors examined blood coagulability in 14 ulcerative colitis, 5 Crohn's disease, and 3 related disease patients, and reported that there was a general tendency toward hypercoagulability in most cases.

In the present study, we have made comparative examinations on blood coagulation in two groups divided into active stage and remission in 35 ulcerative colitis and 19 Crohn's disease patients.

During the active stage of both ulcerative colitis and Crohn's disease, there were increases in fibrinogen content, platelet count, and HT activity in the coagulation screening tests; increases in factor VIII and IX activities; decreases in factor XI activity; and accelerated platelet retention rate, and platelet aggregation rate induced by ADP, collagen, and Ristocetin.

Although a few cases showed hypocoagulability, a definite tendency to hypercoagulability was seen in most cases. During the stage of remission, this hyper- (partly hypo-) coagulability was generally normalized, but many cases still showed a tendency to hypercoagulability. Considering the aspects of blood coagulability, these findings suggest that some cases still have active alterations in the bowel during the clinical stage of remission.

From these results, the following conclusions can be drawn:

1) Most cases of ulcerative colitis and Crohn's disease showed definite signs of hypercoagulability during the active stage. During remission, this hypercoagulability was generally normalized, but many cases remained slightly abnormal. This hypercoagulability may cause thromboembolic complications even during the clinical stage of remission.

2) From the fact that hypercoagulability is an aspect hitherto unknown, blood coagulation study offers very important information concerning severity, prognosis, and surgical indication in these diseases.

3) When marked hypercoagulability and disseminated intravascular coagulation (DIC) syndrome are present, the therapeutic program for ulcerative colitis and Crohn's disease must include anticoagulant therapy (oral anticoagulants, heparin, and/or suppressants of platelet function) in order to achieve favorable effects.

REFERENCES

1. Bargen, J. A. and Barker, N. W.: Extensive arterial and venous thrombosis complicating chronic ulcerative colitis. *Arch. intern. Med.* (Chicago), **58**: 17–31, 1936.
2. Dennis, C. and Karlson, K. E.: Surgical measures as supplements to the management of idiopathic ulcerative colitis. *Surgery*, **32**: 892–912, 1952.
3. Edwards, F. C. and Truelove, S. C.: The course and prognosis of ulcerative colitis. III. Complication. *Gut*, **5**: 1–15, 1964.
4. Sloan, W. P., Bargen, J. A., and Gage, R. P.: Life histories of patients with chronic ulcerative colitis: a review of 2,000 cases. *Gastroenterology*, **16**: 25–38, 1950.
5. Graef, V., Baggenstoss, A. H., Sauer, W. G., and Spittel, J. A.: Venous thrombosis occurring in nonspecific ulcerative colitis: a necropsy study. *Arch. intern. Med.* (Chicago), **117**: 377–382, 1966.
6. Yoshida, Y., Tajima, T., Kuroe, S., Higuchi, K., Aizawa, N., Chiba, M., Kaneshiro, F., and Matsunaga, F.: Ulcerative colitis. *Jap. J. clin. Med.*, **32**: 2121–2128, 1974 (in Japanese).
7. Watanabe, H., Hiwatashi, N., and Yamagata, S.: Clinical observations on ulcerative colitis. *Tohoku J. exp. Med.*, **123**: 197–213, 1977.
8. Kawamura, T., Mori, K., Watanabe, H., Goto, Y., Kokubo, T., Oguma,

S., and Okabe, H.: An autopsy case of ulcerative colitis-associated pulmonary thrombosis. *Igakuno Ayumi,* **14**: 208–213, 1978 (in Japanese).
9. Kobayashi, J., Arakawa, T., Kamata, T., Hino, K., Yui, S., Okuno, T., Sowa, Y., and Kawashima, M.: Ulcerative colitis and blood coagulation and fibrinolytic system. *Jap. J. Gastroenterol.*, **75**: 232–235, 1978 (in Japanese).
10. Mori, K., Watanabe, H., Sakai, H., Suzuki, S., and Goto, Y.: Studies on blood coagulation in ulcerative colitis and Crohn's disease. *J. Therapy*, **61**: 1307–1314, 1978 (in Japanese).

Intra-Arterial Administration of Steroids for Severe Ulcerative Colitis

Shozo Baba, Masahisa Motegi,** Satoru Morioka,* and Kenji Mizutani**

INTRODUCTION

Ulcerative colitis is primarily a benign disease; however, the mortality rate is still high when operated on during the severe attack phase.

According to a collective review done in Japan by Shiratori[1] the mortality rate in emergency operations was 33% in comparison with 6% for elective surgery. Goligher reported similar results.[2] The reasons for such a high mortality are various: malnutrition, large doses of steroid administration for a long duration, the stress of a major operation, etc.

Various attempts have recently been made to eliminate emergency operations as far as possible: e.g., hyperalimentation, elemental diet, intensive intravenous regimens,[3] ascendicostomy,[4] ileostomy–colostomy procedure,[5] etc. With the same purpose of overcoming acute exacerbation, we tried to inject water-soluble prednisolone directly into the mesenteric arteries of severe ulcerative colitis patients.

METHODS AND MATERIALS

According to the Seldinger method, Cook's green catheter was inserted through the femoral artery and routine mesenteric arteriography was taken. After mesenteric angiography, the extent of the lesion was determined, and water-soluble prednisolone was injected through the same catheter. The dosage of prednisolone was 10 to 30 mg into the inferior and/or superior mesenteric artery, depending upon the severity and extent of the lesion.

We have treated 28 cases with 35 steroid injections. By sending questionnaires to collaborating hospitals, 18 cases which were treated in a similar manner were collected. Furthermore, 10 cases were collected from published reports. Analysis was based upon these 56 cases.

---

*Second Department of Surgery, Hamamatsu Medical College, Hamamatsu, Japan
**Division of Gastroenterology, Kanagawa Saiseikai Hospital, Yokohama, Japan

The age distribution ranged from 11 to 71, and the sex ratio was 35 to 21 (male to female). Severity was determined by the criteria of Truelove and others. Among the treated cases, there were 35 severe cases, 5 fulminant cases, and 9 moderate cases. The rest of the cases were excluded because of inadequate documentation.

The efficacy of the treatment was determined not only by subjective symptoms such as the frequency of bowel movement or bloody discharge, but also by objective symptoms such as fever, leucocyte count, Hb, ESR, serum protein, Gordon test if hypoproteinemia was present, and fluoroscopic and endoscopic examinations including biopsy. Patients were kept under close observation for three days to evaluate the efficacy of treatment. In cases in which treatment was ineffective, operations were promptly scheduled. Infusion, transfusion, and other supportive therapies were carried out in most of the cases.

RESULTS

In terms of subjective symptoms, remarkable improvement was seen in bowel movement. Improvement of diarrhea was seen in 85% and a decrease in bloody discharge was seen in 71% of cases. When the therapy was effective, the diarrhea stopped and abdominal pain disappeared within a few hours after injection. Decreases in pulse rate and subsidence of fever were seen in most of the cases. Improvement in ESR was also seen, except for three occasions.

Sixteen cases showed hypoproteinemia under a level of 6.5 g/dl. After the injection therapy, 72% of cases with hypoproteinemia showed remarkable improvement. Notably, the value of serum protein of two cases was as low as 4.8 g/dl and 5.4 g/dl. At this time, the leakage of serum protein was measured by the Gordon test, using ^{131}I-PVP. The leakage of plasma protein was proved in both cases, revealing values of 3.0% (control 0–1.5%) and 1.6% (control 0–1.5%), respectively. After the intra-arterial steroid injection therapy, leakage of plasma protein improved significantly, and serum protein rose to 6.6 g/dl and 7.4 g/dl, respectively. At this point, the Gordon test returned to normal.

A comparison of endoscopic examinations was made before and after intra-arterial injection in 26 cases (Fig. 1). Improvement was seen in 15 cases (57.7%). Seven cases did not show any improvement. The other four cases were difficult to evaluate because of poor descriptions.

Overall response rate in our series, which was calculated by various scoring parameters (Table 1), was 69.2%. Response rate for the initial severe attack reached as high as 80%. Because fluoroscopic examination

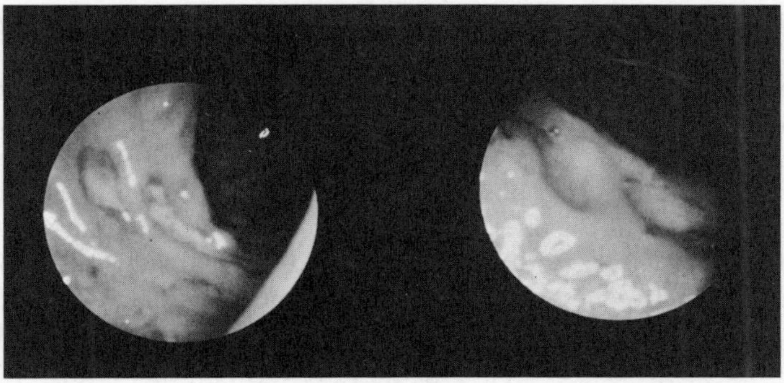

FIG. 1. Endoscopic examination before (left) and after (right) intra-arterial steroid injection.

TABLE 1. Disease Activity Parameters

			Score
Clinical signs and symptoms:	Diarrhea	1–2	0
		3–5	1
		6–10	2
		10–	3
	Blood in stool	occult (−)	0
		(+)	1
		macroscopic (+)	2
	Fever	−37.5° C	0
		37.5–39.0° C	1
		39.0° C–	2
	Abdominal pain	(−)	0
		(+)	1
	Tachycardia	< 100/min	0
		≧ 100/min	1
Laboratory data:	ESR	< 30 mm/hr	0
		≧ 30 mm/hr	1
	Leukocytosis	< 10,000/mm³	0
		≧ 10,000/mm³	1
	Hemoglobin	> 12 g/dl	0
		10–12 g/dl	1
		< 10 g/dl	2
	Albumin	> 3.5 g/dl	0
		< 3.5 g/dl	1
	α_2-Globulin	< 0.8 g/dl	0
		≧ 0.8 g/dl	1

Evaluation of intra-arterial PSL injection therapy
- Markedly effective = decrease in score ≧ 6
- Effective 2–5
- Ineffective 0–1

may aggravate the symptoms in very severe cases, we estimated the extent and severity of the lesions by angiography in such cases.

Analysis was made of selective mesenteric angiographic findings in 22 cases of ulcerative colitis. Loss of normal tapering of the vasa recta was seen in all cases, increase of capillary blush was seen in 20 cases, and early venous filling was observed in 9 cases. Also in these cases, the average diameter of the inferior mesenteric artery was 5.6 mm, which was greater in comparison with the 3.8 mm in 20 normal subjects. In 4 cases, successive selective mesenteric angiography and injections were performed twice during the attack; and improvement in early venous drainage was noted in 3 cases. In the first angiograph, tortuosity and loss of normal tapering of the vasa recta and early venous filling were observed; however, one month after intra-arterial injection, the angiographic picture showed improvements such as the limitation of the lesion in the rectum and the disappearance of early venous drainage. Incidentally, complete remission was seen in this case after the three serial intra-arterial injections, and body weight increased by 10 kg. Follow-up has consisted of administering salazosulfapyridine on and off, and no sign of relapse has been noted for the past 10 years.

Only one case which was treated from the very beginning of the initial attack showed restored haustration in the fluoroscopic examination (Fig. 2); however, no marked improvement was seen in lead pipe pattern in the rest of the treated cases.

We have treated three cases of toxic megacolon (Fig. 3). Two of them re-

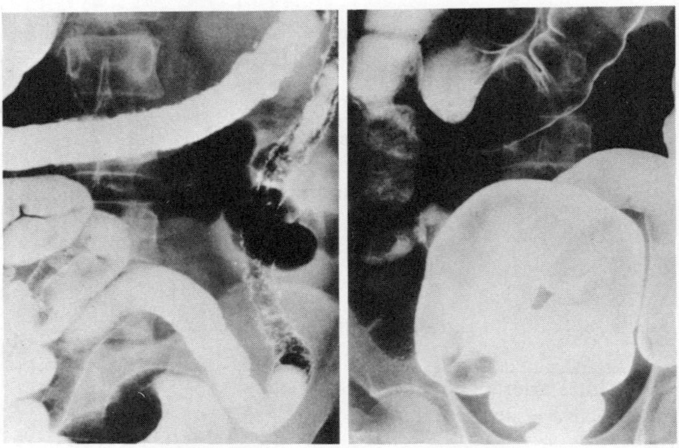

FIG. 2. Left, before treatment; right, after treatment.

sponded to the intra-arterial steroid injection therapy. The response rate was thus 66.7%.

One patient with toxic megacolon (30-year-old male) responded dramatically (Fig. 4). He was febrile (39.0° C) and became toxic despite the administration of a high dosage of oral steroid and steroid enema. The day after the respective intra-arterial injections of 10 mg and 20 mg prednisolone into the inferior and superior mesenteric artery, his temperature tended to become normal and bowel movements of 10 times a day decreased to less than 3 times a day. Bloody stool disappeared one week post-injection. By one month later, he had regained his weight and his hypoproteinemia had also improved; however, two years later, the patient developed severe exacerbation which necessitated surgery. All the toxic megacolon cases had been operated on by the second or third attack of the long-term follow-up; therefore, it is advisable to perform surgery during the remission period obtained by intra-arterial injection therapy.

Two cases underwent emergency surgery because of the ineffectiveness of intra-arterial injection therapy. In six other cases, the patients showed recurrences which did not respond to the second intra-arterial injection and underwent surgery. The remaining 20 cases in which intra-arterial therapy was carried out have been followed up and controlled by routine

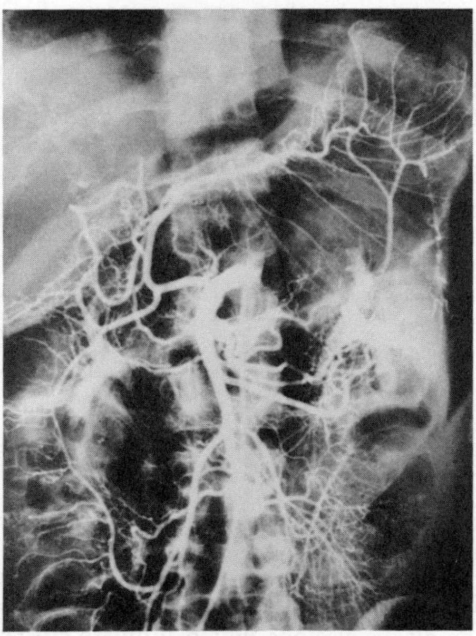

FIG. 3.

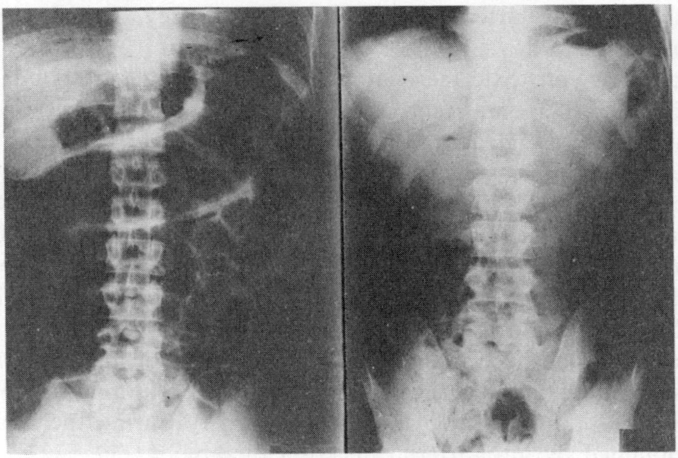

FIG. 4. Left, before treatment; right, after treatment.

medical treatment without operation. The longest follow-up is now 11 years.

Analysis was also made by adding the 28 collected cases from collaborating hospitals and published reports.[6-8] The overall response rate was 67.3%. For initial attacks, the response rate was 81.3%; it was 65.2% for relapse and remission cases, and 40% for the chronic continuous type (Table 2). The extent of lesion does not show much difference as far as response rate is concerned.

TABLE 2. Response to Intra-Arterial Steroid Injection

Type of ulcerative colitis	Response			No. of subjects	Efficacy ratio
	Very effective	Effective	Ineffective		
Initial attack	5	8	3	16	81.3%
Relapse and remission	3	12	8	23	65.2%
Chronic continuous	0	2	3	5	40.0%
Acute fulminant	1	2	2	5	60.0%
(Unknown	0	7	0	7)	

DISCUSSION

Severe ulcerative colitis has been treated both medically[9] and surgically. There are many discussions which indicate surgery for emergency patients. Our report indicates that more than two thirds of severe ulcerative colitis patients may respond to this trigger treatment and overcome the critical period. Elective surgery can thus be followed more safely. Perforation is a contraindication for intra-arterial steroid injection therapy. Therefore, when treating toxic megacolon cases, frequent monitoring of the patient is essential. If there is any sign of progress in the disease, immediate operative procedures should be considered.

The effectiveness of this trigger treatment is short acting; therefore, when a patient overcomes the critical stage, regular supportive therapy, including oral steroids, or an additional second injection a week later might be necessary. The possible defects of this method are: 1) it requires special techniques and expertise in selective angiography; and 2) there is the possibility of developing thrombosis when the patient is in a hypercoagulable state; however, up to the present, such a complication has not been experienced in our series.

The pharmacological activity of steroids on ulcerative colitis is not clearly understood. In ulcerative colitis, Bacaner[10] observed a decrease in mucosal blood flow, inferring the possibility of the presence of arteriovenous shunting. In fact, early venous drainage can be observed frequently by selective angiogram. We performed microangiography of the resected specimens of the colon in ulcerative colitis cases and found the abnormalities in mucosal vascular architecture. Relative mucosal ischemia might thus be contributing to the pathophysiology of ulcerative colitis. Recent reports show the participation of vasoactive substances, such as prostaglandin,[11] bradykinin, histamine, etc., in the development of severe ulcerative colitis.

In terms of the functioning mechanism in the effectiveness of this intra-arterial steroid injection method, the following possibilities can be considered: 1) it works as lysosomal stabilizer of colonic epithelial cells against mucosal ischemia; and 2) it is useful for the improvement of microcirculation. If the normalization of vasomotion is carried out by injecting steroid directly into the mesenteric arteries early in the course of the disease, before irreversible changes have occurred in the colon, it may prove of value.

SUMMARY

After taking selective mesenteric angiograms, intra-arterial injections of water-soluble prednisolone were administered selectively into mesenteric arteries of patients with severe ulcerative colitis. The efficacy of the treatment was evaluated not only by subjective symptoms, but also by such objective signs as fever, serum protein, Gordon test, and fluoroscopic and endoscopic examinations.

The overall response rate of severe ulcerative colitis patients in our series was 69.2%. For initial attack it was 80.0%. Two out of three toxic megacolon cases were successfully treated. Results from other institutions, collected by sending questionnaires, were similar. Patients should be carefully observed, and if there is no response, immediate operative procedures should be considered.

REFERENCES

1. Shiratori, T., *et al.*: Report on Inflammatory Bowel Disease by the Research Group Supported by Ministry of Health and Welfare, 1976.
2. Goligher, J. C., *et al.*: Ulcerative Colitis, 2nd ed. Bailliere, Tindall & Cassell, London, 1968.
3. Truelove, S. C., *et al.*: Intensive intravenous regimen for severe attacks of ulcerative colitis. *Lancet,* **1**: 1067–1070, 1974.
4. Shiratori, T., *et al.*: Ulcerative colitis. *Gekachiryo*, **33(1)**: 46–51, 1975 (in Japanese).
5. Turnbull, R. B., *et al.*: Surgical treatment of toxic megacolon; Ileostomy and colostomy to prepare patients for colectomy. *Am. J. Surg*., **122**: 325–331, 1971.
6. Yamagata, J., *et al.*: A case report of severe ulcerative colitis treated by one shot intraarterial therapy of steroid with remarkable result. *J. Jap. Soc. Coloproct*., **30(5)**: 451, 1977.
7. Osawa, N., *et al.*: Several trials of selective intraarterial therapy in our clinic. *J. Jap. Pract. Surg. Soc.,* **39(1)**: 124–129, 1978.
8. Suzuki, K. and Yokouchi, A.: Pharmacology and clinic with special reference to ulcerative colitis. *Shindan to Chiryo*, **65(1)**: 40–46, 1977 (in Japanese).
9. Norlard, C. C. and Kirsner, J. B.: Toxic dilatation of colon etiology, treatment and prognosis in 42 patients. *Medicine*, **48**: 229-250, 1969.
10. Bacaner, B. M.: Quantitative measurement of regional colon blood flow in the normal and pathological human bowel. *Gastroenterology*, **51**: 764–777, 1966.
11. Sharon, P., *et al.*: Role of prostaglandins in ulcerative colitis. *Gastroenterology*, **75**: 638–640, 1978.

Long-Term Management of Ulcerative Colitis

Derek P. Jewell

Although corticosteroids are highly effective in treating acute attacks of ulcerative colitis, they are of little benefit in maintaining remission, at least in doses which do not induce a high rate of side effects.[1,2] Therefore, corticosteroids should be tailed off once a satisfactory remission has been obtained, and most patients should be off them three months after treatment has begun. The remission is maintained with sulphasalazine and most of this paper will be concerned with this drug.

SULPHASALAZINE

Sulphasalazine was introduced in 1942 by Nana Swartz[3] for the treatment of rheumatoid arthritis and ulcerative colitis, and she subsequently reported its use in 124 cases of ulcerative colitis.[4] It took 20 years before controlled trials showed that the drug was more effective than a placebo in treating mild attacks of ulcerative colitis but was not so effective as corticosteroids.[5-8] Then, in 1965, Misiewicz *et al.*[9] showed that in a dose of 2 g daily, sulphasalazine significantly reduced the relapse rate when used over a 12-month period. Of 33 patients treated with a placebo, 24 of them relapsed during the 12 months compared with only 7 relapses in 34 patients maintained on sulphasalazine. This has now been amply confirmed by another study which showed that the six-month relapse rate was reduced from about 56% to about 12% by sulphasalazine.[10] Therefore, all patients with ulcerative colitis should receive sulphasalazine in order to minimize the risk of further attacks.

The next question concerns how long patients should be maintained on the drug. In the Oxford study,[10] the trial was stratified into two groups according to whether patients entering the trial had had sulphasalazine for less than five years or for longer than this. The results clearly demonstrated

Gastroenterology Unit, Radcliffe Infirmary, Oxford, England, UK that the beneficial effect of sulphasalazine continued over many years. Therefore, it was concluded that patients should be continued indefinitely on the drug and this is now standard practice in Oxford. A rather similar trial from Denmark[11] did not confirm the long-term effect of sulphasalazine, but this might be explained by the fact that only symptomatic relapses were recorded. The Oxford trial[10] assessed disease activity by symptoms, sigmoidoscopy, and rectal biopsy so that asymptomatic relapses were also recorded.

Sulphasalazine contains 5-aminosalicylic acid (5-ASA) linked to sulphapyridine by an azo bond. Only about 10% of the parent compound is absorbed, the rest passing unchanged into the colon where it is split into its two moieties by azoreductase enzymes of the colonic bacteria. Sulphapyridine is readily absorbed and is largely metabolized in the liver. Higher blood levels are found in slow-acetylators, and the total blood levels of sulphapyridine and its metabolites show a direct correlation with side effects (nausea, vomiting, headache, and so on).[11] Most of the 5-ASA released in the colon from sulphasalazine passes out into the feces. Some is absorbed and is excreted into the urine although there is also a small enterohepatic circulation.[13,14]

It has now been shown that the active moiety of sulphasalazine is the 5-aminosalicylic acid. Azad Khan *et al.*[15] showed that 5-ASA was just as effective as sulphasalazine in the treatment of mild active ulcerative colitis but sulphapyridine had little effect. Similar findings were subsequently reported by van Hees *et al.*[16] using suppositories rather than enemas. Since many of the side effects of sulphasalazine are due to the sulphapyridine moiety, there is great interest in the development of alternative pro-drugs which will liberate 5-ASA into the colon. One drug, disodium azodisalicylate, contains two molecules of 5-ASA linked by an azo bond. Its pharmacokinetics are very similar to those of sulphasalazine[17] and it appears to be effective when used in the management of mild attacks of ulcerative colitis.[18] Formal therapeutic trials are now in progress to assess its role as a treatment for active disease and as a maintenance treatment.

Side effects of sulphasalazine are common, and about 10% of patients are unable to tolerate it. Table 1 lists many of the side effects. The gastrointestinal intolerance and headaches can often be overcome by starting with a low dose and gradually increasing it. Patients who show hypersensitivity rashes to sulphasalazine can often be desensitized using daily doses as low as 1 mg.[19] Male infertility has been recently recognized as a complication but it is reversible once the drug has been stopped.[20] The optimal dose for maintenance treatment which provides maximal therapeutic benefit with the least side effects is 2 g daily.[21]

TABLE 1. Side Effects of Sulphasalazine

Dose-related:	General malaise
	Nausea and vomiting
	Anorexia
	Headache
	Crenated red cells, macrocytosis
	Heinz-body hemolytic anemia
Unrelated to dose:	Fever
	Hypersensitivity reactions (including erythema nodosum and erythema multiforme)
	Photosensitivity rashes
	Agranulocytosis
	Male infertility

AZATHIOPRINE

There is no evidence that azathioprine has any role in treating active disease[22] but its role as a maintenance agent is less well defined. In one trial,[22] azathioprine had a marginal benefit in reducing the relapse rate over a one-year period compared with a placebo, but the difference between the two groups just failed to reach statistical significance. More recently, it has been shown that azathioprine may be useful in allowing a reduction in steroid dosage in those patients who are on continuous steroid therapy.[23] Since it is very unusual for patients to need continuous corticosteroid therapy, this is not an infrequent indication for using azathioprine. Nevertheless, azathioprine is worth using in patients who are requiring repeated courses of corticosteroids and in whom surgery is not being considered.

SODIUM CROMOGLYCATE

There is little evidence to support the use of sodium cromoglycate either to treat active disease or maintain a remission. Favorable reports were published on its use in patients with proctitis, using oral and topical administration,[24] and in patients with ulcerative colitis.[25] However, subsequent studies have reported disappointing results with cromoglycate used either for treatment of an attack or to maintain remission.[26–29] Therefore, at a dose of 800 mg daily, the drug cannot be recommended for managing patients with ulcerative colitis. It would still be interesting to know whether a much bigger dose would be more effective.

LONG-TERM FOLLOW-UP

The majority of patients run a chronic intermittent course and will have relapses of their disease. They should be instructed to report to the clinic as soon as symptoms begin so that the attack can be treated early on. It is therefore helpful to see all patients regularly, even though many will only need an annual visit. Patients who are at high risk of developing a colonic cancer should be monitored carefully.

REFERENCES

1. Truelove, S. C. and Witts, L. J.: Cortisone and Corticotrophin in ulcerative colitis. *Brit. Med. J.*, **1**: 387, 1959.
2. Lennard-Jones, J. E., Misiewicz, J. J., Connell, A. M., Baron, J. H., and Avery Jones, F.: Prednisone as maintenance treatment for ulcerative colitis in remission. *Lancet,* **1**: 188, 1965.
3. Swartz, N.: Salazopyrin, a new sulfanilamide preparation. A. Therapeutic results in rheumatoid arthritis. B. Therapeutic results in ulcerative colitis. C. Toxic manifestations in treatment with sulfanilamide preparations. *Acta Med. Scand.*, **110**: 577, 1942.
4. Swartz, N.: The treatment of 124 cases of ulcerative colitis with salazopyrin and attempts at desensitisation in cases of hypersensitiveness to sulpha. *Acta Med. Scand.*, **206 (Suppl.)**: 465, 1948.
5. Dick, A. P., Grayson, M. J., and Carpenter, R. G.: Controlled trial of sulphasalazine in the treatment of ulcerative colitis. *Gut*, **5**: 437, 1964.
6. Baron, J. H., Connell, A. M., and Lennard-Jones, J. E.: Sulphasalazine and salicylazosulphadimidine in ulcerative colitis. *Lancet,* **1**: 1094, 1962.
7. Truelove, S. C., Watkinson, G., and Draper, G.: Comparison of corticosteroids and sulphasalazine therapy in ulcerative colitis. *Brit. Med. J.*, **2**: 1708, 1962.
8. Lennard-Jones, J. E., Longmore, A. J., Newell, A. C., Wilson, C. W. E., and Avery Jones, F.: An assessment of prednisone, salazopyrine and topical hydrocortisone hemisuccinate used as out-patient treatment for ulcerative colitis. *Gut,* **1**: 217, 1960.
9. Misiewicz, J. J., Lennard-Jones, J. E., Connell, A. M., Baron, J. H., and Avery Jones, F.: Controlled trial of sulphasalazine in maintenance therapy of ulcerative colitis. *Lancet,* **1**: 185, 1965.
10. Dissanayake, A. S. and Truelove, S. C.: A controlled therapeutic trial of long-term maintenance treatment of ulcerative colitis with sulphasalazine. *Gut*, **14**: 923, 1973.
11. Riis, P., Anthonison, P., Wulff, H. R., Folkenborg, O., Bonnevie, O., and Binder, V.: The prophylactic effect of salazosulphapyridine in ulcerative colitis during long-term treatment. A double-blind trial of patients asymptomatic for one year. *Scand. J. Gastroent.*, **8**: 71, 1973.
12. Das, K. M., Eastwood, M. A., McManus, J. P. A., and Sircus, W.: Adverse reactions during salicylazosulphapyridine therapy and the relation with drug metabolism and acetylator phenotype. *New Eng. J. Med.*, **289**: 491, 1973.
13. Peppercorn, M. A. and Goldman, P.: Distribution studies of salicylazosulfapyridine and its metabolites. *Gastroenterology*, **64**: 240, 1973.

14. Azad Khan, A. K., Aronson, J. K., and Truelove, S.C.: The disposition and metabolism of sulphasalazine in man. *Brit. J. Clin. Pharmac.*, **13**: 523, 1982.
15. Azad Khan, A. K., Piris, J., and Truelove, S. C.: An experiment to determine the active therapeutic moiety of sulphasalazine. *Lancet*, **2**: 892, 1977.
16. Van Hees, P. A. M., Bakker, J. H., and van Tongeren, J. H. M.: Effect of sulphapyridine, 5-aminosalicylic acid, and placebo in patients with idiopathic proctitis: a study to determine the active therapeutic moiety of sulphasalazine. *Gut*, **21**: 632, 1980.
17. Willoughby, C. P., Aronson, J. K., Agback, H., Bodin, N. O., Andersson, E., and Truelove, S. C.: Distribution and metabolism of disodium azodisalicylate: a potential therapeutic agent for ulcerative colitis. *Gut* (in press).
18. Jewell, D. P. and Truelove, S. C.: Disodium azodisalicylate in ulcerative colitis. *Lancet*, **2**: 1168, 1981.
19. Holdsworth, C. D.: Sulphasalazine desensitisation. *Brit. Med. J.*, **282**: 110, 1981.
20. Toovey, S., Hudson, E., Hendry, W. F., and Levi, A. J.: Sulphasalazine and male infertility—reversibility and possible mechanisms. *Gut*, **22**: 445, 1981.
21. Azad Khan, A. K., Howes, D. T., Piris, J., and Truelove, S. C.: Optimum dose of sulphasalazine for maintenance treatment in ulcerative colitis. *Gut*, **21**: 232, 1980.
22. Jewell, D. P. and Truelove, S. C.: Azathioprine in ulcerative colitis: Final report on a controlled therapeutic trial. *Brit. Med. J.*, **2**: 627, 1974.
23. Kirk, A. P. and Lennard-Jones, J. E.: Controlled trial of azathioprine in chronic ulcerative colitis. *Brit. Med. J.*, **1**: 1291, 1982.
24. Heatley, R. V., Calcraft, B. J., Rhodes, J., Owen, E., and Evans, B. K.: Disodium cromoglycate in the treatment of chronic proctitis. *Gut*, **16**: 559, 1975.
25. Mani, V., Lloyd, G., Green, F. H. Y., Fox, H., and Trunberg, L. A.: Treatment of ulcerative colitis with oral disodium cromoglycate. *Lancet*, **1**: 439, 1976.
26. Buckell, N. A., Gould, S. R., Day, D. W., Lennard-Jones, J. E., and Edwards, A. M.: Controlled trial of disodium cromoglycate in chronic persistent ulcerative colitis. *Gut*, **19**: 1140, 1978.
27. Dronfield, M. W. and Langman, M. J. S.: Comparative trial of sulphasalazine and oral sodium cromoglycate in the maintenance of remission in ulcerative colitis. *Gut*, **19**: 1136, 1978.
28. Willoughby, C. P., Piris, J., Heyworth, M., and Truelove, S. C.: Comparison of disodium cromoglycate and sulphasalazine as maintenance therapy for ulcerative colitis. *Lancet*, **1**: 119, 1979.
29. Binder, V., Elsborg, L., Greibe, J., Hendriksen, C., Hoj, L., Birger Jensen, K., Kristensen, E., Madsen, J. R., Mamer, B., Riis, P., and Williamson, L.: Disodium cromoglycate in the treatment of ulcerative colitis and Crohn's disease. *Gut*, **22**: 55, 1981.

Elemental Diets in the Treatment of Crohn's Disease

Tsuneyoshi Yao, Kensaburo Imamura,** and Koichi Fujita**

INTRODUCTION

Although there have been many reports on the therapeutic value of elemental diet (ED) in Crohn's disease,[1–6] its effectiveness without concomitant drugs and long-term follow-up have not been satisfactorily clarified. Furthermore, its effects on radiographic signs have not been reported. In this report, 21 consecutive patients with Crohn's disease treated solely with ED were studied to determine the effects of ED as a primary therapy in Crohn's disease. Its short-term effects on symptoms, nutritional state, pertinent laboratory findings, and radiographic signs were studied. In addition, the long-term course after discontinuation of ED was studied.

MATERIALS AND METHODS

During a period of two and half years from June 1979 to December 1981, a total of 23 patients with Crohn's disease were admitted to the First Department of Internal Medicine, Fukuoka University Hospital. All but two patients who were intolerable with longstanding use of a feeding tube were subjected to treatment with ED. The subjects of the present study were 21 patients treated with ED, 12 males and 9 females. The average age was 23.2 ± 8.5 yr, ranging from 12 to 44 years. Eleven had enteritis and 10 enterocolitis. Eleven of them had no history of previous treatment for Crohn's disease. Three had been on steroids and one on metronidazole. Two had been treated with IVH. The remaining

*First Department of Internal Medicine, School of Medicine, Fukuoka University, Fukuoka, Japan
**Second Department of Internal Medicine, Faculty of Medicine, Kyushu University, Fukuoka, Japan

four, one with enteritis and three with enterocolitis, had undergone operation.

Elemental diet used was ED-AC produced by Ajinomoto Company, Japan. The ingredients are as follows: carbohydrates (dextrin) 79.4%, amino acids 17.6%, lipids 0.66% (soy bean oil 0.64%, lecitin 0.02%), electrolytes 2.0%, others 0.2%, and vitamins 1,646.9 ppm. The ingredients are quite similar to those of Vivonex. ED-AC was given through an Argyle feeding tube introduced via the nasal route in the vicinity of Treitz' ligament. Because the reconstituted diet is hyperosmolar, its concentration was gradually increased to full strength over four days to reduce side effects such as diarrhea and abdominal colic. The daily maintenance dose of calories was 2,100 to 2,700 kcal (40–60 kcal/kg body weight). The average period of treatment with ED was 8.1 $\pm$ 2.9 wk, ranging from 4 to 15 weeks. Oral intake was prohibited during the treatment except for water and some pieces of candy. Drugs had been gradually withdrawn by ten days after commencement of the treatment in all cases.

Changes in symptoms and nutritional state, signs of inflammation such as ESR and CRP, and radiographic signs before and just after discontinuation of ED were studied. In addition, follow-up study was done after treatment. Four patients took another course of treatment with ED and one took IVH during the follow-up period. In those patients, the follow-up period was divided at the time of recommencement of ED or IVH and the results of the follow-up studies were evaluated separately. Ten patients had several complications: marked stenosis with proximal dilatation in five, external fistula in two, internal fistula in two, and abdominal abscess in one patient. The results, except for radiographic signs, were analyzed separately in patients having complications and in those without complications.

RESULTS

Changes in symptoms, nutritional state, ESR and CRP, and radiographic signs before and after the first treatment with ED

Symptoms. All 16 patients who had had abdominal pain and 6 with fever were relieved of these symptoms. Complete amelioration of diarrhea could not be achieved in 4 of 16 patients who had complained of this symptom, 2 of whom were operated cases.

Nutritional state. Body weight, serum albumin, and serum cholesterol showed improvement (Table 1). The increase in serum albumin was statistically significant. These improvements seemed more prominent in patients without complications, although the differences were not statistically significant.

TABLE 1. Changes in Nutrition before and after the First Treatment with ED

		Before ED	After ED
Body weight (% of ideal weight)	Complication (−) ($n = 11$)	81.9 ± 8.3	91.2 ± 12.2
	Complication (+) ($n = 10$)	78.2 ± 7.7	84.0 ± 6.2
Serum albumin (g/dl)	Complication (−)	3.2 ± 0.7**	4.1 ± 0.4**
	Complication (+)	3.4 ± 0.8*	3.9 ± 0.4*
Serum cholesterol (mg/dl)	Complication (−)	120.0 ± 18.4	140.2 ± 38.1
	Complication (+)	105.8 ± 29.5	124.0 ± 30.0

*$p < 0.05$, **$p < 0.001$.

ESR and CRP. In all patients without complications, ESR became normalized and CRP negative (Table 2). Improvement of ESR was statistically significant in those patients. In patients with complications, ESR remained abnormal in three and CRP continued positive in two patients. Although a tendency toward improvement of ESR was recognized in those patients, it was not statistically significant.

TABLE 2. Changes in ESR and CRP before and after the First Treatment with ED

	ESR (mm/hr)			CRP
	Before ED	After ED	No. of normalized cases	No. of normalized cases
Complication(−) ($n = 11$)	34.7 ± 24.6*	4.9 ± 2.8*	11	11
Complication (+) ($n = 10$)	28.1 ± 19.5	14.2 ± 16.1	7	8

*$p < 0.001$.

From these results it was considered that the therapeutic effects of ED on symptoms, nutritional state, and ESR and CRP were more prominent in patients without complications.

Radiographic signs. Analysis was made on radiographic signs obtained by double-contrast study (Figs. 1 and 2). Both patient groups with and without complications were collectively analyzed since there was no obvious difference between the two. A comparative study of small intestinal lesions before and after ED could be done in thirteen patients with enteritis and that of colonic lesions in five patients with enterocolitis (Table 3). Stenosis remained unchanged or became aggravated. Three patients with stenosis eventually underwent an operation due to chronic intestinal obstruction within eleven weeks after initiation of ED because stenotic lesions had become more marked with the treatment.

Narrowing remained mostly unchanged, although a few cases showed

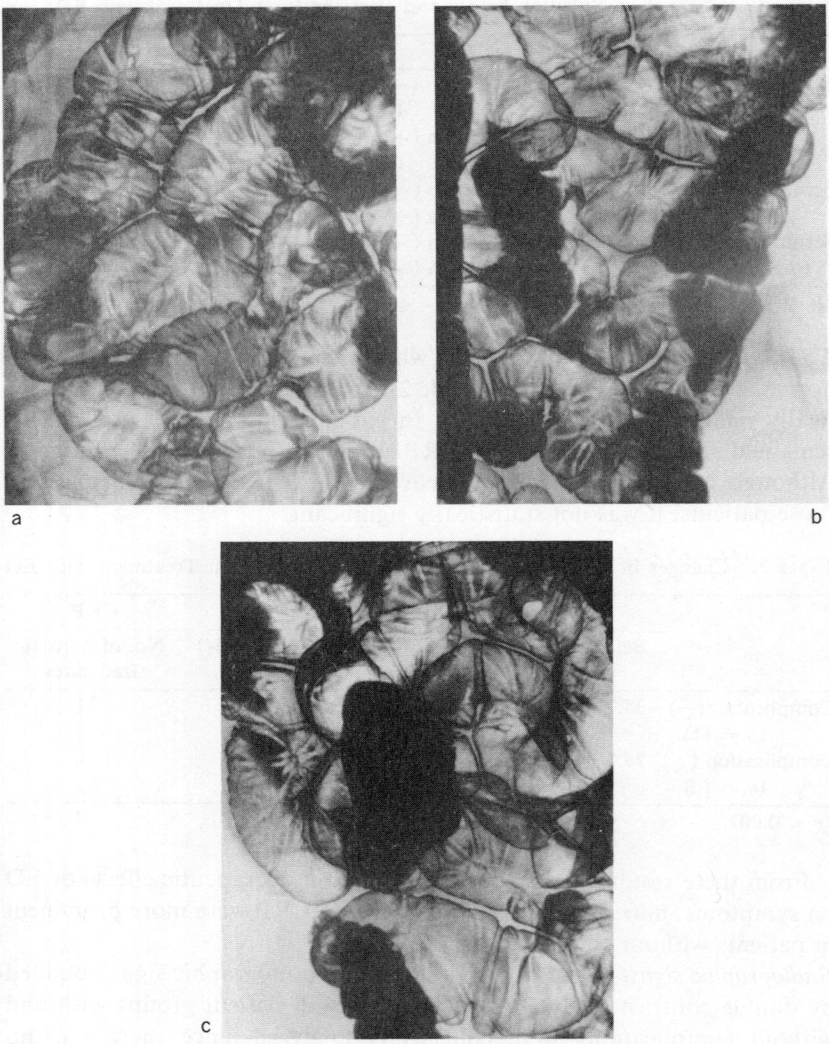

a b c

FIG. 1. a) Double-contrast study of the small intestine taken before initiation of ED showing active longitudinal ulcers.

b) Double-contrast study of the patient shown Fig. 1a taken at the end of ED. The width of longitudinal ulcers decreased compared to that of Fig. 1a.

c) Double-contrast study of the patient shown in Figs. 1a and 1b taken 11 months after discontinuation of ED. Aggravation was not recognized.

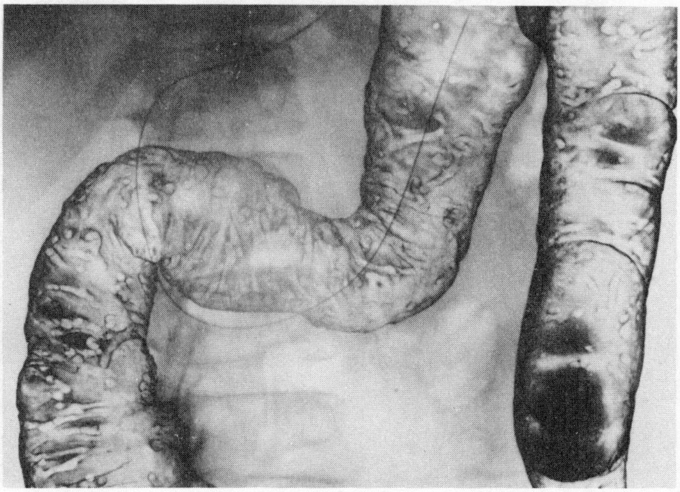

FIG. 2a. Double-contrast study taken during treatment with ED, showing marked inflammatory polyps.

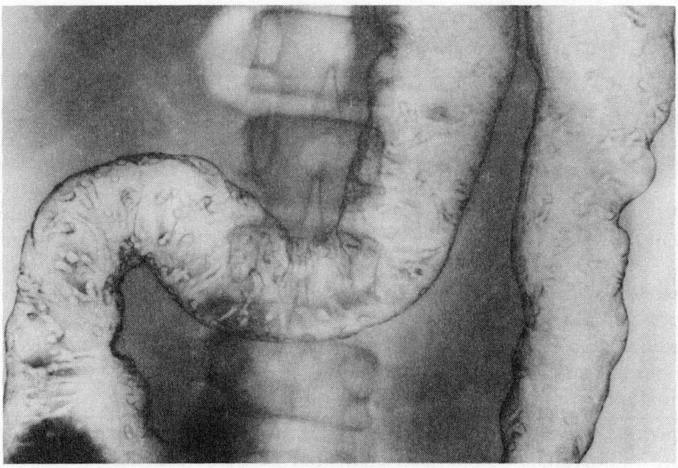

FIG. 2b. Double-contrast study of the patient shown in Fig. 2a taken just after the ED. Inflammatory polyps decreased in number.

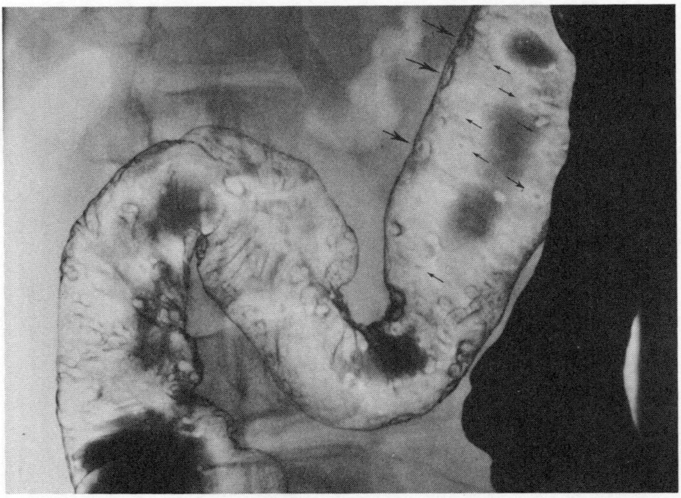

FIG. 2c. Double-contrast study of the patient shown in Figs. 2a and 2b taken 11 months after discontinuation of ED. Recurrence of aphtoid ulcers was revealed (arrows). Inflammatory polyps were not aggravated.

TABLE 3. Changes in Radiographic Signs before and after ED

	Small intestine ($n = 13$)		Colon ($n = 5$)	
	Before ED	After ED	Before ED	After ED
Stenosis	2 cases	Unchanged 2	5 cases	(Aggravated 3) Unchanged 2
Narrowing	13	Aggravated 2 Unchanged 10 Improved 1	5	Aggravated 1 Unchanged 3 Improved 1
Cobblestone and/or infl. polyp	11	Improved 11	5	Improved 5
Longitudinal ulcer	11	Improved 11	1	Improved 1
Serpiginous and/or aphthoid ulcer	8	Improved 8	3	Improved 3 (scarred)

( ): operated during or after the treatment with ED due to intestinal obstruction. Therefore radiographic comparison could not be made exactly.

improvement or aggravation. Cobblestoning and inflammatory polyps became less noticeable in most patients. Longitudinal ulcers showed improvement in all patients. Most serpiginous and aphthoid ulcers were healed.

From these results, ED seemed to improve various types of ulcers, cobblestoning, and inflammatory polyps. However, stenosis was aggravated, presumably due to the development of fibrosis associated with the healing process.

Long-term course after discontinuation of ED

Two out of 11 cases without complications and 5 out of 10 cases with complications eventually underwent an operation. Six out of these 7 patients were excluded from follow-up study since they underwent an operation within three months after discontinuation of ED. Accordingly, follow-up study was done on 10 patients without complications and 5 with complications. Five of 10 patients without complications took another treatment with ED and one took IVH treatment within 12 months after discontinuation of the first treatment with ED. Their follow-up period was divided at the time of commencement of the second ED or IVH.

The average period of follow-up after the first ED was 10.3 ± 3.7 mo (7–12 mo) in patients without complications and 7.8 ± 5.2 mo (4–18 mo) in those with complications. Furthermore, seven patients took a third treatment with ED or IVH after discontinuation of the second ED. In these patients, the follow-up period was divided at the time of commencement of the third ED or IVH.

The average period of follow-up after the second ED was 17.6 ± 4.8 mo (9–23 mo) in five patients without complications, and was five and six months in two patients with complications. Salazopyrin was prescribed to all but two patients during the follow-up period, and one was on steroids for eight months.

Symptoms. As shown in Table 4, 80% of patients without complications had been kept free from symptoms until six months after the first and second ED. However, symptoms had developed again in one third of the patients by twelve months. Most of the patients with complications

TABLE 4. Follow-Up Study: Symptoms

		Period of follow-up (mo)			
		–3	–6	–12	–24
Complication (−)	After 1st ED (n = 10)	0/10	2/10	4/10	0/0
	After 2nd ED (n = 5)	1/5	1/5	0/5 (1)	1/4 (1)
Complication (+)	After 1st ED (n = 5)	3/5	4/5	1/1	1/1
	After 2nd ED (n = 2)	1/2	2/2		

Patients with symptom/patients followed up.
( ): Number of patients with steroids.

began to suffer from symptoms again by six months after discontinuation of the first and second ED.

Body weight. In patients without complications, a tendency to increase body weight was found during a follow-up period of ten months (Table 5). Furthermore, after the second ED, body weights which had recovered to a normal range were not reduced during further follow-up for eighteen months. However, in patients with complications, a tendency toward reduction in body weight after the second ED was recognized.

TABLE 5. Follow-Up Study: Body Weight

		Period of follow-up	% of ideal body weight	
			End of ED	End of follow-up
Complication (−)	After 1st ED ($n = 10$)	10.3 ± 3.7	88.2 ± 8.9	94.8 ± 9.5
	After 2nd ED ($n = 5$)	17.6 ± 4.8	100 ± 10.1	99.2 ± 8.3
Complication (+)	After 1st ED ($n = 5$)	7.8 ± 5.2	85.8 ± 6.9	83.4 ± 8.1
	After 2nd ED ($n = 2$)	5.5 ± 0.5	94.4 ± 0.5	86.7 ± 0.7

TABLE 6. Follow-Up Study: CRP

		Period of follow-up (mo)			
		–3	–6	–12	–24
Complication (−)	After 1st ED ($n = 10$)	8/10	9/10	9/10	0/1
	After 2nd ED ($n = 5$)	3/5	3/5	3/5	2/4
Complication (+)	After 1st ED ($n = 5$)	5/5	3/3	1/1	1/1
	After 2nd ED ($n = 2$)	2/2	2/2		

Patients with positive CRP/patients followed up.

CRP. As shown in Table 6, 70% of patients without complications revealed positive CRP by three months after discontinuation of ED. In patients with complications, all showed positive CRP by three months after discontinuation of ED.

Changes in radiographic signs. Because of the small number of patients in whom X-ray examinations were performed at a regular interval during the follow-up period, a precise analysis of changes in radiographic signs could not be done. Patients with single or multiple treatments with ED or IVH are combined in Table 7.

TABLE 7. Follow-Up Study: Changes in Radiographic Sign

Radiographic sign	Small intestine (n = 7)			Colon (n = 4)		
	End of ED	After 8–30 mo		End of ED	After 6–16 mo	
Stenosis	1 cases	Unchanged	1	3 cases	Aggravated	1
					Unchanged	2
Narrowing	7	Aggravated	2	4	Aggravated	2
		Unchanged	5		Unchanged	2
Cobblestone and/or infl. polyp	6	More remarkable	3		Unchanged	2
		Improved	3		Improved	2
Longitudinal ulcer	7	Recurred	5	1 (scar)	Unchanged	1
		Unchanged	1			
		Improved	1			
Serpiginous and/or aphthoid ulcer	3	Recurred	2	3 (scar)	Unchanged	2
		Disappeared	1		Recurred	1

Generally, stenosis and narrowing remained unchanged or became aggravated. Cobblestone appearance or inflammatory polyps which had improved during the first ED revealed indefinite changes throughout the follow-up period, i.e., some were further improved and some were further aggravated, but not to the same extent as before treatment. Most ulcers recurred after discontinuation of ED; however, the severity was less than that before treatment. Aggravated ulcers, cobblestoning, and inflammatory polyps were mostly improved again by repeated ED or by IVH.

DISCUSSION

Although there have been some reports on the therapeutic effects of ED in Crohn's disease, most of the reported patients treated with ED were severe cases for whom an operation was indicated.[1–4)] Russell[5)] stated that ED may be most effective for those patients having severe diarrhea, internal fistula, and perianal fistula. O'Morain *et al.*[6)] employed treatment with ED for four weeks in 32 exacerbations in 27 cases with Crohn's disease. This treatment was dramatically effective in 29 out of 32 exacerbations in both clinical status and pertinent laboratory data such as hemoglobin, ESR, and serum albumin. However, in their study, the number of patients treated solely with ED was only eight. In the present study no patients were taking drugs during treatment with ED. Our study showed an outcome similar to that of O'Morain *et al.*,[6)] namely, not only relief of symptoms but improvement in nutritional state and laboratory data were obtained. These results may suggest that ED can bring forth remission in patients with Crohn's disease.

In four patients who had been on steroid therapy until initiation of ED, complete secession from steroids could be achieved within ten days of treatment with ED. This also suggests that ED may be effective in secession from steroids.

The therapeutic effects of ED were more pronounced in patients without complications. CRP became positive again by six months after discontinuation of ED in most of the cases with or without complications. However, more than two thirds of the patients without complications had been kept free from symptoms for more than six months. On the contrary, most patients with complications began to suffer from symptoms again by six months after discontinuation of ED. From the results, it is felt that ED should be indicated more frequently for patients without complications than for those with complications, despite the frequent employment of ED in severe cases with complications in most of the previous reports.

There have been no reports on radiographic changes in ED treatment. Although stenosis and narrowing were aggravated in some cases, our study showed that cobblestone appearance and various types of ulcers were improved by ED and, moreover, that they were never again aggravated as severely as the pre-treatment state throughout the follow-up period. These results suggest that treatment with ED may improve not only symptoms, nutrition, and laboratory findings but histological findings as well. Namely, treatment with ED may heal ulcers and cause subsidence of mucosal and submucosal edema and subsequently improve cobblestone appearance and inflammatory polyps. Stenosis was intractable to the treatment, presumably due to fibrotic change. This may have been further aggravated by the development of fibrotic change associated with the healing process of ulcer and cobblestone appearance.

We do not think, of course, that treatment with ED solely suffices every patient with Crohn's disease. In fact, we have experienced some patients whose disease recurred shortly after discontinuation of ED or IVH and in whom remission could have soon been achieved with steroids. Although one has to take care of the catabolic state with long-term steroid therapy, the nutritional state is well maintained for a long period by ED, as has been shown in this study. Therefore, an appropriate combination of ED and steroids may be necessary for some patients with Crohn's disease.

In conclusion, it is considered from the present study that ED may be very effective as a primary therapy in patients with Crohn's disease without complications.

SUMMARY

Twenty-one patients with Crohn's disease treated solely with ED were studied.

1) Symptoms, ESR, and nutritional state were remarkably improved.

This improvement was more remarkable in patients without complications than in those with complications.

2) Follow-up study after discontinuation of ED showed that symptoms recurred sooner in patients with complications than in those without complications.

A further increase in body weight after discontinuation of ED was recognized in patients without complications; however, in patients with complications a tendency toward reduction in body weight was found.

3) Although some stenosis and narrowing were aggravated, ulcer and cobblestone appearance were remarkably improved. Some ulcers and cobblestoning were aggravated after ED was discontinued; however, there was none which became as severe as the pre-treatment state.

From these results it is considered that ED is very effective as a primary therapy in patients without complications.

REFERENCES

1. Votik, A. J., Echava, V., Feller, J. H., *et al.*: Experience with elemental diet in the treatment of inflammatory bowel disease. *Arch. Surg.*, **107**: 329–339, 1973.
2. Axelsen, C. and Jarnum, S.: Assessment of therapeutic value of an elemental diet in chronic inflammatory bowel disease. *Scand. J. Gastroent.*, **12**: 89–95, 1977.
3. Goode, A., Hawkins, T., Feggetter, J. G. W., *et al.*: Use of an elemental diet for long-term nutritional support in Crohn's disease. *Lancet*, 1976.
4. Rocchio, M. A., Cha, C. M., Haas, K. F., *et al.*: Use of chemically defined diets in the management of patients with acute inflammatory bowel disease. *Amer. J. Surg.*, **127**: 469–475, 1974.
5. Russell, R. I.: Progress report. Elemental diets. *Gut*, **16**: 68–79, 1975.
6. O'Morain, C., Segal, A. W., and Levi, A. J.: Elemental diets in treatment of acute Crohn's disease. *Brit. Med. J.*, **281**: 1173–1175, 1980.

The Therapeutic Effect of Elemental Diet on Crohn's Disease

Nobuo Hiwatashi, Yasutoshi Konno,* Kazundo Kobayashi,**
Yoshio Goto, and Hikaru Watanabe***

SUMMARY

Fourteen patients with Crohn's disease were treated by continuous nasogastric infusion with elemental diet (2,400 kcal/day) for 28–136 days. No other food was allowed. Increases in serum albumin and body weight were observed in all patients. In 11 of the 14 patients, ESR and CRP came within normal range; CDAI decreased below 150 in 12 patients. Inflammation and ulceration disappeared or became smaller, morphologically. However, internal fistulas and stenosis were almost unchanged in longstanding patients. This study suggests that ED is very effective for early or acute Crohn's disease when it does not have irreversible complications.

INTRODUCTION

Sulfasalazine and prednisone have generally been used as the standard medical treatment in Crohn's disease. However, the therapeutic effects of these drugs have not been satisfactory to date, and there have been few cases which have had improvement of radiological and endoscopic findings by the medical treatment.

Restriction of oral intake, malabsorption, and protein loss serve to aggravate the malnutrition in patients with Crohn's disease. Therefore, in this study we treated the patients with Crohn's disease with elemental diet (ED) for the purposes of bowel rest and intensive nutritional restitution; and we investigated the therapeutic effect of ED on Crohn's disease as primary therapy.

*Third Department of Internal Medicine, Tohoku University School of Medicine, Sendai, Japan
**Division of Gastroenterology, National Sendai Hospital, Sendai, Japan

PATIENTS

Fourteen patients with Crohn's disease were treated with ED (Table 1). They were hospitalized at the Tohoku University Hospital or our co-worker's hospital from September 1980 to December 1981. The diagnosis of Crohn's disease was based on the criteria established by the Research Committee for Crohn's Disease of the Japanese Society of Gastroenterology.[1] These patients consisted of 11 males and 3 females Their range of ages was from 14 to 46 years, and their mean age was 23 years. In terms of the extent of lesions, 11 patients had ileocolitis, 2 had ileitis, and one had colitis. Ileal resections had been performed on 2 patients. The periods from onset of symptoms to ED therapy were from 1 to 15 years, and the mean was 5 years. Before the treatment with ED, 5 patients had been treated with sulfasalazine, 2 patients with prednisone and sulfasalazine, and one with metronidazole. Only one of them obtained remission. The other 6 patients were untreated for Crohn's disease.

TABLE 1. Patient Profiles ($n = 14$)

Sex		Age (years)	Extent of lesions			Period from onset of symptoms (years)
Male	Female		Ileitis	Ileocolitis	Colitis	
11	3	14–46 (mean 23)	2	11	1	1–15 (mean 5)

METHODS

The elemental diet used was Elental (Morishita Co., Osaka). Elental is composed of amino acids, very little fat, electrolytes, vitamins, trace elements, and as the major energy source, dextran.[2] ED was administered through a nasogastric feeding tube at a constant rate during the entire day. With a gradual increase in the concentration of ED, a maintenance dose of 2,400 kcal/day was administered from the fifth day.[3] The duration of ED therapy was decided by the clinical symptoms and laboratory data; it lasted from 28 to 136 days, with an average of 56 days. During the period of ED therapy, no other food was allowed. Intralipid was given intravenously, and no other drug was given except for two patients who had been treated with prednisone. The therapeutic value of ED was judged by the Crohn's Disease Activity Index (CDAI), as elaborated by the National Cooperative Crohn's Disease Study.[4] Remission was defined as below 150 on the CDAI. Radiological and endoscopic examinations were done before ED therapy and within one week from cessation of ED. Findings before and after ED therapy were compared.

RESULTS

Clinical and nutritional responses

The elemental diet induced remarkable clinical improvement in all patients (Table 2). CDAI decreased from 237 to 73 during ED therapy, and became less than 150 in all but two patients. ESR and CRP were normalized in 11 patients. Serum protein and albumin increased from 6.2 to 7.1 g/dl and from 3.1 to 4.4 g/dl, respectively. Serum cholesterol levels increased significantly, but serum triglyceride levels did not show any fixed tendency. Body weight approached ideal weight, and the average weight gain was 6.8 kg.

TABLE 2. Clinical and Laboratory Results of Treatment with Elemental Diet

Parameters	n	Before ED (mean)	After ED (mean)	Significance[a]
CDAI	14	237	73	$p < 0.01$
ESR (mm/h)	14	41	13	$p < 0.01$
CRP	14	2.8 +	0.3 +	$p < 0.01$
Serum total protein (g/dl)	14	6.2	7.1	$p < 0.01$
Serum albumin (g/dl)	14	3.1	4.4	$p < 0.01$
Serum cholesterol (mg/dl)	13	137	159	$p < 0.05$
Serum triglyceride (mg/dl)	12	101	131	n.s.
Body weight/ideal weight (%)	14	80.9	92.6	$p < 0.01$

[a]Using Wilcoxon's signed rank sum test.

Changes in radiological findings

Lesions of the small intestine. Changes in radiological findings before and after ED treatment were compared in 10 cases (Table 3). Long longitudinal ulcers, which are very characteristic findings of Crohn's disease in Japan,[1] had been found in all cases. Of the total 15 longitudinal ulcers, 10 ulcers became scars (Fig. 1), 3 became smaller, and 2 did not change. Of the 3 cobblestone appearances, one became a scarred zone with pseu-

TABLE 3. Changes in Radiological Findings in the Small Intestine (10 Cases)

Before ED		After ED	
Longitudinal ulcer	(15 lesions in 10 cases)	→ Scar	(10)
		→ Smaller	(3)
		→ No change	(2)
Cobblestone appearance	(3 cases)	→ Scarred zone	(1)
		→ Pseudopolyps	(1)
		→ Improvement	(1)
Irregular ulcer	(1 case)	→ Scar	(1)
Fissuring ulcer	(1 case)	→ Disappearance	(1)
Stenosis	(1 case)	→ No change	(1)

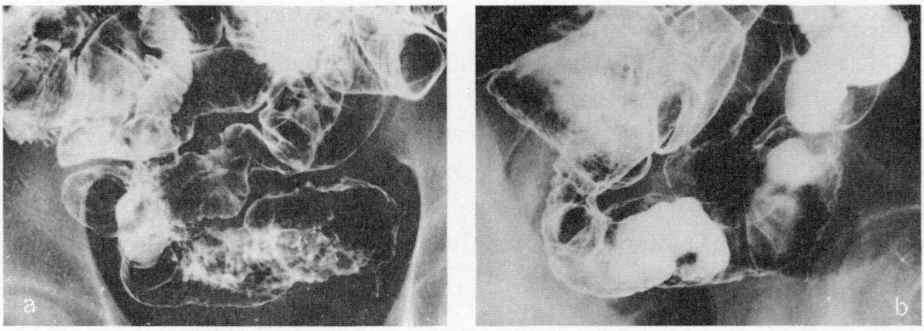

FIG. 1. Crohn's ileitis. A 20-year-old male.
a) Before treatment. Longitudinal ulcers and cobblestone appearance with fissuring ulcers are found in the terminal ileum.
b) After treatment. Longitudinal ulcers have changed into areas of eccentric rigidity; most of the area of cobblestone appearance has changed into pseudopolyps, but a part of it remains. Fissuring ulcers have disappeared.

dopolyps and converging folds which went in multiple directions (Fig. 2). Another one changed into pseudopolyps, and the remaining one showed improvement. Irregular ulcers became scars and fissuring ulcers disappeared. Stenosis in one case remained the same.

Lesions of the large intestine. Twelve cases were investigated (Table 4). Of the 9 cobblestonings in 8 patients, 7 lesions became pseudopolyps (Fig. 3), and another 2 lesions showed a tendency to improvement. All of

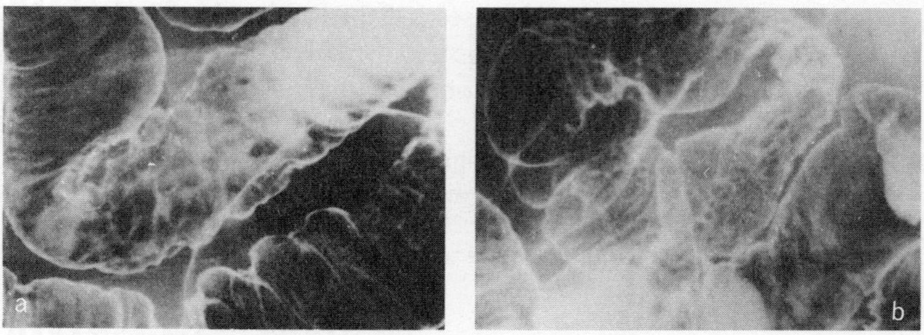

FIG. 2. Crohn's ileocolitis. A 17-year-old male.
a) Before treatment. Cobblestone appearance and a longitudinal ulcer are found in the ileum.
b) After treatment. Findings mentioned above have changed into a scarred zone with pseudopolyps and converging folds.

TABLE 4. Changes in Radiological Findings in the Large Intestine (12 Cases)

Before ED		After ED	
Cobblestone appearance	(9 lesions in 8 cases)	→ Pseudopolyps	(7)
		→ Improvement	(2)
Fissuring ulcer	(6 cases)	→ Disappearance	(6)
Longitudinal ulcer	(2 cases)	→ Scar	(2)
Irregular ulcer	(4 cases)	→ Pseudopolyps	(3)
		→ Scar	(1)
Aphthoid ulcer	(3 cases)	→ Disappearance	(3)
Internal fistula	(4 cases)	→ Closure	(2)
		→ No change	(2)
Narrowing or stenosis	(6 cases)	→ Improvement	(2)
		→ No change	(3)
		→ Worsening	(1)

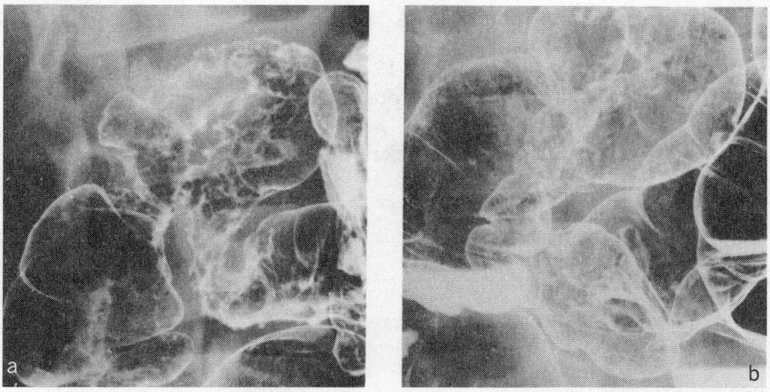

FIG. 3. Crohn's ileocolitis. A 17-year-old male.
a) Before treatment. Cobblestone appearance with fissuring ulcers is found from the transverse colon to the mid-ascending colon.
b) After treatment. Cobblestone appearance has changed into pseudopolyps. Fissuring ulcers have disappeared.

the fissuring ulcers found in 6 cases disappeared. Longitudinal, irregular, and aphthoid ulcers became scars or disappeared (Fig. 4). Internal fistulas had been found in 4 cases before ED treatment. Two of them, in which fistula formation had been developing for a short time, had closure of the fistulas, whereas 2 longstanding cases did not (Fig. 5). Although narrowing or stenosis had been found in 6 cases, improvement was observed in only 2 cases.

Changes in endoscopic findings

Ten cases were examined by fiberoptic colonoscopy both before and

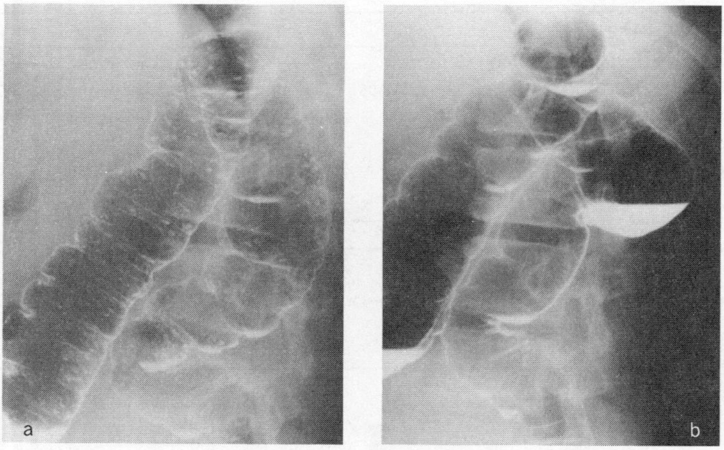

FIG. 4. Crohn's ileocolitis. A 17-year-old male.
a) Before treatment. Numerous aphthoid ulcers are observed in the left side of the colon.
b) After treatment. These ulcers have disappeared.

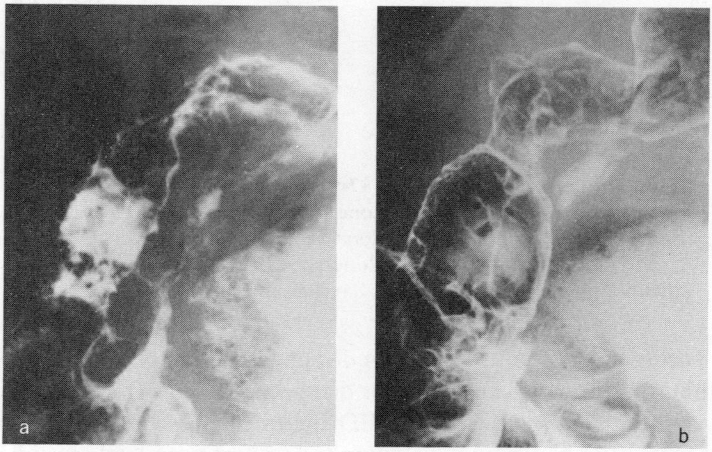

FIG. 5. Crohn's ileocolitis. A 37-year-old male.
a) Before treatment. Cobblestone appearance with stenosis is found in the right side of the colon. There is an internal fistula between the hepatic flexure and the cecum.
b) After treatment. Cobblestone appearance has changed into pseudopolyps and converging folds. Stenosis has improved, but the fistula still remains.

after ED treatment (Table 5). Cobblestone appearances of the large intestine had been observed in 8 cases. In 6 of them, intercommunicated ulcers disappeared and cobblestonings changed into pseudopolyps (Fig. 6). Intercommunicated ulcers became smaller and shallower in one case. In the remaining one case, raising mucosa became flat and intercommunicated ulcers changed into a few aphthoid ulcers (Fig. 7). Stenosis with cobblestone appearances showed a tendency to improvement. Most of the longitudinal ulcers became scars (Fig. 8) or became remarkably smaller.

TABLE 5. Changes in Endoscopic Findings (10 Cases)

Before ED			After ED	
Cobblestone appearance	(8 cases)	→	Pseudopolyps	(6)
		→	Improvement	(1)
		→	Aphthoid ulcer	(1)
Longitudinal ulcer	(5 cases)	→	Scar	(4)
		→	Smaller	(1)
Irregular ulcer	(2 cases)	→	Scar	(1)
		→	Smaller	(1)
Discrete round ulcer	(4 cases)	→	Pseudopolyps with converging folds	(4)
Aphthoid ulcer	(4 cases)	→	Disappearance	(3)
		→	Reduction	(1)
Stenosis	(2 cases)	→	Improvement	(2)

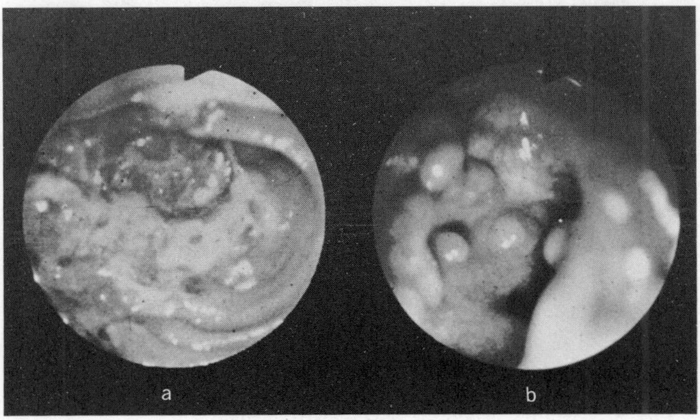

FIG. 6. Crohn's ileocolitis. A 17-year-old male.

a) Before treatment. Cobblestone appearance is found in the transverse colon. We could not insert a fiberscope beyond this area because of stenosis.

b) After treatment. Cobblestone appearance has changed into pseudopolyps. Stenosis has improved.

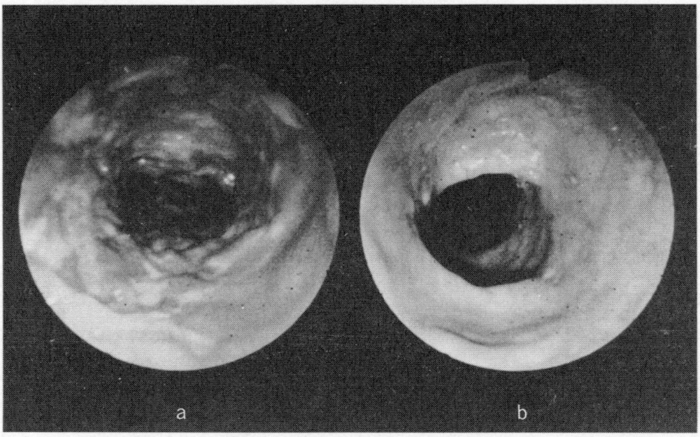

FIG. 7. Crohn's ileocolitis. A 23-year-old male.
a) Before treatment. Cobblestone appearance is seen in the descending colon.
b) After treatment. The cobblestoning has disappeared and mucosa has become flat. A few aphthoid ulcers remain.

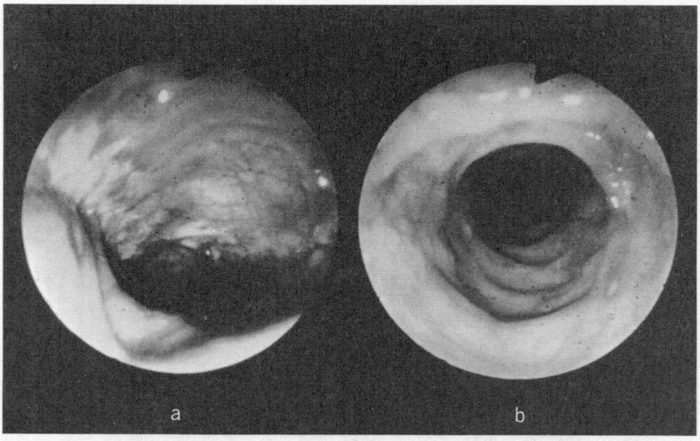

FIG. 8. Crohn's ileocolitis. A 23-year-old male.
a) Before treatment. A longitudinal ulcer is found in the descending colon.
b) After treatment. The ulcer has disappeared and changed into a longitudinal scar with converging folds.

Discrete irregular or round ulcers disappeared or changed into pseudopolyps with converging folds. Aphthoid ulcers disappeared almost entirely (Fig. 9).

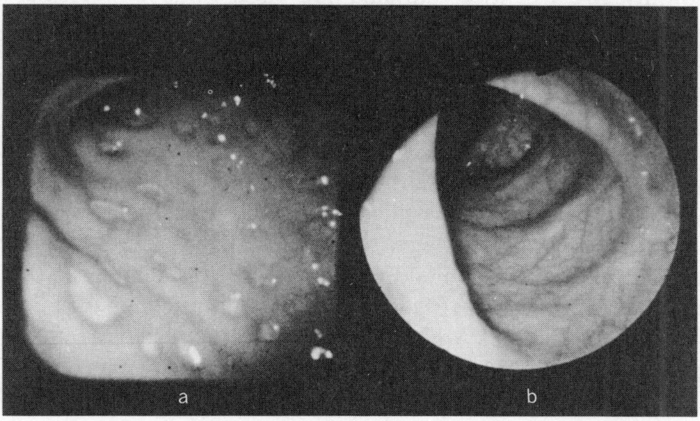

FIG. 9. Crohn's ileocolitis. A 17-year-old male.
a) Before treatment. Numerous aphthoid ulcers are seen in the descending colon.
b) After treatment. These ulcers have disappeared completely.

Complications

Although two patients had slight elevations of transaminase and one had continuous diarrhea, they were not severe.

Follow-up study

All patients were given 3–4 g of sulfasalazine daily and began to eat orally after cessation of ED. In 2 patients, who were above 150 on the CDAI, their symptoms flared up immediately. Of the 12 patients who went into remission, 5 patients relapsed 3–6 months after beginning oral ingestion. The other 7 patients, most of whom had short periods between the onset of symptoms and ED therapy or had limited extents of lesions, are still in clinical remission 9–23 months later. None of the 14 patients has had surgical operations up to the present.

COMMENTS

Twelve of 14 patients in this study went into remission. In those patients, not only did improvement of clinical symptoms and normalization of serological tests occur, but disappearance or remarkable improvement of morphological findings were also observed. It was found that ED treatment was more effective than the standard medical treatment as primary therapy in Crohn's disease. The therapeutic effect of ED is very good when administered to patients without stenosis or fistulas shortly after the onset of symptoms. Most of these patients had good clinical courses after the beginning of oral ingestion. On the other hand, beginning oral ingestion tends to induce relapse of symptoms in longstanding patients who have some complications. Consequently, ED treatment of Crohn's disease should be undertaken in the early or acute stages in patients who have no irreversible complications. Additionally, after this therapy has induced improvement of the general condition and simultaneously decreased disease activity, standard medical treatment should be continued.

The same therapeutic effect as with ED is expected from total parenteral nutrition (TPN). However, in addition to general differences, we think ED is better than TPN for two reasons. First, ED is easy to manage and can be administered at home when a relapse occurs. Second, as Crohn's disease is in hypercoagulability,[5)] such an increase in platelet count or platelet hyperfunction, thrombus formation is prone to occur with TPN.

In our continuing investigations, we would like to observe the long-term clinical courses of the patients and to determine whether ED is able to modify the usual progression of Crohn's disease.

REFERENCES

1. The Japanese Research Committee for Crohn's Disease (Chairman: S. Yamagata): Crohn's disease in Japan. *Gastroenterologia Japonica*, **14**: 366, 1979.
2. Ogoshi, S., *et al.*: Enteral hyperalimentation with elemental diet. I. With reference to an new elemental diet. *Geka*, **40**: 913, 1978 (in Japanese).
3. Ogoshi, S., *et al.*: Enteral hyperalimentation with elemental diet. II. With reference to how to administer an elemental diet. *Geka*, **40**: 991, 1978 (in Japanese).
4. Best, W. R., *et al.*: Development of a Crohn's disease activity index. National Cooperative Crohn's Disease Study. *Gastroenterology*, **70**: 439, 1976.
5. Mori, K., *et al.*: Studies on blood coagulation in ulcerative colitis and Crohn's disease. *Tohoku J. exp. Med.*, **132**: 93, 1980.

A Trial of New Home-Hyperalimentation for Short Bowel Syndrome

——Its Therapeutic Application for Inflammatory Bowel Disease

Kei Matsueda, Noritsugu Umeda, Emi Shimojo, Ryuichi Sakagami, Masakazu Takazoe, Kazuhiro Mori, Etsuo Hoshino, Akira Muraoka, and Ryosuke Shoda

The incidence and prevalence of Crohn's disease have been increasing in recent years in our country, and we are seeing more complicated forms of Crohn's disease. Among such complications, short bowel syndrome (SBS) is one of the most serious because not only its treatment but also its rehabilitation are quite difficult. So far, rehabilitation of such patients can be achieved by home-hyperalimentation (H-HA) using total parenteral nutrition (TPN).

However, H-HA by TPN has disadvantages in practicality, safety, and cost-effectiveness which make it more difficult for a patient with SBS to be socially rehabilitated. Therefore, we tried to develop a better H-HA for SBS.

The aim of this study was to investigate the efficacy of a newly developed H-HA for SBS and to evaluate the feasibility of its therapeutic application for inflammatory bowel disease (IBD).

MATERIALS AND METHODS

We developed a new approach for SBS which consists of the following two steps: the first step is "Induction Treatment (I-Rx)" and the second is "Maintenance Treatment (M-Rx)" (Table 1). As I-Rx, a small-sized feeding tube was inserted either in the stomach or in the duodenum, and

TABLE 1. New Approach to Short Bowel Syndrome

1. Induction Rx:	Continuous administration of elemental diet by infusion pump
2. Maintenance Rx:	Overnight administration of elemental diet by self-intubation ↓ New home-hyperalimentation

Section of Gastroenterology, National Medical Center Hospital, Tokyo, Japan

continuous administration of elemental diet (ED) was performed by infusion pump. The infusion rate was kept low (60–100 ml/hr) to avoid GI symptoms, but it provided adequate calories as a total daily dose. After the patient's nutritional status was stabilized, the feeding tube was extubated during daytime but it was self-intubated at bedtime, and overnight administration of ED was performed as M-Rx which provided 1,200–1,600 kcal/day. This treatment did not disturb the patients' social life because they were free from the feeding tube during daytime. We used this M-Rx as a new H-HA.

Using such methods, we performed the following two studies:

1) Two cases of SBS secondary to mesenteric thrombosis were treated with I-Rx and M-Rx, then nutritional assessments were carried out and the efficacy was compared with TPN.

2) We also applied the same treatment to patients with IBD (6 with Crohn's disease and 2 with ulcerative colitis), and evaluated its therapeutic efficacy on the IBD itself as well as complications such as protein-calorie malnutrition (PCM), vitamin D deficiency, and fistula formation.

RESULTS

Patients with SBS

SBS case 1 (Table 2) was a 40-year-old male who had subtotal gastrec-

TABLE 2. SBS Case 1 (Y. S., 40-year-old male)

PHI:

Jan. 1977	Subtotal gastretcomy with B-II anastomosis for multiple gastric ulcers.
May 1977	Admitted with acute abdomen. Massive small bowel necrosi due to mesenteric thrombosis was found. Massive small bowel resection with jejuno-ascending colostomy was performed. Only 1 m of small intestine from the lig. of Treitz was retained.

The patient developed massive diarrhea (4–6 *l*/day) post-operatively and lost a lot of body weight (59 → 45 kg).

PMH and family H: Non-contributory

P/E on admission:

Height 168 cm. Body weight 44.6 kg. Triceps skin fold 6 mm. Arm muscle circumference 18 cm.

Laboratory data:

CBC: Hgb 5.9, Hct 19.8, WBC 5.7×10^3, Lymph. 54%.

Chem.: T-protein 4.5 g/dl, Albumin 1.6 g/dl, Chol. 102 mg/dl, Na^+ 144 mEq/*l*, K^+ 3.2 mEq/*l*, Ca^{++} 7.3 mg/dl.

Fecal volume: 4–6 *l*/day

Steatorrhea: 40 g/day

Rx: 1) Restriction of fat intake
2) MCT oil
3) Enteral hyperalimentation

tomy and massive small bowel resection because of gastric ulcer and mesenteric thrombosis. Figure 1 illustrates the patient's intestinal anastomosis; only 1 m of small bowel was left, and he developed severe diarrhea and weight loss. Physical examination on admission showed severe malnutrition. Laboratory data indicated severe PCM and his fecal volume was 4–6 *l*/day with 40 g of steatorrhea per day. As I-Rx, continuous administration of ED was performed by infusion pump (Fig. 2, left). As M-Rx, overnight administration of ED was performed by self-intubation (Fig. 2, right). The self-intubation was quite safe and easily performed, and in fact, this patient claimed that it was much easier than

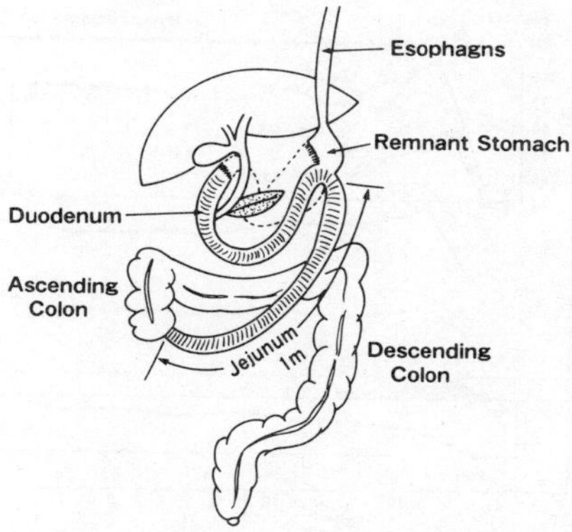

FIG. 1. SBS case 1: schema of intestinal anastomosis.

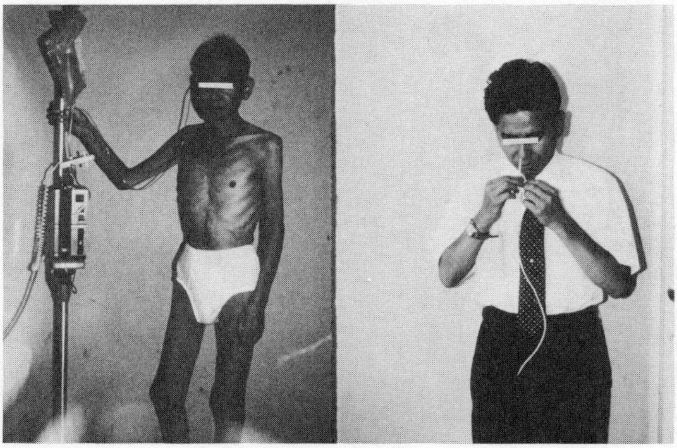

FIG. 2.

brushing his teeth. Figure 3 demonstrated the patient's clinical course. With the M-Rx, a positive nitrogen balance was maintained, and total protein and body weight increased from 4.5 to 7.5 g/dl and from 44 to 56 kg, respectively. After normalizing all nutritional parameters, the patient was placed on the M-Rx which could maintain normal nutrition. Therefore, the M-Rx was used as H-HA. Figure 4 shows his nutritional status before and after the treatment, demonstrating tremendous nutritional improvement. He has been successfully rehabilitated for more than three years with the new H-HA.

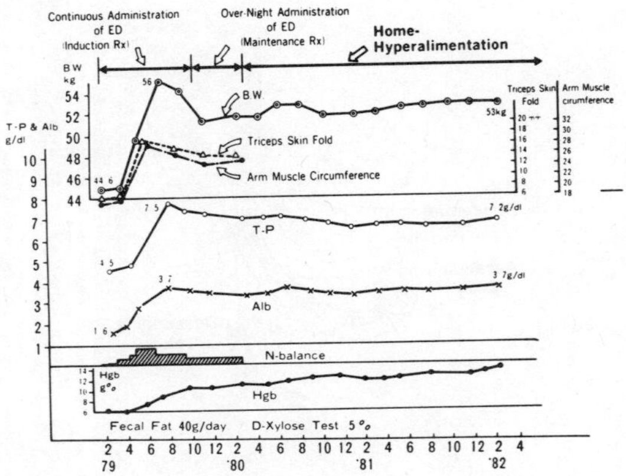

FIG. 3. SBS case 1: clinical course.

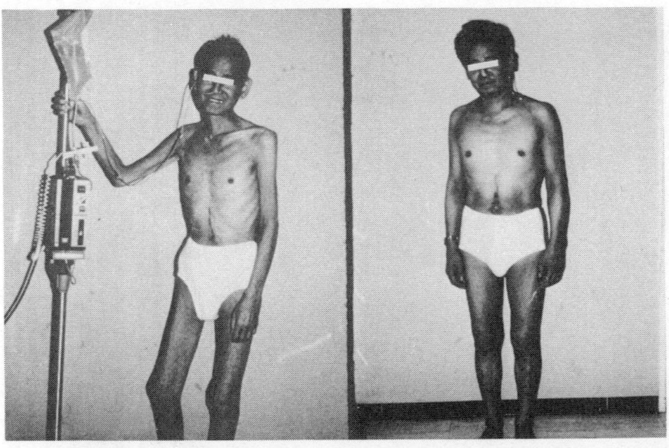

FIG. 4. SBS case 1: nutritional status before (left) and after (right) the treatment.

The second case of SBS (Table 3) was a 24-year-old male who had massive small bowel resection because of mesenteric thrombosis. Only 40 cm of small intestine was left (Fig. 5). Laboratory data indicated severe PCM, and the patient had 50 g of steatorrhea per day. He was treated in the same manner as the first case; his clinical course is shown in Fig. 6.

TABLE 3. SBS Case 2 (H. F., 24-year-old male)

Dx: 1) Anti-thrombin III deficiency
Mesenteric thrombosis
Massive small bowel resection
2) Short bowel syndrome
Operation: See Fig. 5
Laboratory data:
T-protein 4.1 g/dl, Albumin 2.8 g/dl, Chol. 54 mg/dl.
Fecal volume: 1–1.5 *l*/day
Steatorrhea: 50 g/day

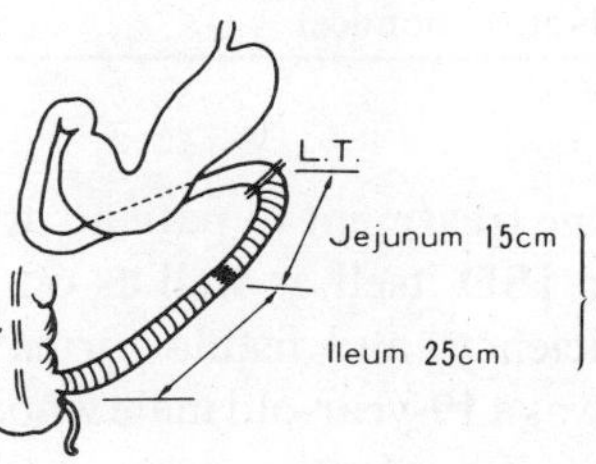

FIG. 5. SBS case 2: operation.

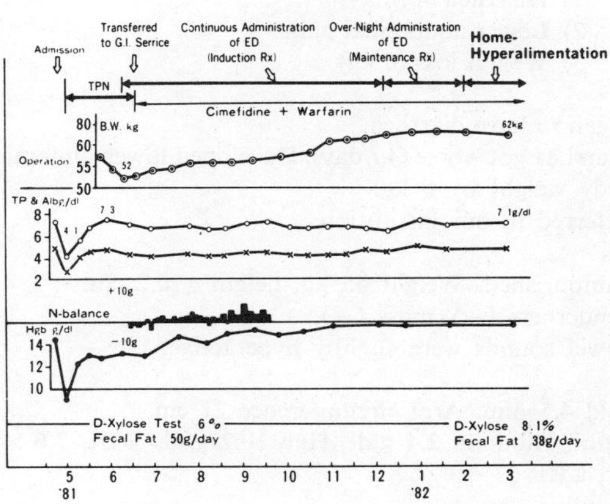

FIG. 6. SBS case 2: clinical course.

With the I-Rx, nitrogen balance was kept positive and every nutritional parameter improved dramatically; he was then placed on the M-Rx to maintain normal nutritional status. Therefore, the M-Rx was also used as H-HA. Again, this patient has been successfully rehabilitated for more than eight months with our H-HA.

The efficacy of our new H-HA was compared with that of conventional H-HA using TPN, and the results are shown in Table 4. The new H-HA is much more practical, safer, and more economical than the conventional one.

TABLE 4. Home-Hyperalimentation: Comparison of the Two Methods

	TPN	Our method (self-intubation with elemental diet)
Practicality	Need special technique	Practical
Safety	Increased risk	Safe
Cost-effectiveness	Not economical	Economical

Patients with IBD

We also applied the same treatment to patients with IBD and evaluated its therapeutic efficacy on IBD itself as well as on its complications such as PCM, vitamin D deficiency, and fistula formation. Among the IBD patients, case 1 (Table 5) was a 19-year-old male who had severe PCM due to

TABLE 5. IBD Case 1 (K. Y., 19-year-old male)

Chief complants: 1) Diarrhea (4 *l*/day)
2) Lower abdominal pain
3) Weight loss (6 kg)

PHI:
Sept. 1980 Began to have diarrhea.
Dec. 1980 Diarrhea got worse (4 *l*/day). Developed lower abdominal pain and lost body weight by 6 kg.
June 1981 Referred to our institution.

P/E:
Moderately malnourished. Weight 45 kg, height 170.2 cm.
Abdomen: Tenderness (−), mass (−).
Bowel sounds were slightly hyperactive.

Laboratory data:
Triceps skin fold 4.5 mm. Arm circumference 21 cm.
T-protein 5.8 g/dl, Albumin 2.4 g/dl, Hgb 10.2 g/dl, WBC 7.6×10^3,
ESR 59 mm/hr, CRP (++).

Dx: 1) Crohn's colitis
2) Protein-calorie malnutrition

Crohn's colitis. As shown in Fig. 7, with the I-Rx nitrogen balance was kept positive, good weight gain was observed, and all symptoms disappeared. He also had vitamin D deficiency; serum 25(OH)D was 2.0 ng/ml, but it became normal (10.6 ng/ml) during the treatment. Marked improvement of the GI lesions occurred, as was shown in Fig. 7.

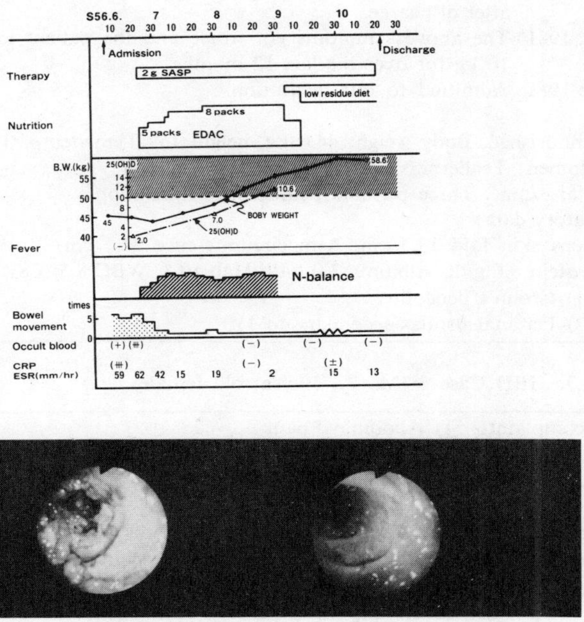

FIG. 7. IBD case 1: clinical course (since June 1981) and fiberscopy of intestine before (left) and after (right) the treatment.

The second case of IBD (Table 6) was an 18-year-old female who had three perianal fistulae with severe PCM. She was found to have Crohn's ileocolitis. With the I-Rx, nitrogen balance was kept positive, and nutritional parameters became normal. She also had vitamin D deficiency, but serum 25(OH)D jumped up to 12 ng/ml during the treatment. The three perianal fistulae closed completely during the treatment. However, she was placed on the new H-HA for a while to prevent recurrence of the fistulae. Now, she is doing well without the H-HA (Figs. 8a and 8b).

The third case of IBD (Table 7) was a 19-year-old female who was admitted to another institution, and peritoneal biopsy was performed which induced an enterocutaneous fistula. Then, she was referred to our institution and was found to have severe Crohn's ileitis with enterocu-

TABLE 6. IBD Case 2 (C. F., 18-year-old female)

Chief complaints: 1) Diarrhea and lower abdominal pain
2) Fever
3) Weight loss (10 kg)

PHI:

Mar. 1980 Diarrhea, abdominal pain, and fever developed. Admitted to a local hospital. Dx was "dehydration" but etiology? Symptoms continued even after discharge.

Apr. 1981 The above symptoms got worse and the patient lost body weight by 10 kg for over the last 12 months.

June 1981 Admitted to our institution.

P/E:

Malnourished. Body weight 44.0 kg, height 159.0 cm, temp. 37.5°C.
Abdomen: Tenderness (+) at the ileocecal region
Rectal exam.: Three perianal fistulas with indulation

Laboratory data:

Triceps skin fold 13.5 cm. Arm circumference 22.5 cm.
T-protein 6.6 g/dl, Albumin 3.0 g/dl, Hgb 10.3, WBC 8.5, ESR 45, CRP 4+.

Dx: 1) Crohn's ileocolitis
2) Perianal fistulas secondary to 1)

TABLE 7. IBD Case 3 (M. Y., 19-year-old female)

Chief complaints: 1) Abdominal pain
2) Fever
3) Weight loss (6 kg)

PHI:

Began to have intermittent abdominal pain at the age of 16.

June 1981 Abdominal pain got worse and fever and weight loss developed.

July 1981 Admitted to N. University Hospital but Sx and general conditions deteriorated.
Peritoneal Bx: 500 ml of acites (?) was drained.

Aug. 1981 Transferred to our institution.

P/E:

Severely malnourished. Weight 36 kg, height 162.5 cm.
Abdomen: Mild metallic bowel sounds. Diffuse peri-umbilical tenderness (+).
Suture scar (+) at left mid-quadrant of abdomen.

Laboratory data:

Triceps skin fold 11 mm. Arm circumference 17 cm.
T-protein 7.1 g/dl, Albumin 2.9 g/dl, Hgb 10.9, WBC 14.4,
ESR 58 mm/hr, CRP 4.5+.

Dx: 1) Crohn's ileitis
2) S/P enterocutaneous fistula

taneous fistula. With the I-Rx, tremendous nutritional improvement occurred and the fistula closed completely (Figs. 9a and 9b). She was placed on the H-HA to prevent the recurrence of the fistula. However, after discontinuing it, flare-up of the ileitis occurred and an internal fistula

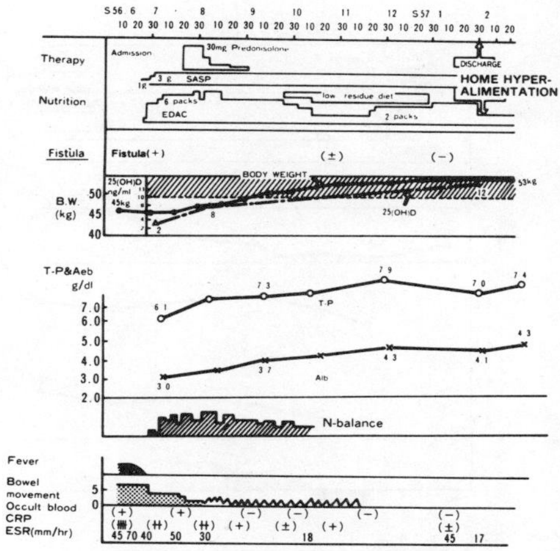

FIG. 8a. IBD case 2: clinical course (since June 1981).

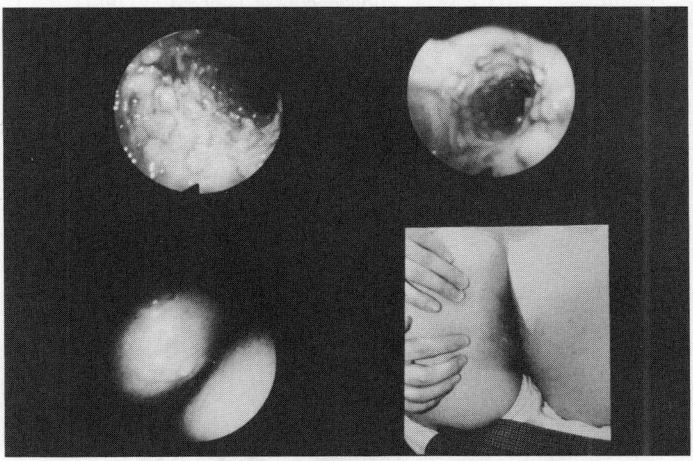

FIG. 8b. IBD case 2: fiberscopy of intestine before (upper left) and after (upper right) the treatment and perianal fistulae (lower).

developed. Then she was re-placed on the I-Rx, and so far she has been successfully rehabilitated with the new H-HA, although she has still the internal fistula.

Table 8 summarizes the results obtained from the six patients with Crohn's disease who were treated with enteral hyperalimentation. Four of the six patients had completed our treatment: each of them had marked

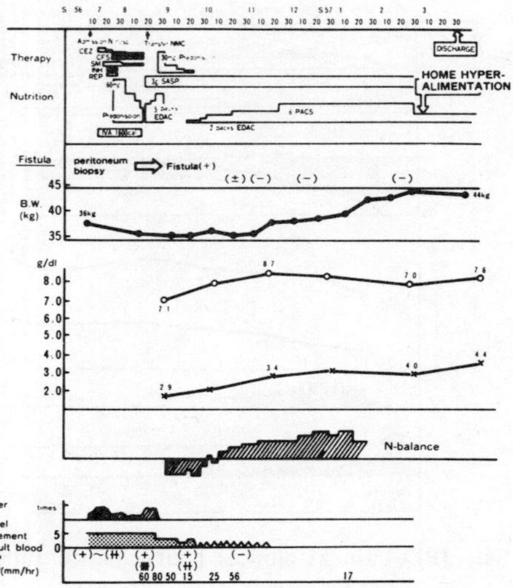

FIG. 9a. IBD case 3: clinical course (since July 1981).

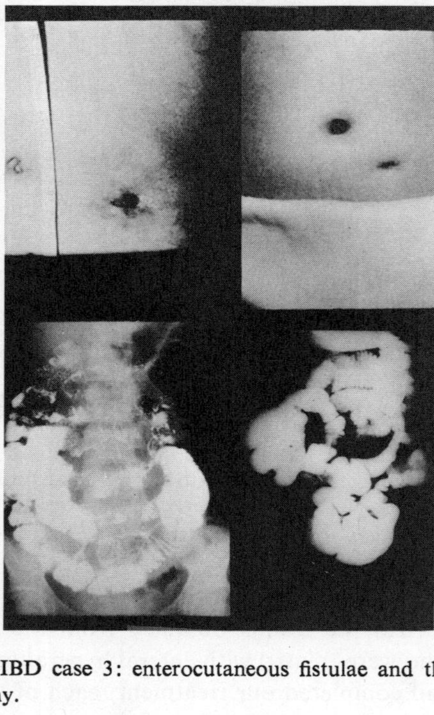

FIG. 9b. IBD case 3: enterocutaneous fistulae and their roentgenography.

TABLE 8. Therapeutic Efficacy of Enteral Hyperalimentation

Case	Age and sex	Diagnosis	Effect of enteral hyperalimentation to:							
			GI lesions	Complications						
				Malnutrition					Vitamin D deficiency	Fistula
				N-Bal	Weight (kg)	T-P (g/dl)	Alb (g/dl)	Triceps skin fold (mm)		
1) K. Y.	21/male	Crohn's colitis	Markedly improved	(+)	↑ 13.0	↑ 1.4	↑ 1.4	↑ 5.0	Resolved	—
2) C. F.	18/female	Crohn's ileo-colitis	Markedly improved	(+)	↑ 8.5	↑ 1.6	↑ 1.2	↑ 10.5	Resolved	Resolved
3) M. Y.	19/female	Crohn's jejuno-colitis	Markedly improved	(+)	↑ 8.5	↑ 0.5	↑ 1.5	↑ 3.0	—	Resolved
4) T. K.	28/female	Crohn's colitis	Markedly improved	(+)	↑ 3.5	↑ 1.5	↑ 1.3	—	—	—
				(Average)	↑ 8.4	↑ 1.3	↑ 1.4	↑ 6.2		
5) A. S.	17/female	Crohn's ileo-colitis	Markedly improved	(+)	1.5	2.4	0.6	—	—	Abscess (+) almost resolved
6) C. T.	20/female	Crohn's ileitis	Improving	(+)	2.5	1.5	1.3	—	—	—

improvement of GI lesions and nutritional status. For example, average weight gain was 8.4 kg, total protein increased by 1.3 g/dl on the average, and vitamin D deficiency found in 2 cases was resolved completely. Two patients had fistula formation but it was also closed. Two other patients are still on the treatment, but they show similar improvement. One of them had fistula with abscess formation, but it has almost been resolved with the I-Rx.

CONCLUSIONS

For SBS, continuous administration of ED (60–100 ml/hr) by infusion pump (I-Rx) was quite an effective measure to reverse malnutrition. Furthermore, overnight administration of ED by self-intubation (M-Rx) was confirmed to be a very supportive measure for rehabilitating patients with SBS because 1) self-intubation is quite safe and easily performed, 2) overnight administration of ED does not disturb the patient's normal social life, and 3) it provides the patients with enough calories to maintain nutrition (1,200–1,600 kcal/night). Therefore, the M-Rx can be used as new H-HA, and it was confirmed to be much more practical, safer, and more economical than TPN. It could also make the patients with SBS easier to socially rehabilitate.

For IBD, the I-Rx was also confirmed to be effective for Crohn's disease itself, especially GI lesion, and for complications such as PCM, vitamin D deficiency, and fistula formation. The M-Rx or our new H-HA was also confirmed to be quite a supportive measure for rehabilitating complicated Crohn's disease such as fistula formation.

Intravenous Hyperalimentation in Crohn's Disease

Osamu Fukui, Nobuteru Kikkawa, Masami Murai, Hitoshi Sasai, and Shigeru Mizuno

A clinical study of intravenous hyperalimentation (IVH) in Crohn's disease was conducted.

SUBJECTS AND METHODS

A total of 17 patients with Crohn's disease (10 males and 7 females) were treated at the Osaka National Hospital from 1975. The patients treated ranged from 16 to 29 years in age, the average age being 22.1 years old. The diseased parts were one case upper GI tract, 2 cases small bowel, 10 cases both small and large bowels, and 4 cases large bowel. The complaints were chiefly fever, stomachache, diarrhea, viscous bloody excrements, and general prostration, accompanied by ulcer and perforation, formation of thiselo, etc. Of the 17 patients, 10 patients were given treatment and 7 patients received surgical treatment as well. In the course of treatment, fever, inflammation of the bladder, severe emaciation, etc., were observed; and IVH was conducted ten times on five patients.

IVH was performed this way: a catheter was inserted from the ordinary subclavian vein by percutaneous puncturing and left in the upper vena cava. The composition of the nutrients administered to the superior vena cava was adjusted according to Dudrick's original method,[1] and so was his method of examining data of the patients. Calories used per day were from 1,250 to 2,800. The duration ranged from 7 days to 94 days.

RESULTS

All the patients who received IVH therapy gained weight and showed improvements in total protein with ESR and CRP returning to normal conditions, but X-ray and endoscopic examination indicated little change

Division of Gastroenterology, Osaka National Hospital, Osaka, Japan

TABLE 1. Clinical Effects of IVH Therapy in Crohn's Disease

Case No.	Age and sex	Clinical symptom	Average cal/day	Duration (days)	Side effect	Body weight	Total protein	ESR	CRP	X-ray and endoscopic effect	Clinical effect
2	25/m	Obstruction	1,870	35	Hyperglycemia	↑	↑	↓↓	↓	Yes	Disappearance of obstructive signs
		Obstruction	1,250	18	None	~	↑	↓	~	?	Disappearance of obstructive signs → operation
3	29/f	Emaciation	2,320	37	Zn-deficiency	↑↑	↑↑	↓	↓	No	Improvement of general condition
5	30/m	Fistula	2,870	94	None	↑↑	↑	↓	?	?	Healing of fistula → operation
6	22/m	Colo-vesical fistula	2,870	46	Zn-deficiency	↑↑	↑↑	↑	↓↓	No	Healing of colo-vesical fistula
		Emaciation	2,870	38	None	↑↑	↑↑	↓	↓	No	Improvement of general condition
7	21/m	Emaciation	2,580	35	Zn-deficiency, hyperglycemia	↑	↑	↓	~	Yes	Improvement of general condition
		Colo-vesical fistula	2,440	50	Liver function damage	↑	↑	↓	↓↓	No	Healing of cystitis
		Obstruction	1,900	7	None	~	~	↓	~	?	Disappearance of obstructive signs
		Obstruction	1,900	7	None	~	~	↓	~	?	Disappearance of obstructive signs

in all the patients except for two in whom a slight remission was observed. Side effects (stomatitis due to zinc deficiency disease and dermatitis) were observed three times in those whose duration of IVH treatment was more than 35 days, but were alleviated when zinc was replenished. Temporary hyperglycemia and hypoglycemia were observed in one patient each, and infection of the insertion area was found in two (Table 1).

The clinical effects of IVH were that improvement or remission was observed four times in three patients, remission in fistula in three patients, and general improvement in all the patients. The effects produced were evaluated according to Crohn's disease activity index (CDAI)[2,3] (Fig. 1). CDAIs before IVH and after three weeks were compared. In the seventh CDAI, improvement was observed in all the cases.

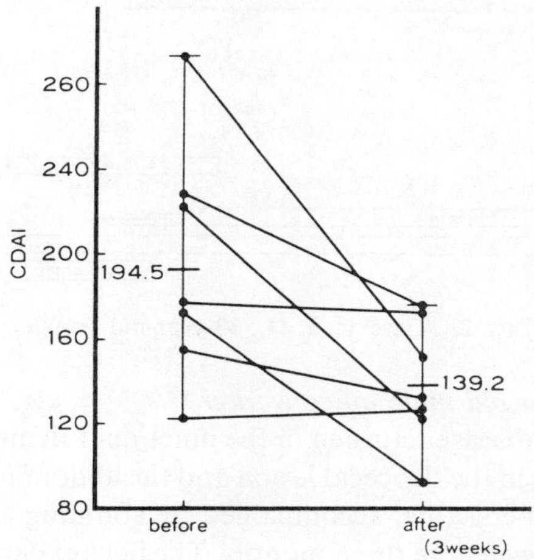

FIG. 1. Effect of IVH on Crohn's disease activity index.

CASE PRESENTATIONS

The following are two cases in which IVH proved to be very effective:

Case 1: A 33-year-old housewife

Since the end of 1976, she had been treated for Crohn's disease of the large bowels and was improving. But around the time of December 1978, she had fever, diarrhea, viscous femafecia, and anorexia with edema all over the body, especially in the lower thighs, with pleural effusion and ascites as well. When she was admitted into hospital in March 1979, she had edemata all over the body, a medium degree of abdominal dropsy, and pleural effusion that came under the left lungfield collar bone.

Examination data indicated an increase in ESR and CRP, hypoalbuminemia, and anemia. SASP and corticosteroids were administered. In addition, IVH of 2,400 kcal/day was given, and 200 ml of blood was transfused eight times. After two weeks, pleural effusion and abdominal dropsy faded quickly, with a decrease in edema and a marked improvement in clinical symptoms. In this case, IVH worked well (Fig. 2).

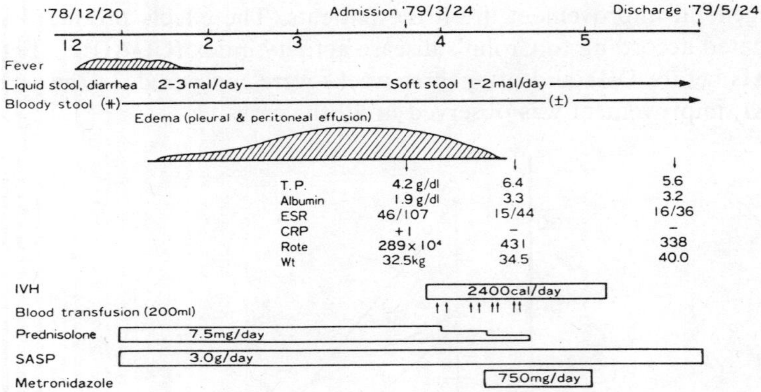

FIG. 2. Case 1: S. O., 33-year-old female.

Case 2: A 27-year-old male office worker

In this case the disease returned in the junctional ileum with a sausage-like mass forming in the ileocecal lesion and the abdominal pain becoming colicky and then persisting, accompanied by vomiting and fever. He lost 10 kg of his body weight in three months. The ileus expanded, and another operation was considered.

As treatment before the operation, IVH was started to improve the general symptoms (Fig. 3). In the IVH treatment, the patient was given no food so as to empty the bowels, to change the bacteria in the bowels, and to put out edemata on intestinal mucous membrane. Then, Denis' tube was inserted deep into the small bowel and while drainage was being done, a nutrient with some 1,800 kcal was supplied by IVH. Three days after IVH was started, the stricture symptoms in the bowels quickly faded along with the abdominal pain from pressure. The steadily increasing weight showed that the patient's condition was returning to normal. On the 18th day, barium was injected through the Denis' tube for roentgenography and the marked improvement in stricture was confirmed. On the 20th day, the Denis' tube was pulled out, and the replenishing of 2,050 kcal/day by IVH was continued until the 35th day when the catheter was pulled

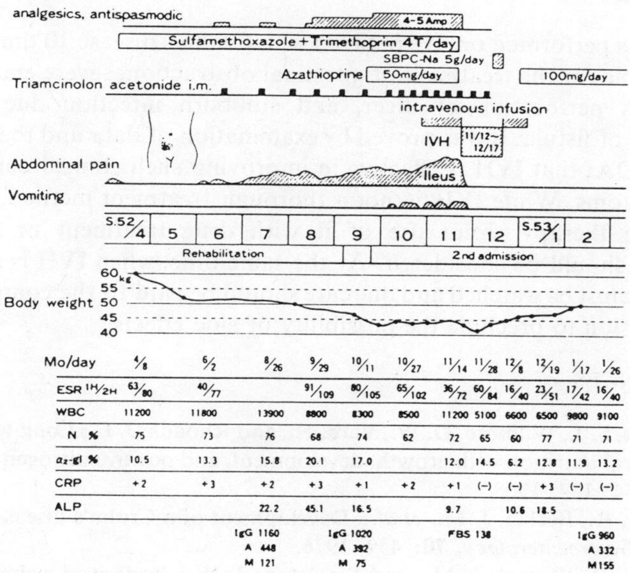

FIG. 3. Case 2: M. Y., 27-year-old male.

out. After that, the method of administration was switched to oral. The patient's condition and weight continued to improve. This patient thus recovered through conservative treatment alone.

DISCUSSION AND CONCLUSION

As shown, IVH is the best way to improve the general condition of serious alimentary deficiency caused by acute exacerbation and ileus. It involves bringing the intestinal tube to a complete rest and replenishing electrolytes, vitamins, etc., and restoring a positive nitrogen balance extrabuccally. Therefore, this treatment is useful in improving serious Crohn's disease accompanied by ileus symptom, complications caused by the formation of fistula, abscess, etc. However, no complete treatment effect can be expected. We believe that IVH is an adjunctive therapy and is effective in improving the general symptoms and condition of the patient before operation.

In performing IVH, due care has to be paid to such side effects as bleeding in the puncturing of the artery for catheter insertion, aeropelura, the formation of thrombus, infection, sepsis, and the composition of nutrients, especially the balance of dextrose minor elements.

SUMMARY

IVH was performed on five patients with Crohn's disease 10 times. IVH is applicable for the treatment of intestinal obstruction, severe emaciation as well as perforation of ulcer, and stubborn infection due to the formation of fistula. It was proved by examination of data and the evaluation of CDAI that IVH is effective in improving such clinical conditions and symptoms. While IVH is not a thorough treatment method, it is an adjunctive therapy. Joint use of it with drug treatment or surgical treatment should be considered. At the same time, when IVH is applied, infection must be watched and due care should be paid to the composition of transfusion to preclude the possibility of side effects.

REFERENCES

1. Dudrick, S. J., Wilmore, D. W., Vara, H., and Rhoada, J. E.: Long-term total parenteral nutrition with growth, development, and positive nitrogen balance. *Surg.*, **54**: 134, 1968.
2. Best, W. R., Beckel, J. M., *et al.*: Development of a Crohn's disease activity index. *Gastroenterology*, **70**: 439, 1976.
3. Best, W. R., Beckel, J. M., and Singleton, J. W.: Rederived values of the eight coefficients of the Crohn's disease activity index (CDAI). *Gastroenterology*, **77**: 843, 1979.

Prognosis and Treatment for Patients with Crohn's Disease

Richard G. Farmer

Crohn's disease of the small intestine was originally described in 1932 by Crohn, Ginzberg, and Oppenheimer[1] from the Mount Sinai Hospital in New York. Their report encompassed many of the complications and clinical features of the disease and, in fact, is still appropriate as a clinical review. In 1954, Van Patter, Bargen, and their colleagues[2] from the Mayo Clinic reported 600 cases of regional enteritis in a massive article in *Gastroenterology*. They reaffirmed the clinical features and the observation that the disease was limited to areas of the digestive tract proximal to the ileocecal valve. A "modern" era of understanding Crohn's disease was entered in 1960 upon publication, by Lockhart-Mummery and Morson[3] from St. Marks Hospital in London, of a report of 25 cases of Crohn's disease involving the colon. They noted that their patients had "localized or diffuse inflammation of the large intestine whom we believe to have the same disease as that described by Crohn, Ginzberg and Oppenheimer in 1932." They proposed avoidance of the term regional enteritis and use of the eponym Crohn's disease to avoid confusion and to assist in the differentiation from ulcerative colitis. However, confusion in terminology continued to exist for the next decade with multiple terms being applied to Crohn's disease, especially if the colon were involved. These included granulomatous colitis, ileocolitis, transmural colitis, right-sided colitis, as well as regional enteritis and ileitis. An interesting historical observation is that, during this time, the incidence of Crohn's disease appeared to increase rapidly; initially this was thought to be due to an increased recognition of the disease, but subsequently it was established that the incidence was truly rising. Twenty years ago, a center in the U.S.A. or Western Europe involved in seeing large numbers of patients with inflammatory bowel disease saw five or six cases of ulcerative colitis to every

Chairman, Division of Medicine, Department of Gastroenterology, Cleveland Clinic Foundation, Cleveland, Ohio, U.S.A.

case of Crohn's disease (regional enteritis). Today that trend has almost completely reversed, for reasons which are unexplained. Nevertheless, the clinical phenomenon of an increasing number of patients with Crohn's disease is recognized worldwide.

PATHOLOGY

Crohn's disease is a transmural pathological process which can involve any portion of the gastrointestinal tract, but has a particular predilection for the ileum. The characteristic gross and the microscopic pathological features include submucosal lymphedema and serositis, giving the gross appearance of a thickened segment of intestine, and discontinuous involvement with "skip areas" often near areas of significant stenosis ("string sign"). Mucosal changes may also be discontinuous, and submucosal lymphedema can give a "cobblestone" appearance to the mucosa. Discrete ulceration may also occur, but the typical diffuse uniform granularity and friability of the mucosa of ulcerative colitis is seldom seen. There is a propensity for microscopic fissuring which may lead to fistula formation. Despite its popularity as a histologic feature, granulomas are found in only about 50% of cases. In 1968, we[4)] described the above-mentioned features which were in agreement with those described by Morson and his colleagues.[3)] Recently, we have reviewed a consecutive series of 336 pathological specimens reaffirming our original histologic criteria.[5)] There were 121 patients with a diagnosis of ulcerative colitis and 245 with Crohn's disease. Pathological features are described in Table 1.

TABLE 1. Comparative Pathological Features of Ulcerative Colitis and Crohn's Disease

Pathological features	Ulcerative colitis	Crohn's disease
Transmural inflammation	1+	4+
Serositis	1+	4+
Granulomata	±	2+
Lymphedema	±	4+
Fissuring	±	3+
Crypt abscesses	4+	2+
Mucosal dysplasia	2+	±

4+ = 75–100%; 3+ = 75%; 2+ = 25–50%; 1+ = 5–25%; ± = 0–5%.

CROHN'S DISEASE DEFINITIONS

During a 1979 workshop on Crohn's disease in Cape Town, South Africa, a working group devised the following definitions: Crohn's disease is a chronic inflammatory process primarily affecting the alimentary tract.

Its most common presenting symptoms include diarrhea, weight loss, and crampy abdominal pain.

The disease involving the bowel may be classified as: 1) continuous diseases localized to a) the small intestine, b) the ileocolic region, and c) the large intestine; and 2) discontinuous disease involving one or combinations of the above with/without lesions elsewhere.

The pathological confirmation of the diagnosis of Crohn's disease can be achieved in the resected specimen by the findings of the signs shown in Table 2.

TABLE 2. Pathological Findings in and Pathological Features of Crohn's Disease

Gross pathological findings
Major (i.e., characteristic)
Sinuses
Fistulae
Asymmetrical bowel involvement
Fissure ulcers
Skip lesions
Minor (i.e., frequently found but less specific)
Narrowing of the bowel lumen
Thickening of mucosal folds
Cobblestone appearance of the mucosal pattern
Other ulcers—usually discrete and superficial
Pathological features
Macroscopic findings
Serosal injection and/or adhesions
Strictures
Fistulae
Cobblestone mucosal pattern
Ulcers—superficial discrete, fissure, longitudinal
Microscopic findings
Thickening of the bowel wall
Lymphoid aggregates
Transmural inflammation
Granuloma
Submucosal fibrosis
Muscular hypertrophy

CLINICAL FEATURES

In the original papers concerning small intestine Crohn's disease[1,2] the symptoms of diarrhea, abdominal pain, and weight loss were emphasized. In the features described by Lockhart-Mummery and Morson[3] for colonic Crohn's disease, diarrhea was the predominant symptom, and perianal lesions were found in 17 of their 25 cases. Weight loss was also a significant symptom, although abdominal pain and rectal bleeding were much less frequent. Also, they emphasized that a completely normal sigmoidoscopic examination was possible for patients with Crohn's disease of the colon (again a significant differential point from ulcerative colitis: in virtually all cases of ulcerative colitis the sigmoidoscopic examination is abnormal and there is no perianal disease). Additionally, Crohn's disease of the colon may affect only a portion of the colon with "skip" lesions present.

In 1975, we reported a series of 615 consecutive patients with Crohn's disease[6)] and advanced the concept of the "clinical pattern." Emphasis was placed on the initial and primary manifestation of the disease, recognizing that in some cases there is extension of disease to involve widespread portions of the intestinal tract. Nevertheless, our studies indicated that the clinical features could be categorized based on the primary location of disease. The clinical patterns shown in Table 3 were recognized.

TABLE 3. Clinical Patterns of Crohn's Disease

	No. of patients
Ileocolic (involvement of the right colon and terminal ileum)	252 (41.0%)
Small intestine (without colon involvement)	176 (28.6%)
Colon (without small intestine involvement)	166 (27.0%)
Anarectal (without other demonstrable involvement initially)	21 (3.4%)

Cleveland Clinic Series, 615 patients, Ref. 6.

Almost 90% of our patients had a combination of diarrhea, abdominal pain, and weight loss in varying degrees of severity, with diarrhea being the predominant symptom. Rectal bleeding was a statistically significant differentiation between colonic disease and other locations. Rectal fistulae were statistically more common with ileocolic and colonic pattern. Among statistically significant complications were: 1) perianal fistulae, internal fistulae, and intestinal obstruction with ileocolic pattern; 2) perianal fistulae, toxic megacolon, and arthritis with the colon pattern; and 3) intestinal obstruction with the small intestine pattern. The mean age of the patients was 32 years at the time of diagnosis, and only 17% had symptoms for less than six months (reflecting our referral population). Symptoms had been present for up to four years for 68% of our patients. The largest percentage of patients having a short duration of symptoms was in the colon pattern.

In evaluating a patient with Crohn's disease, these criteria are useful: 1) the location and extent of disease, 2) the severity of symptoms and findings, 3) the duration of disease, and 4) the overall impact on the patient, nutritionally and functionally.

LOCATION AND EXTENT OF DISEASE

As we emphasized in our 1975 paper,[6] the anatomic location of disease plays a significant role in the clinical features, prognosis, indication for surgery, and subsequent clinical course of the patient with Crohn's disease. The National Cooperative Crohn's Disease Study[7] also affirmed this phenomenon and Table 4 lists the important differences in symptomatology among patients with various locations of disease. Thus, as can be seen, diarrhea is the most common symptom in all categories followed by abdominal pain and weight loss. The latter was more associated with extensive small bowel or colonic disease and also reflected increased severity of disease as well. Our experience clearly indicated their perianal manifestations were more a feature of ileocolic and colonic disease than of small intestine disease and that extraintestinal manifestations were more a feature of colonic than either ileocolic or small intestine involvement.

TABLE 4. Initial Symptoms (Crohn's Disease) Related to Disease Location

	Cleveland Clinic 615 Cases Farmer *et al.*, 1975[6]			NCCDS 569 Cases Mekhjian *et al.*, 1979[7]	
	Ileocolic	Small intestine	Large intestine	Total	Large intestine
Diarrhea	4+	4+	4+	4+	4+
Abdominal pain	3+	3+	3+	4+	4+
Bleeding	1+	1+	2+	2+	3+
Weight loss*	1+	1+	1+	4+	4+
Perianal disease	2+	±	2+	2+	2+
Arthritis	±	±	1+	1+	1+

4+ = greater than 75% of cases; 3+ = 50–75%; 2+ = 25–50%, 1+ = 5–25%; ±, 5% or less.
*Defined as loss of 20% of body weight.

With regard to location of disease, our study[6] as well as a subsequent study of Crohn's disease in children[8] indicated that approximately 40% of patients have involvement of the distal ileum and proximal colon, that about 25–30% of patients have involvement of the small intestine alone, and that about 25% of patients have involvement of the colon without more proximal disease. These observations have been verified by others[7,9] (Table 5). Studies concerned with extraintestinal manifestations[6,10] have also shown the preponderance of colonic disease. The most common manifestations are those of monarticular synovitis usually involving the large joints; erythema nodosum and pyoderma gangrenosum may also occur. As noted in our study of childhood Crohn's disease[8] growth retardation can be an important systemic feature for children, particularly with prepubertal onset.

TABLE 5. Crohn's Disease: Initial Site of Involvement

Series	Small Intestine	Ileocolic	Colon	Other
Stockholm (Ref. 9)	41%	41%	17%	1%
NCCDS (Ref. 7)	30%	55%	14%	1%
Cleveland Clinic (Ref. 6)	29%	41%	27%	3%

Location of disease is also a significant factor in the subsequent development of complications and particularly those leading to surgery[6] (Table 6). For patients with small intestine or ileocolic location of disease, complications are frequently more "local," whereas chronicity, malnutrition, and so-called medical intractability are more often associated with colonic location of disease.[11] Intestinal obstruction is particularly associated as an indication for surgery for patients with small intestine disease, and intestinal obstruction and/or internal fistula with development of abscess are the most common indications for surgery with disease located in the ileocolic region.[6] Perianal manifestations of Crohn's disease are more likely to be associated with colonic or ileocolic disease than more proximal location (while perianal disease may be the initial location,[6] it is frequent that colonic involvement ensues). While more proximal small intestine involvement could logically be associated with severe malnutrition and systemic features, this location of disease is unusual. Likewise, gastroduodenal Crohn's disease is not a common location, although when present is associated with rather characteristic symptoms (post-prandial fullness, pain, vomiting, and weight loss). Location of disease is probably the single most important clinical determinant of the course of Crohn's disease in a given patient.

TABLE 6. Crohn's Disease: Clinical Features and Complications

	Ileocolic	Small Intestine	Colon	Statistically significant
Perianal disease	38%	14%	36%	yes
Internal fistula	34%	17%	16%	yes
Intestinal obstruction	44%	35%	17%	yes
Growth retardation	13%	3%	3%	no
Pyoderma	1.6%	0%	3%	no
Arthritis	3.6%	4%	16%	yes
Spondylitis	1.6%	0.6%	5%	no
Megacolon	2%	0%	11%	yes

Cleveland Clinic Series, 615 patients, Ref. 6.

CROHN'S DISEASE ACTIVITY INDEX

Development of an activity index to assess the clinical severity of Crohn's disease has been a problem for many years. Although it has been shown that the primary symptoms of Crohn's disease are abdominal pain, diarrhea, and weight loss,[6,7] these symptoms are somewhat variable and are not entirely accurate in the assessment of disease activity. Not only is the assessment of disease activity important in the day-to-day management of patients with Crohn's disease, it is also significant in clinical trials. Thus, the National Cooperative Crohn's Disease Study (NCCDS) developed a quantifiable disease index.[12] However, this disease index did not provide all of the necessary solutions to this problem and has been re-evaluated.[13] It must be emphasized that the NCCDS Crohn's Disease Activity Index (CDAI) (Table 7) was developed primarily for evaluation of a randomized prospective clinical trial, and not for day-to-day clinical usage. Nevertheless, one might surmise that these two goals are not mutually exclusive of each other, and there have been attempts to put the CDAI to clinical use. Two problems have arisen: first, the CDAI is a mixture of subjective and "objective" data, and the weighing of the various factors makes considerable difference in the quantification of it; second, it is reasonably cumbersome and it requires a fair amount of time to complete the required forms.

Partly because of these two factors and partly because of the stimulus provided by the CDAI, others have attempted to develop activity indices

TABLE 7. Crohn's Disease Activity Index (CDAI)[12,13]

1. Liquid or very soft stools (number in 1 week): none; 1–4; 5–9; 10–19; 20–49; and 50–98
2. Abdominal pain (sum of 7 daily ratings): 0 = none; 1 = mild; 2 = moderate; 3 = severe
3. General well-being (sum of 7 daily ratings): 0 = generally well; 1 = slightly below par; 2 = poor; 3 = very poor; 4 = terrible
4. Symptoms or findings presumed related to Crohn's disease
   1) Arthritis or arthralgia
   2) Skin or mouth lesions, pyoderma gangrenosa or erythema nodosum
   3) Iritis or uveitis
   4) Anal fissure, fistula, or perirectal abscess
   5) Other bowel-related fistulae, such as enterovesical, etc.
   6) Febrile episode exceeding 100°F during past week
5. Taking Lomotil or opiates for diarrhea: 0 = no; 1 = yes
6. Abnormal mass: 0 = absent; 2 = questionable
7. Hematocrit: (47 minus hematocrit), males; (42 minus hematocrit), females
8. Body weight: $100 \times \{1 - (\text{body weight/standard weight})\} \gtrless 11.2\%$

for patients with Crohn's disease. Lloyd-Still and Green[14] have developed a "clinical score" for children with inflammatory bowel disease (IBD) which brings in such factors as school attendance, growth and development, and laboratory and X-ray findings. The Dutch group[15] have developed an activity index with 18 variables based on the evaluation of data from 63 patients. However, this activity index has not been widely accepted, again because of its cumbersome and multi-variable nature. A French group[16] has developed what they called "Laboratory Supplementation of Crohn's Disease Activity Index" in which they used such studies as the C-reactive protein, sedimentation rate, and orosomucoid levels to supplement the clinical evaluation of patients with Crohn's disease.

Perhaps the most widely used of the newer activity indices is that developed by Harvey and Bradshaw[17] called "A Simple Index of Crohn's Disease Activity" (Table 8). This has the advantage of being strictly clinical and of enabling the clinician to modify the variable factors on each evaluation of the patient. However, this index may be too "simple" in view of the complexity of Crohn's disease itself.

TABLE 8. The Simple Index of Crohn's Disease Activity[17]

1. General well-being: 0 = very well, 1 = slightly below par, 2 = poor, 3 = very poor, 4 = terrible
2. Abdominal pain: 0 = none, 1 = mild, 2 = moderate, 3 = severe
3. Number of liquid stools per day
4. Abdominal mass: 0 = none, 1 = dubious, 2 = definite, 3 = definite and tender
5. Complications: arthralgia, uveitis, erythema nodosum, apthous ulcer, pyoderma gangrenosum, anal fissure, new fistula, abscess (score 1 per item)

Our work in the assessment of patients with Crohn's disease has indicated the significance of the "clinical pattern"[6] in which the anatomic location of disease plays an important role in the clinical course, prognosis, complications, and indication for surgery for patients with Crohn's disease. In addition, symptoms from Crohn's disease may not be due to disease activity as such, but may be due to fibrosis, stenosis, and partial intestinal obstruction. Thus, at the time of operation and resection of the stenotic segment, there may be little or no actual inflammation, and the pathologist may find marked fibrosis and stenosis but without significant evidence for inflammatory change or granulomas. This creates yet an additional problem in the assessment of the "disease activity" for patients with Crohn's disease.

In light of all of these observations, an international study group has been formed to develop a new disease activity index for patients with Crohn's disease (Table 9). Those involved with the development of the previous indices are active in the current study group, and computer modeling and testing of the variables are currently underway. Whether or not this disease activity index will be modified by subsequent computer generated data remains to be seen. Nevertheless, the attempt to quantify the disease activity of Crohn's disease is worthwhile, and is an ongoing project. However, the quantifiability of such an index, its clinical usefulness and reproducibility, and its widespread acceptance by both clinicians and clinical investigators remain to be seen.

TABLE 9. Clinical Assessment of Disease Activity in Crohn's Disease (International Study Group on Crohn's Disease)

1. Bowel habits—frequency and consistency of stools
2. Abdominal pain—severity, persistence, and changes
3. Body weight—changes since last examination
4. The physician's assessment of the patient's sense of well-being (subjective and functional evaluation)
5. Hemoglobin and hematocrit changes since last examination, and/or abnormalities
6. Oral temperature
7. Presence of an abdominal mass (or question thereof)
8. Presence of abdominal tenderness
9. Perianal and/or abdominal fistula
10. Systemic manifestations (arthritis, etc.), growth curves in children

SEVERITY OF DISEASE

In considering a patient with Crohn's disease, and the contradistinction to that of ulcerative colitis, relatively simple parameters such as the degree of rectal bleeding and the extent of mucosal inflammation as seen on proctosigmoidoscopy are not possible in the majority of cases. Therefore, other evidence of clinical severity must be utilized in assessing the patient's current status as well as in the difficult area of assessment of response to therapy. In addition, "objective" features are often absent or relatively non-specific. One can utilize the healing or observable changes in perineal fistulae, abdominal masses, and the weight of the patient, but otherwise clinical features may be difficult to assess for changes. Use of colonoscopy[18)] in Crohn's disease is more helpful in the initial evaluation of the patient and the differential diagnosis, rather than as a sequential evaluation mechanism. Since dysplasia is an extremely rare phenomenon in Crohn's disease, the use of endoscopy for this purpose, as it is used in ulcerative colitis, is not helpful. The presence of anemia and hypoalbuminemia are helpful, but generally correlate with the nutritional status of the patient and often do not provide additional clues beyond those observed in the clinical evaluation of the patient. The presence of fever and extraintestinal manifestations may be helpful in indicating activity of disease. However, the most useful clinical judgments are the assessment of the patient's major symptoms, usually progressive diarrhea, abdominal pain, and weight loss. As emphasized by Fazio,[19] toxic megacolon is now more frequent in Crohn's disease than ulcerative colitis.

An additional factor of importance, and particularly in the assessment of response to therapy, is the problem posed by cicatrical narrowing of the gut, particularly in the distal small intestine or ileocecal region. The patient may have little or no actual inflammatory process going on at a given time but may experience symptoms of progressive abdominal pain and distension associated with scarring and narrowing of the intestinal lumen. Thus, response to medical therapy may be poor, creating the impression that there is medical "intractability" or leading to a fruitless search for additional therapy when the problem can be alleviated by resection of the area in question. Thus, assessment of the "fibrotic" manifestations is important, and can be accomplished if one recognizes a relative lack of inflammatory and systemic features in the patient with progressively developing intestinal obstruction.

DURATION OF DISEASE

In Crohn's disease, again in striking contrast to the patient with ulcerative colitis, the problem of duration of disease relates to 1) the location of disease, 2) the systemic and nutritional effects, and 3) whether or not an operation has occurred. Since experience has shown that about two thirds of patients with Crohn's disease will require an operation at some time during the course of their illness, this latter is of great significance in assessing the long-term status of the patient.[6,9,20] In fact, recurrences following surgery in Crohn's disease have been shown to be among the most important of the long-term features of Crohn's disease and have been the subject of intense interest in recent years.[21,22] Recurrences are most characteristically associated with original location of disease in the ileocolic region and previous resection. Virtually all recurrences occur just proximal to the anastomosis at the site of the previous resection. Thus, it is generally considered that presence of recurrence as such is not an indication for surgery, but that if subsequent complication should occur (usually stenosis with partial obstruction) it may lead to another operation.

EFFECT ON THE PATIENT

Because the symptoms of Crohn's disease frequently are chronic, multiple, and often resistant to therapy, the effect on the patient can be extremely negative from several points of view. The patient may function suboptimally, in a nutritional, social, or economic sense, and if a child or adolescent, fail to grow. These negative features may create or exacerbate psychological or interpersonal relationship problems creating an added burden for the patient. If it is implied by the physician or another person that psychological factors are implicated in the cause of the disease, this can enhance feelings of guilt which make these other phenomena somewhat perpetuating. There has been recent emphasis on the "quality of life" for patients with Crohn's disease, and our study of childhood onset[8] showed that 10 years after onset of illness about two thirds of patients considered that they were functioning suboptimally. Since many patients are afflicted with Crohn's disease at a time in their lives in which they are attempting to develop social and economic independence, and are rendered more dependent by the illness, all of these factors can have a significantly negative impact. The need for therapy and compliance with it as well as a variety of nutritional deficiencies and other symptoms can easily cause the patient to develop a "sick role" behavior pattern. Thus, it stands to reason that patients with Crohn's disease certainly should be encouraged to try to maintain patterns of activity and nutrition that are as normal as is possible under their given set of circumstances. Because many patients with Crohn's disease will require surgery,[7,9,20] and often an ileostomy will be involved,[11,20] the problems can be compounded. Further, recurrences following surgery[21] may simply restart the cycle again. Steroid side effects can be an additional problem. Therefore, it is certainly obvious that the physician must play a role in helping the patient with these myraid problems.

EXTRAINTESTINAL MANIFESTATIONS

The so-called systemic or extraintestinal manifestations of Crohn's disease have been recognized but poorly understood for many years. Our study[6] showed that the most common of these was arthritis, with a statistically significant involvement of the colonic pattern occurring in 16% of patients. An additional 5% with colonic Crohn's disease had spondylitis, while 3% each had pyoderma gangrenosum and growth retardation. Patients with ileocolic and small intestine patterns had "systemic" features less frequently, with 4% having arthritis. A significant complication was that of toxic megacolon, occurring in 11% of patients with colonic pattern, only 2% of patients with ileocolic pattern, and no patient with initial small intestine pattern. Toxic megacolon was characterized by Fazio[19] as follows: 1) the presence of toxicity, including tachycardia, fever, leukocytosis and hypoalbuminemia; 2) the presence of dilatation of the colon 5 cm or greater; 3) associated features of abdominal distension, tenderness, anemia, hypotension, and electrolyte imbalance.

We have recently evaluated the extraintestinal manifestations of Crohn's disease and compared them with those in ulcerative colitis for a group of over 800 patients with childhood onset of inflammatory bowel disease.[23] The complications and extraintestinal manifestations in the two groups are described in Tables 10 and 11. As can be seen, the clinical complications were quite different between the two diseases, with statistically significant differences for most features and complications. This only re-emphasizes the clinical differences between the two diseases. On the other hand, the extraintestinal manifestations, with the single exception of growth retardation, were similar in both groups.

TABLE 10. Complications in Inflammatory Bowel Disease: Childhood Onset[23]

	Crohn's disease (505 patients)	Ulcerative colitis (333 patients)	
Complications	71.5%	33.8%	$p < 0.001$
Perianal disease	27.1%	1.8%	$p < 0.001$
Intestinal obstruction	24.4%	3.3%	$p < 0.001$
Internal fistula	16.4%	0.9%	$p < 0.001$
Growth retardation	7.9%	2.1%	$p < 0.001$
Megacolon	6.3%	3.0%	$p < 0.05$
Chronicity	14.9%	21.9%	$p < 0.01$
Surgery	62.8%	35.6%	$p < 0.01$

TABLE 11. Extraintestinal Manifestations of Inflammatory Bowel Disease: Childhood Onset[23]

	Crohn's disease (505 patients)	Ulcerative colitis (333 patients)	
Arthritis	7.3%	7.2%	$p < 0.9$
Pyoderma	1.4%	1.8%	$p < 0.4$
Iritis	0.1%	0.9%	$p < 0.3$
Liver disease	0.6%	1.5%	$p < 0.3$
Erythema nodosum	2.8%	3.3%	$p < 0.8$

CROHN'S DISEASE IN CHILDHOOD AND ADOLESCENCE

We have conducted a long-term follow-up study of 522 patients seen between 1955 and 1974 at the Cleveland Clinic, with onset of Crohn's disease under the age of 21.[8] Follow-up information was obtained for 98.4% of the patients, and the mean follow-up for the entire series was over seven years with a greater than five-year follow-up for 67% of the patients. Nearly 60% of the patients were ages 16 to 20 at onset of disease. Operation had been performed for 69% of the patients and 2.4% (13 patients) had died. Most of the deaths occurred postoperatively and were associated with sepsis and hypoalbuminemia.

One of the most important aspects of the long-term prognosis for patients with Crohn's disease is the patient's assessment of his quality of life. In this study of 522 patients with childhood onset of Crohn's disease,[8] patients were asked to assess the cumulative effect of the illness and treatment and to make a statement regarding their current state of health. Responses were categorized in three ways: good—ability to function in a nearly normal manner with minimal interference from illness and its sequela; poor—severe effect on life style requiring medication and frequent hospitalization; fair—suboptimal but adequate functioning (i.e., chronic illness and partial disability). We observed that only 23% of patients considered their quality of life to be good, 67% were functioning at suboptimal level, and 6% described their state of health as poor, 2.4% of the patients had died. These findings only underscore the importance of the aspect that chronic illness plays in the lives of patients with Crohn's disease and again reiterates that therapeutic measures must take this into account.

A striking similarity between patients with Crohn's disease and ulcerative colitis is the high association of similar diseases within the family. In a recent report of data obtained by interviews from 838 patients with IBD having an onset under the age of 21,[24] we found that 280 (33%) had a positive family history for inflammatory bowel disease. These included 29% of the patients with ulcerative colitis and 35% of the patients with Crohn's disease. Included were 16% of the patients with IBD in the immediate family, with an almost equal distribution between Crohn's disease and ulcerative colitis. A similar percentage of parents and siblings were affected: 9.8% and 9% of parents and 6% and 7.5% of siblings for patients with ulcerative colitis and Crohn's disease, respectively. While these data may or may not have environmental or genetic implications, they certainly have implications regarding the impact on the family of having multiple members afflicted with inflammatory bowel disease. These data only reiterate the important point of physicians' awareness of the natural history of inflammatory bowel disease and the various prognostic factors involved, as these are questions which patients invariably ask.

OPERATION IN CROHN'S DISEASE

Operations for patients with inflammatory bowel disease (IBD) are frequently necessary. Often there is much confusion in the mind of the patient about the type of operation needed, and great concern expressed over the possible need for an ileostomy or other stoma. Additionally, patients often have the impression that if a disease is present it should be removed and thus hope for a "simple" solution to an often complex problem. Because of this, close cooperation between the physician and surgeon is essential to the optimal management of a patient undergoing surgery for IBD. Multiple factors must be considered before the decision for operation can be finally determined: need for the operation based on the clinical situation; the state of nutrition of the patient; the presence or absence of infection; use of steroids or other therapy and its possible effects; potential postoperative problems, such as the short bowel syndrome; and the patient's psychological state of readiness for the operation. All of this is, of course, moot if the problem is a life-threatening emergency and the operation must be performed as such. However, in most cases, the decision for operation in a patient with IBD can be approached somewhat logically. Therefore, the more information available to the physician, and the better he understands the nature of the operation, the better the approach to management of the patient will be.

In our previous study of indications for surgery for 500 patients with Crohn's disease,[20] we found that approximately two thirds of patients with Crohn's disease will undergo operation. The figure is far lower for patients with ulcerative colitis. In studies of childhood onset of IBD of more than 800 children with ulcerative colitis and Crohn's disease whom we have followed for over 10 years,[8,23] we have found that approximately two thirds of the patients with Crohn's disease have undergone operation compared with one third of the patients with ulcerative colitis. In fact, many patients with ulcerative colitis have become reasonably free of symptoms, and the patient has not been particularly receptive to the idea that an operation might possibly be necessary. This has complicated the problem of cancer surveillance for patients with ulcerative colitis, and studies attempting to determine which patients are at greatest risk for developing cancer in long-term ulcerative colitis are underway.

The problem for patients with Crohn's disease, on the other hand, is often quite different from that of those with ulcerative colitis. The problem for a patient with Crohn's disease is that of recurrent symptoms, malnutrition, diarrhea, abdominal pain, and often chronic ill health. Thus, although there are many similarities between the indications for surgery, and even the types of surgery, for patients with ulcerative colitis and Crohn's disease there are many differences as well.

For the patient with Crohn's disease, there may be problems with chronic intermittent disease, requirements for medication, malnutrition, and ability to function, but complications are often based on location of the disease process. In our previous study,[20] we compared the location of disease to the indication for surgery and established that there were statistical differences for surgical indications (Table 12).

TABLE 12. Crohn's Disease: Comparison of Disease Location to Indication for Surgery

Indication for surgery	Disease location		
	Colon	Small intestine	Ileocolic
Perianal disease	+	−	+
Intestinal obstruction	−	+	+
Internal fistula and abscess	−	+	+
Toxic megacolon	+	−	−
Poor response to medical therapy	+	−	−

Thus, disease location in Crohn's disease was found to be highly characteristic of certain complications leading to the need for operation. Patients with colonic Crohn's disease experience malnutriton, chronic disease, and debility more frequently than do those with ileocolic or small intestine location of disease. In these latter two circumstances, localized complications such as intestinal obstruction or localized fistula with abscess are the most frequent indications for the need for operation. Although development of intestinal carcinoma in Crohn's disease is quite unusual, it may occur in patients with long-standing partial ileal obstruction or in bypassed loops of the small intestine. Nevertheless, the problem of cancer surveillance in Crohn's disease is not as numerically significant as in ulcerative colitis.

A significant problem in Crohn's disease is that of chronic disease and malnutrition, particularly because operation and removal of the colon (or other disease segment) is not as predictably beneficial as it is in ulcerative colitis. Although recurrences in Crohn's disease are more frequent following small bowel resection with anastomosis, recurrences can occur following any type of operation in Crohn's disease.[22)] Therefore, assessment of the patient with malnutrition, complications or side effects from steroid therapy, and failure to function socially and economically may be more difficult to determine than that of the patient with ulcerative colitis. The indication and timing of operation for the patient with colonic Crohn's disease and chronic debility usually require the greatest degree of understanding and cooperation in the decision-making process among the physician, surgeon, and patient.

However, our experience with Crohn's disease had indicated that most patients who undergo surgery do so for a specific complication, and particularly if the anatomic location is that of the small intestine or the ileocolic region.[20] Statistically significant indications for surgery for ileocolic Crohn's disease include 1) internal fistula, 2) intestinal obstruction, and 3) perianal disease. Intestinal obstruction was the most frequent indication for patients with small intestine disease, with fistula and abscess second. Those with the colonic pattern had a more frequent occurrence of chronic disease heralding the need for surgery as well as toxic megacolon, perianal disease, and internal (sigmoid) fistula as additional frequent indications.

The frequency of need for operations for patients with Crohn's disease can hardly be overemphasized. In both our studies during the years 1966 to 1972,[6] and in our longer-term study of children with Crohn's disease,[8] we observed that over two thirds of patients with Crohn's disease will require an operation if they are followed for 10 years. In fact, in the Stockholm series,[9] 84% of patients with Crohn's disease had undergone an operation at some time during the 20-year period. In a comparison of the clinical course of ulcerative colitis (proctocolitis) and Crohn's disease of the colon,[11] Lennard-Jones and co-workers emphasized that "the chance of requiring operation among patients with Crohn's colitis was 72% within six years of first admission to the hospital compared with 44% among patients with proctocolitis." Likewise, they noted that "the two diseases tend to follow a different course" and that proctocolitis (ulcerative colitis) was found to be more acute, whereas Crohn's colitis often required admission for chronic symptoms, a finding also in agreement with our study.[20]

Two unusual features of Crohn's disease which are worthy of mention are hyperoxaluria and ureteral obstruction. If in excess of 50 cm of terminal ileum is resected, the patient may develop hyperoxaluria and renal stones on the basis of increased dietary oxalate absorption, characteristically in conjunction with some degree of steatorrhea.[25] Hyperoxaluria may also occur with extensive inflammation of the ileum, but is usually associated with resection. Ureteral obstruction is typically on the right side (44 of 48 cases seen at the Cleveland Clinic occurred on the right side)[26] and is usually found with inflammatory mass secondary to ileocolic Crohn's disease (with or without a perforation, internal fistula, and abscess). Because renal function can be severely compromised and hydronephrosis can occur, this complication is especially dangerous as it may be difficult to detect clinically in its early state.

RECURRENCES

One of the most important problems in dealing with Crohn's disease is that of postoperative recurrences, especially so because of the high incidence of need for operation in the first place. The Cape Town classification[27] defined a recurrence in Crohn's disease as the "appearance of the objective signs—defined radiologically, endoscopically or pathologically—of Crohn's disease in the bowel of the patient who previously had a resection of all microscopically diseased tissue." This was contrasted with a relapse of Crohn's disease after a symptom-free interval, in patients with known disease, providing that other non-related causes of these symptoms have been excluded. Use of colonoscopy following resection for detecting a recurrence,[18,21] can be a valuable method for detecting a recurrence, as can endoscopy through a stoma. Since most recurrences occur just proximal to the anastomosis and since most patients requiring surgery have had a resection with anastomosis,[20] attention to recurrences at this site (usually an ileocolic anastomosis) has been emphasized. In a recent review of recurrences following surgery for Crohn's disease, Lee and Papaioannou[21] noted that a number of studies have shown crude recurrence rates of between 30% and 60% ten years following resective surgery. They quoted Hellers[9] as having observed an overall crude recurrence rate of 42% with an incidence of 30% for patients following colectomy and ileostomy. While there is no question that the recurrence rate appears to be higher following a resective procedure with anastomosis (be it ileocolic or ileorectal anastomosis), there is a significant recurrence rate following stomal procedures as well.[11] It is difficult to predict those patients at highest risk for developing recurrences, but there are attempts at doing this. In an ongoing study, we are following over 550 patients with more than 10 years after diagnosis and have found that almost 70% have required one operation and one half of those operated have had a recurrence requiring yet another resection. We have attempted to correlate this to initial location of disease (clinical pattern) as well as initial indications for surgery. Our data thus far suggest that the presence of ileocolic disease is associated with a higher requirement for operation in the first place as well as a higher recurrence rate than other anatomic locations.[22] Further, if the original indication for surgery was an internal fistula in the ileocecal region, this patient is at highest risk for developing a subsequent recurrence requiring yet a further operation. These data continue to be analyzed.

In our recent study on recurrence,[22] we concluded that the initial distribution of disease (the "clinical pattern") determines the subsequent clinical course and emphasized that ileocolic disease more frequently requires resection. The incidence of recurrent ileocolic disease was significantly greater than that of disease involving either the small intestine or the large intestine alone and was also unrelated to the initial length of large intestine involved.

MEDICAL THERAPY IN CROHN'S DISEASE

Although there have been no dramatic breakthroughs in the medical therapy of Crohn's disease in recent years, there has been renewed interest brought about by the National Cooperative Crohn's Disease Study.[7] Medical treatment continues to have as mainstays sulfasalazine and prednisone.[28,29] Because of concern over steroid side effects, use of sulfasalazine and other agents has been evaluated, but systemic steroids continue to be the single most effective agents for Crohn's disease.[28,29] Data from the National Cooperative Study indicated that sulfasalazine was likely to be beneficial for patients with colonic Crohn's disease.[30] Immunosuppressive agents have been controversial but have been used as anti-inflammatory agents as well as an immunosupressive agents, as well as for their "steroid-sparing" effect. Although some studies have been encouraging in the use of immunosuppressives,[31] the prevailing opinion is that of caution.[28,29]

The role of nutrition in Crohn's disease can be a significant one because of long-standing symptoms, chronic diarrhea, malnutrition, or extensive small intestine involvement. Thus, in the past, a high-protein low-residue diet was frequently prescribed, and patients were quite concerned over their dietary and nutritional intake. It is more common currently to recommend a "normal" dietary intake by the patient with as few restrictions as possible in terms of diet and activity. Thus, there has been a general relaxation of dietary restrictions recently. However, patients who are significantly malnourished (20% or greater below their ideal weight) or whose symptoms are difficult to control medically present a difficult nutritional problem. The use of hyperalimentation has been widespread in Crohn's disease in the past several years, and we have evaluated its use as a "primary" form of therapy or "adjunctive" in anticipation of subsequent surgery.[32] It has clearly been in the latter category that hyperalimentation has been most useful, with an average duration of about three weeks. With the development of home hyperalimentation, patients who were refractory to previous forms of therapy have an additional source of treatment, albeit expensive and fraught with multiple difficulties. Other forms of nutritional supplement have also been attempted, with varying results.

The use of "supportive" therapy for patients with Crohn's disease can be valuable, but can also compound rather than improve many of the problems. This is particularly true for antidiarrheal agents as well as tranquilizers. The most frequently used antidiarrheal agents in the United States are Diphenoxylate and Loparamide, and the managing physician needs to be aware of over-dependence on such agents by patients. Similarly, "sick role behavior" can accelerate the use of tranquilizers and make their use a problem as well. The use of anticholinergics has been somewhat controversial in the past because of the possibility of the development of toxic megacolon, but their judicious use can help with the bothersome symptom of abdominal cramping and can avoid the use of narcotics or other specific analgesic medications.

Specific vitamin and mineral deficiencies may occur, but there is widespread use of multiple vitamin preparations for patients with Crohn's disease whose value is largely unproved. Similarly, replacement of iron and folic acid deficiencies may sometimes be necessary. The use of vitamin B12 (always parenterally) may need to be considered if the disease affects 50 cm or more of terminal ileum, or if a similar amount has been resected. However, with the ability to evaluate the size of red cells, vitamin B12 levels, and other sophisticated means of measurement, reliance on morphologic changes and neurologic abnormalities is no longer as much of a problem as previously. Thus, physicians should take an overall view of the patient and the disease rather than simply treating symptoms or prescribing a steroid agent without appropriate supportive therapy.

GEOGRAPHICAL DISTRIBUTION OF INFLAMMATORY BOWEL DISEASE

Geographic distribution of IBD is centered in the United States, United Kingdom, and Scandinavia. Epidemiological studies have been carried out more in Scandinavia[9)] and the United Kingdom[33)] than in the United States or Western Europe. The incidence is lower in Southern Europe, and presumably also in Eastern Europe, and is uncommon in South America. In both South Africa and Australia, among the white population, both ulcerative colitis and Crohn's disease are found. It is well known that blacks and Orientals have a disproportionately lower incidence of both ulcerative colitis and Crohn's disease, and Jews have a disproportionately higher incidence. However, the exact magnitude of the Jewish incidence, particularly in the United States, is not known. In Japan, ulcerative colitis is now more common than previously, but as yet Crohn's disease is rare. The geographical patterns of a "Western civilization" and a "northern" climate have invited considerable speculation and interest, particularly to explain the increasing incidence of Crohn's disease. Dietary and other ethnic considerations also have come to attention. It is interesting to note that the increased incidence of Crohn's disease may have reached a plateau[9)] in the late 1970s. Whether or not this trend will continue is not known because centers such as the Cleveland Clinic with a known interest and referral patterns continue to have an increasing number of cases annually (Table 13).

TABLE 13. Number of Patients with Inflammatory Bowel Disease in a Given Year (Cleveland Clinic)

Year	Crohn's disease	Ulcerative colitis	Proctosigmoiditis*
1960	33	122	18
1965	127	169	15
1970	315	171	43
1975	875	356	146
1978	1034	338	120

*Separate from ulcerative colitis; includes proctitis.

SUMMARY

Regardless of epidemiological, geographical, or pathological considerations, the major impact of IBD is on the patient and the family. Thus, awareness of these aspects will greatly facilitate the physician's ability to deal with the patient and the diseases. Crohn's disease, especially, has become one of the most important chronic disease affecting young persons in the U.S.A. and Western Europe. Its many complications, tendency for recurrences and remissions, and frequent need for operations all can have a significant impact on the patient. An understanding of these factors by the physician coupled with a sympathetic, appropriate, and comprehensive approach to the patient can be of great assistance in dealing with the symptoms of Crohn's disease as well as with the disease itself.

REFERENCES

1. Crohn, B. B., Ginzburg, L., and Oppenheimer, G. D.: Regional ileitis: A pathological and clinical entity. *JAMA*, **99**: 1323–1329, 1932.
2. Van Patter, W. N., Bargen, J. A., Dockerty, M. B., Feldman, W. H., Mayo, C. W., and Waugh, J. M.: Regional enteritis. *Gastroenterology*, **26**: 347–350.
3. Lockhart-Mummery, H. E. and Morson, B. C.: Crohn's disease (regional enteritis) of the large intestine and its distinction from ulcerative colitis. *Gut*, **1**: 87–105, 1960.
4. Farmer, R. G., Hawk, W. A., and Turnbull, R. B.: Regional enteritis of the colon: A clinical comparison with ulcerative colitis. *Am. J. Digestive Dis.*, **13**: 501–514, 1968.
5. Farmer, R. G., Hawk, W. A., and Turnbull, R. B.: Clinical and pathological correlations in inflammatory bowel disease: A reaffirmation of histologic criteria for diagnosis. *Cleve. Clin. Quarterly*, **46**: 35–37, 1979.

6. Farmer, R. G., Hawk, W. A., and Turnbull, R. B.: Clinical patterns in Crohn's disease: A statistical study of 615 cases. *Gastroenterology*, **68**: 627–635, 1975.
7. Mekhjian, H. S., Switz, D. M., Melynk, C. S., Rankin, G. V., and Brooks, R. K.: Clinical features and natural history of Crohn's disease. *Gastroenterology*, **77**: 898–906, 1979.
8. Farmer, R. G. and Michener, W. M.: Prognosis of Crohn's disease with onset in childhood and adolescence. *Dig. Dis. Sci.*, **24**: 752–757, 1979.
9. Hellers, G.: Crohn's disease in Stockholm County, 1955–1974. A study of epidemiology, results of surgical treatment and longterm prognosis.
10. Rankin, G. B., Watts, H. D., Melnyk, C. S., and Kelley, M. L., Jr.: National Cooperative Crohn's Disease Study: Extra intestinal manifestations and perianal complications. *Gastroenterology*, **77**: 914–920, 1979.
11. Lennard-Jones, J. E., Ritchie, J. K., and Zohrab, W. J.: Proctocolitis and Crohn's disease of the colon. A comparison of the clinical course. *Gut*, **17**: 477–482, 1976.
12. Best, W. R., Becktel, J. M., and Singleton, J. W.: Development of a Crohn's Disease Activity Index: National Cooperative Crohn's Disease Study. *Gastroenterology*, **70**: 439–444, 1976.
13. Best, W. R., Becktel, J. M., and Singleton, J. W.: Rederived values of the eight coefficients of the Crohn's Disease Activity Index (CDAI). *Gastroenterology*, **77**: 843–846, 1979.
14. Lloyd-Still, J. D. and Green, O. C.: A clinical scoring system for chronic inflammatory bowel disease in children. *Digestive Dis. and Sci.*, **24**: 620–624, 1979.
15. Van Hees, P. A. M., Van Eleren, P. H, Van Lier, H. J. J., and Van Tongeren, J. H. M.: An index of inflammatory activity in patients with Crohn's disease. *Gut*, **21**: 279–286, 1980.
16. Andre, C., Descos, L., Landais, P., and Fermanian, J.: Laboratory supplementation of Crohn's Disease Activity Index. *Lancet*, **2**: 594–595, 1980.
17. Harvey, R. G. and Bradshaw, J. M.: A simple index of Crohn's disease activity. *Lancet*, **1**: 514, 1980.
18. Waye, J. D.: Endoscopy in inflammatory bowel disease. *Clinics in Gastroenterology*, **9**: 279–296, 1980.
19. Fazio, V. W.: Toxic megacolon in ulcerative colitis and Crohn's colitis. *Clinics in Gastroenterology*, **9**: 389–408. 1980.
20. Farmer, R. G., Hawk, W. A., and Turnbull, R. B.: Indications for surgery in Crohn's disease: An analysis of 500 cases. *Gastroenterology*, **71**: 245–250, 1976.
21. Lee, E. C. G. and Papaioannou, N.: Recurrences following surgery for Crohn's disease. *Clinics in Gastroenterology*, **9**: 419–438, 1980.
22. Lock, M. R., Farmer, R. G., Fazio, V. W., *et al.*: Recurrences and reoperation for Crohn's disease. The role of disease location in prognosis. *New Eng. J. Med.*, **304**: 1586–1588, 1981.
23. Michener, W. M., Whelan, G., Greenstreet, R. L., and Farmer, R. G.:

Comparison of the clinical features of Crohn's disease and ulcerative colitis with onset in childhood or adolescence. *Clev. Clin. Quarterly,* **49**: 13–16, 1982.
24. Farmer, R. G., Michener, W. M., and Mortimer, E. A.: Studies of family history among patients with inflammatory bowel disease. *Clinics in Gastroenterology,* **9**: 271–278, 1980.
25. Farmer, R. G., Mir Madjlessi, S. H., and Kiser, W. S.: Urinary excretion of oxalate, calcium, magnesium and uric acid in inflammatory bowel disease: Relationship to urolithiasis. *Cleve. Clin. Quarterly,* **41**: 109–117, 1974.
26. Siminovitch, J. M. P. and Fazio, V. W.: Ureteral obstruction secondary to Crohn's disease: A need for ureterolysis? *Am. J. Surg.,* **139**: 95–98, 1980.
27. Lee, E. C. G.: Crohn's Workshop. A Global Assessment of Crohn's Disease. HM & M (Publishers), London, 1981.
28. Riis, P.: A critical survey of controlled studies in the treatment of ulcerative colitis in Crohn's disease. *Clinics in Gastroenterology,* **9**: 351–370, 1980.
29. Singleton, J. W.: Medical treatment of inflammatory bowel disease. *Medical Clinics of North America,* **64**: 1117-1134, 1980.
30. Summers, R. W., Switz, D. M., Sessions, J. T., *et al.*: National Cooperative Crohn's Disease Study: Results of drug treatment. *Gastroenterology,* **77**: 847–869, 1979.
31. Present, D. H., Korelitz, B. I., *et al.*: Treatment of Crohn's disease with 6-Mercaptopurine. A long-term randomized double-blind study. *New Eng. J. Med.,* **302**: 981–987, 1980.
32. Fazio, V. W., Harford, F. J., Jr., and Farmer, R. G.: Total parenteral nutrition for Crohn's disease—role as primary therapy. *Italian J. Gastroenterology,* **11**: 80–82, 1979.
33. Langman, M. J. S.: Epidemiology of Crohn's disease. In: Crohn's Workshop. A Global Assessment of Crohn's Disease (ed. E. C. G. Lee), pp. 162–169. HM & M (Publishers), London, 1981.

Discussion: Medical Treatment

Richard G. Farmer and Hikaru Watanabe, Chairmen

Dr. Jewell: These are interesting results, Dr. Inoue, which show that you can induce remission in your patients very effectively. The problem, as you said, is how to maintain the remission. I think definition becomes important here. I would like to know how you define mild, moderate, severe, and fulminant, and how remission is defined. Is remission based on symptoms, endoscopic appearances, or histological appearances?

Dr. Inoue: Dr. Truelove's criteria were utilized for the definition of severity. As for the definition of remission, in our Department it is based on endoscopic findings. At a point where there was no more contact bleeding we defined endoscopic remission.

Dr. Morita: Dr. Mori, you mentioned systemic coagulability. What about local coagulability or coagulation factors?

Dr. Mori: I think this point is very important in the etiology of hypercoagulability and we should study this point, but at this time we have only studied systemic hypercoagulability. Now we are going to study the relationship with tissue coagulability and local coagulability. We have not yet obtained any conclusion from the present results.

Dr. Jewell: Thank you for giving us such a thorough study. The data are very similar to those of previous studies. Thromboembolic disease is a major cause of death in these patients, but nowadays it is uncommon. However, when thromboembolic disease occurs, it is safe to treat patients with heparin. I would like to ask you whether you were implying that DIC occurred in your patients because of the hypercoagulable state. Might not a septicemic or endotoxic episode in the postoperative period be a more likely cause?

Dr. Mori: We have not yet studied the etiology or reason of the hypercoagulability. However, the existence of a hypercoagulable state as a background of this disease and endotoxemia or the increase of immune complex in the blood have been observed, and then the patient tends to have DIC develop. This is what we observed in actual cases.

Dr. Jewell: Dr. Baba presented very interesting results, and I am impressed by the dramatic response to intra-arterial steroids. However, the results are very similar to those obtained with intensive intravenous therapy. Therefore, intravenous therapy would seem preferable unless there is an indication to perform mesenteric angiography.

Dr. Baba: When I showed the first effective case to Dr. Goligher, he said that only one case could not bring forth any conclusions. So, I have collected 50 cases up to this time. As a result, as shown here, it is not so superior when compared to intensive intravenous therapy. I would like to choose the cases tried in order to decide the exact indication by myself.

Dr. Farmer: I would like to ask what the indications for the angiography are.

Dr. Baba: I analyzed cases of toxic megacolon in Japan and noted that about 60% of cases had a predisposing factor such as barium enema. Mesenteric angiography might tell us the extent of the lesion, so we started angiography in order to eliminate barium enema in the active stage. Fortunately, we had good angiographists at that time.

Dr. Imamura: I want to ask Dr. Baba two questions: 1) Are repeated treatments of intra-arterial infusions of prednisolone sometimes employed? 2) One might think that a larger dose of prednisolone would be more effective. What is your opinion?

Dr. Baba: I don't know about the dosage, but, in terms of the second injection, I think the response rate is a little lower. On the other hand, I gave two injections for one attack in five cases. I think this is a sort of trigger treatment in which continuous infusion doesn't make much difference.

Dr. Chiba: Dr. Jewell, in the follow-up of patients with ulcerative colitis, it is well known that there are two kinds of patients. One group consists of the patients who relapse often and come to the hospital regularly, and the others are those who don't relapse often or whose symptoms subside gradually. The latter group of patients doesn't come to the hospital. You showed that maintenance with sulphasalazine is effective in keeping patients well. Do you include in your data the patients who continue the stage of remission and don't come to the hospital?

Dr. Jewell: In our Oxford studies I have shown you that attendance of patients was 100%.

Dr. Yoshida: When patients on sulphasalazine relapse, do you increase the dose or give steroids? When the same patients go into remission, do you give the maintenance sulphasalazine again?

Dr. Jewell: When patients relapse on sulphasalazine, we give corticosteroids both systemically and topically. When the patients go into remission, then we trail off the steroids but continue the sulphasalazine.

Dr. Muto: I don't think you mentioned about the management of a very mild chronic continuous disease. I have a patient who is being treated with 20 mg of prednisolone. When we try to taper off steroids, the symptoms come back. So we have to treat the patient the same way for one or two years with the side effects of steroids. How do you recommend treating such patients?

Dr. Jewell: I think that is the ideal situation for trying azathioprine in a dose of about 2.0 to 2.5 mg per kg. Some of them will do reasonably well and you will be able to taper off the corticosteroids. Otherwise they are very difficult. I think sometimes if the quality of life is being severely hampered, that is a very strong indication for considering surgery.

Dr. Riddell: Two quick questions: 1) Do pregnant patients relapse following parturition? 2) Is there a subgroup of colitis with an excess of IgE-containing plasma cells that might respond to cromoglycate?

Dr. Jewell: We have experienced 150 pregnancies in patients with ulcerative colitis. We didn't have one case in which either the disease began during parturition, nor did we have a severe relapse. So, a severe relapse or a first attack of disease in parturition is not a common problem.

Next, commercially available antibodies of IgE may cross-react with IgG or IgM in plasma cells. If properly absorbed, no IgE-containing plasma cells can be found. Eosinophils which autofluoresce and mast cells that may have IgE on the surface may be incorrectly interpreted as IgE-positive plasma cells. Therefore, the evidence of the existence of a subgroup seems to be extremely weak.

Dr. Matsueda: Ulcerative proctitis seems to be refractory to sulphasalazine. What can you do for such patients?

Dr. Jewell: Our experience is much like yours. As I said earlier, I think it is quite likely that the majority of patients with proctitis are a different entity from those with proctocolitis. I don't know what to do with the patients with proctitis who continue to have symptoms. You can treat them with anything—steroids, azathioprine, etc.—and produce no response. So they are an awful problem. I have no answer.

Dr. Farmer: I would like to ask you about the data on which you make the statement that indefinite use of sulphasalazine is indicated. It seems that most of the studies talked about relapses after 6 to 12 months. What about the patient who has not relapsed for three to five years? Why cannot you then stop the therapy despite the implications of those 6 to 12-month studies?

Dr. *Jewell*: In the Oxford study the patients were divided into two groups. In those patients who had had the disease for more than 3 years, often up to 10 years, many of those on sulphasalazine for 8 to 10 years have been well; of those still 50% relapsed within the following six months if they went on dummy preparation. I think that seems to be the evidence.

It is fair to say that a study in Denmark along similar lines came to rather different conclusions. They concluded that if the patients remain free from relapse for two years, I think it was, it was safe to take them off of sulphasalazine. This is very different from the Oxford data. I think the difference is the problem of defining remission, because the Danish study defined remission purely on the basis of symptoms rather than on histological remission or relapse.

Dr. *Ito*: I have the same experience as Dr. Matsueda. Some patients with proctitis were difficult to control. Is there any evidence that a group of proctitis patients who resist medical treatment with sulphasalazine and local steroids have an increased tendency of proximal extension of the disease compared with those who easily respond to medical treatment?

Dr. *Jewell*: Usually about 10% extend proximally—quite a small proportion.

Dr. *Farmer*: That is not necessarily the group that extends. It is our experience also that about 10% extend. But the 10% is not necessarily the same 10% that falls into this category of a poor response later. The poor responders we have seen later do not seem to extend; they just don't seem to go into complete remission.

Dr. *Chiba*: Is there any institution which tried to employ your 5-day intensive intravenous regimen? What were the results of those treated?

Dr. *Jewell*: The regimen is widely used in the U.K. at the moment. Talking to other people that use it, they get very similar results. In the original report and subsequent follow-up report from Oxford, tetracycline was used. I changed to metronidazole for a number of reasons. We are about halfway through a controlled study at the moment to determine whether metronidazole is effective or not.

Dr. *Inoue*: I would like to know your opinion about the effect of azathioprine in minimizing the relapse in the cases in which sulphasalazine cannot be used because of the side effects.

Dr. *Jewell*: Azathioprine has no effect on acute disease, but in chronic disease it may affect a few patients. But I don't think it is useful in everybody. We reserve it for those patients who are having continuous relapse and who, for one reason or another, are not going to surgery. That is how to use it.

There is very little to say about pregnancy insofar as pregnancy is quite safe for patients with ulcerative colitis. And women need not be afraid of getting pregnant because the disease does not affect with the course of the pregnancy, nor is it correlated with an increased number of fetal abnormalities. Furthermore, the pregnancy itself does not have a deleterious effect on the disease. So pregnancy is safe. The next question is "Are the drugs safe?" The answer is yes. Neither prednisolone nor sulphasalazine in our series in Oxford, both in colitis and Crohn's disease, nor in other series has been shown to adversely affect the fetus. There has been some concern about sulphasalazine and neonatorum jaundice, but this was based on theoretical considerations which have by now been shown to be incorrect. So we treat our patients who are pregnant just like any other patients without colitis, but we keep a very close watch on them so any early signs of relapse can be treated effectively without delay.

Dr. Asakura: Dr. Farmer, would you kindly tell us how you treat patients with Crohn's disease in your clinic?

Dr. Farmer: There are frequently multiple forms of therapy, which can include nutritional therapy and other support therapy. Three or four major drugs are used in the drug therapy of Crohn's disease. The most commonly used therapeutic agent is prednisone. The usual dose in a moderate case—with the CDAI of 200 or so—is approximately 40 mg of prednisone or its equivalent with a tapering down to 20 mg, and perhaps continuing the 20 mg-dosage for somewhere between six months and two years. I think that patients are kept on steroids for a longer period of time with Crohn's disease than they are with ulcerative colitis.

There have been many attempts to try and get around the danger or the risk of steroid side effects such as the use of ACTH on a once- or twice-a-week basis, the use of 20 or 40 mg of prednisone on an alternate-day basis, and the use of 2 g dose of sulphasalazine sometimes with prednisone and sometimes without prednisone. This has led to an enormous difficulty in controlled clinical trials and the lack of scientific data is a big problem. The National Crohn's Cooperative Study did not answer the question about steroid side effects.

As far as azathioprine and metronidazole are concerned, both of these are advances in the therapy, but the difficulty is a definition of the end point. This is a very difficult thing to do and it is particularly difficult to randomize, to control, and to have the data similar everywhere.

Dr. Yao: The recurrence rate after the first operation is reported to be about 50% in Western countries. Is that so, or is it more frequent? In the past few years I have treated about 50 patients with Crohn's disease with hyperalimentation, and I experienced three patients who showed complete remission for 2–4 years from their symptoms, sedimentation rate or C-reactive protein, and X-ray findings. Do you have such patients?

Dr. Farmer: The 50% recurrence rate is the first question. And the second question is the treatment with hyperalimentation.

As far as the recurrence rate is concerned, I think that it is important, if you can, to define the reason for surgery in the first place, and that this should be done by both the physician and the surgeon. It is not simply the presence of disease or the presence of symptoms, but the objective findings that there is a complication which has occurred and that this is agreed to by the physician and the surgeon. This is easier said than done, but nevertheless, if one tries to discipline oneself to ask if there is a surgical indication, what the surgical indication is, if the surgical indication is an obstruction, and if so, how do we define obstruction in some sort of objective way? Is it a fistula, and if so, is it a fistula with an abscess, or is it simply serositis with an inflammatory mass? All of these can at least be assessed because in a relatively short period of time with steroid therapy an inflammatory mass will subside or will improve. If the surgeon is aware of the case, and if a problem develops such as a fistula or a toxic megacolon, the surgeon is aware of the problem and can operate on a more urgent basis if necessary. So I think that this type of management requires a team effort, and with the technology of hyperalimentation, another important member of the team is the one working with hyperalimentation. Even though there is a 50% recurrence rate, I do not think that should deter you from recommending an operation or doing an operation, if the operation is indicated. The point that I would make is that in most cases in Crohn's disease the indication for surgery is one that can be defined, rather than simply the fact that the patient has symptoms. I do not think that we should say "Let us not operate because there might be a 50% recurrence rate." What we should say is "Let us not operate because there is not an indication for operation."

Now in determining the indications for operation, we have to look at or have to try and get some assessment of the index or the degree of disease activity. That is where it would be useful if we could come up with a number, like a CDAI of 250 is worse than a CDAI of 150. Unfortunately that isn't necessarily the case. What we are attempting to do in these international workshops is to come up with some agreement where some statistic, or some shorthand, or some numbers could be applied so that some sort of objectivity can be used. The laboratory data, other than the serum albumin and the blood counts, unfortunately are not helping us. The blood sedimentation rate and other non-specific reactants have really not proved to be very helpful in terms of helping to make a clinical decision regarding the need for surgery. I think that to try and analyze the various factors including the duration and the location of the disease is more important than worrying about whether or not there may be a 50% recurrence rate under these particular circumstances.

As far as hyperalimentation is concerned, as we followed up patients for five years after their original hyperalimentation, we have not found that the hyperalimentation altered the long-term prognosis. It has been very rare in our experience that the use of hyperalimentation actually prevented the need for surgery. Most of the time it undoubtedly helped the patient to get through the surgery, helped the patient in a nutritional sense, and was what we now refer to as adjunctive therapy. The two or three circumstances in which we have found hyperalimentation to be the best are in patients with diffuse small intestine disease; but more importantly, in patients with chronic obstruction, chronic fistula formation, and abscess, usually the ileocolic disease in which there is a significant element of malnutrition. Thus a chronic indication for surgery in a patient who is malnourished is probably the most common indication for hyperalimentation at the present time. The other frequent indication is that of total colon Crohn's disease in which the patient does indeed have a poor response to medical therapy and one is trying to help to build the patient up nutritionally. We have not found, as we had hoped eight years ago, that it would be a major breakthrough that would enable us not to require surgery.

In the circumstances that you described with the use of home hyperalimentation, we also have found this to be tremendously beneficial, much like the patients with chronic renal dialysis. And in fact there is a home dialysis program, the chronic ambulatory peritoneal dialysis, which is very similar to what you described. So, I think that's a special circumstance for which this is an excellent treatment and a great technologic breakthrough.

Dr. Muto: I have a feeling that if a patient has a high dose of steroids, then he might have a high risk of complications after the surgery, particularly leakage.

Dr. Farmer: The question has to do with the fact that most patients who have an operation are on large-dose steroids and whether this affects the surgery in an adverse way.

In a referred center patients will come from a fairly great distance and Cleveland Clinic patients come from a radius of approximately 300 miles. Many times we get the patients when they have already been treated with high-dose steroids, and they are referred to us with well-developed complications. In many cases the patient will be referred directly to the surgeon in the first place, and the gastroenterologist will come into the case later on. Therefore, the surgeon who works in our environment is accustomed to dealing with complicated cases and it is not unusual for him to encounter the type of cases you're talking about frequently.

The best example of this, I would say, is toxic megacolon. Our mortality in the toxic megacolon cases in the last 10 years has gone down dramatically, partly because of this team effort.

I do feel that based on whatever data we have available, for example the National Crohn's Cooperative Study, certainly is a strong point for steroid therapy. Very similar is the short-term steroid therapy advocated by Dr. Jewell and Dr. Truelove. One third of our patients do not require surgery, but two thirds do require surgery. Therefore, if we had some way where we could predict which patient might or might not require surgery based on certain clinical features, we might be more willing to try newer forms of therapy. I would say that based on our data, we have not had excessive mortality or morbidity based on previous medical therapy, including steroid.

Dr. Matsueda: The effects of hyperalimentation are complicated. The reason is that doing hyperalimentation and doing proper hyperalimentation are different. If you do a proper one you may get better results. On the other hand, severe ileitis cannot be operated on because it will produce short bowel syndrome. For such patients, we would like to perform our new home hyperalimentation. I wish you could use this procedure in the U.S.A. to see whether it works or not.

Dr. Farmer: I think your point is very well taken. In having seen the development of hyperalimentation during the time I have been interested in inflammatory bowel disease, the technology became available and we had sick patients, and therefore we used the technology. We recognized this as a problem right away and we formed a hyperalimentation committee with physicians, surgeons, and nutritionists on it to try and anticipate exactly the problem you were talking about. What we are attempting to do is to try to apply as much logic as we can; but it still is not easy because of all of the various factors that you have to take into account.

Dr. Yao: Is it the role of the internist to try to have the patient lead a normal social life for as long as possible and to prolong the patient's life?

Dr. Farmer: The problem in Crohn's disease is not as much mortality over the long run, but problems in the relatively short run. There are many patients whom we now see who had Crohn's disease 25 years ago, and where the disease had "burned out." And they are able to function reasonably well. The goal of therapy, although certainly to prevent mortality, is not like in ulcerative colitis where it is most important to maintain surveillance for years. The surveillance for Crohn's disease dosen't have to be quite this rigid as long as you have a rapport with the patient. Then they will come back to see you periodically. But we do not have to do, for example, the colonoscopic surveillance that we do in ulcerative colitis. So given two patients 10 years later, the problems are often quite different. The internist should be in charge of all of this.

Dr. Baba: Could you tell us your idea of how to treat anal complications?

Dr. Farmer: John Alexander Williams in Birmingham, who is a surgeon, emphasizes that whatever one does with anal Crohn's disease, it should be conservative. I think that the emphasis on conservatism in therapy of anal Crohn's disease has become well recognized in the recent past. Certainly one of the things that one tries to avoid is an operation on the sphincter itself that might damage the sphincter. I think usually we try to use as conservative a therapy as possible, both medically and surgically.

Now whether or not metronidazole fits into this conservative therapy is, in my opinion, still open to question; but it may, and if it does, this would be a very positive step forward in terms of treatment of this particular complication. I can't help but feel that even though bacteriologic studies have not been particularly fruitful in this intra-anal disease, and that if metronidazole is effective, it must have some bacteriologic implication which may mean that we are going full circle and coming back to what we started talking about in terms of the bacteriology of Crohn's disease.

VI. SURGICAL TREATMENT

Present Status of Surgical Treatment of Ulcerative Colitis in Japan

——An Enquête Study

Hiroshige Nakano, Tsuneo Shiratori,* and Tetsuichiro Muto***

INTRODUCTION

The incidence of ulcerative colitis in Japan is definitely lower than that in Europe and the U.S.A., and it is considered a relatively rare disease in Japan. The morbidity and incidence of this disease in Japan are 1.86 and 0.312 per 100,000 population,[1] respectively, but the respective values are 19.9 and 6.5 in Britain,[2] and 42.0 and 3.5 in the U.S.A.[3]

Under such conditions, the medical and surgical treatment of ulcerative colitis has progressed in great strides over the past 30 years in Western countries where various treatments have been given and long-term follow-up studies have been done in many cases.

In Japan, therapeutic results have appeared to approach those of the Western countries since 1973, or about 10 years ago, when the Ulcerative Colitis Research Committee of the Ministry of Health and Welfare was organized. However, no conclusions have been proposed yet because the number of cases is small and follow-up study has not been long.

This paper will be concerned with re-analyzing the data obtained by the Research Committee of the Ministry of Health and Welfare and with reporting the present state of surgical treatment for ulcerative colitis in Japan.

SUBJECTS AND METHODS

A questionnaire was conducted on patients who received surgical treatment by the Ulcerative Colitis Research Committee of the Ministry of Health and Welfare (Chairman: Shuji Tsuchiya) in 1975 and by the Inflammatory Bowel Disease Research Committee of the said ministry (Chairman: Tsuneo Shiratori) in 1982.

*First Department of Surgery, Nara Medical University, Kashihara, Nara, Japan
**Department of Surgery, Faculty of Medicine, University of Tokyo, Tokyo, Japan

The subjects consisted of 269 patients in total. The period of follow-up for these patients was from 1 month to 16 years, averaging 5.1 years.

RESULTS

Table 1 shows the year at onset for patients who were treated surgically for ulcerative colitis. The male-female ratio in 261 cases was 140 : 121. By year, the frequency of the incidence increases from 1967 to 1971 and declines thereafter.

TABLE 1. Year of Onset for Patients Treated Surgically for UC

Year	Male	Female	Total (%)
1945–1965	34	33	67 (26)
1966	3	2	5 (2)
1967	10	10	20 (8)
1968	15	5	20 (8)
1969	18	11	29 (11)
1970	12	11	23 (9)
1971	12	13	25 (10)
1972	9	11	20 (8)
1973	8	8	16 (6)
1974	5	7	12 (5)
1975	6	4	10 (4)
1976	4	1	5 (2)
1977	2	2	4 (2)
1978	2	1	3 (1)
1979	0	2	2 (1)
Total	140	121	261

Unknown: 8 cases.

Table 2 shows the age-sex distribution at the time of operation. Surgical operations were performed on patients of various age groups, namely from a 7-year-old child to a 77-year-old. The percentage of operations done was particularly high in patients in their 20s to 40s, i.e., 182 (68%) of 267 cases in this age range.

When the extent of lesion, relapse rate, and mortality rate were examined in the 269 cases, they could be divided into three groups: total colitis 179 cases (67%), left-sided colitis 48 cases (18%), and proctitis 12 cases (4%), as shown in Table 3. The relapse rates and mortality rates in these cases were 26% and 10%, respectively; they were 27% and 12%, respectively, in the cases of total colitis.

Table 4 shows the stage at operation, relapse rate, and mortality rate. There were many cases in which surgical operation was performed in the active stage (191 cases [71%] compared with 71 cases [26%] in the remission stage).

TABLE 2. Sex and Age Distributions at the Time of Operation

Age	Male	Female	Total (%)
7–10	1	2	3 (1)
11–20	13	7	20 (7)
21–30	42	23	65 (24)
31–40	35	33	68 (25)
41–50	22	27	49 (18)
51–60	12	10	22 (8)
61–70	11	12	23 (9)
71–77	6	11	17 (6)
Total	142	125	267

Unknown: 2 cases.

TABLE 3. Extent of Lesion.

Lesion	No. of cases	Relapse (%)	Died (%)
Total colitis	179	49 (27)	22 (12)
Left-sided colitis	48	11 (23)	4 (8)
Proctitis	12	4 (33)	1 (8)
Right-sided or segmental colitis	11	4 (36)	0 (0)
Unknown	19	3 (16)	0 (0)
Total	269	71 (26)	27 (10)

TABLE 4. Stage at Operation

Stage	No. of cases	Relapse (%)	Died (%)
Active	191	53 (28)	22 (12)
Remission	71	17 (24)	5 (7)
Unknown	7	1 (14)	0 (0)
Total	269	71 (26)	27 (10)

When the relapse rate and mortality rate in these stages are examined, the relapse rate is almost equal in the active and remission stages, but the mortality rate in the active stage is about two times higher than that in the remission stage.

Table 5 shows the severity at operation, relapse rate, and mortality rate. Cases operated are mostly moderate to severe cases. The results of the above cases show that a high relapse rate is observed in the moderate group and that a high mortality rate is observed in the severe group.

Table 6 shows the type of disease classified by clinical course, the relapse rate, and mortality rate. There are three types: relapsing-remitting type, 161 cases (60%); chronic-continuous type, 60 cases (22%); and acute fulminating, 20 cases (7%). The highest percentage was observed in

TABLE 5. Severity at Operation

Severity	No. of cases	Relapse (%)	Died (%)
Mild	38	8 (21)	2 (5)
Moderate	123	42 (34)	8 (7)
Severe	92	18 (20)	16 (17)
Unknown	16	1 (6)	1 (6)
Total	269	71 (26)	27 (10)

TABLE 6. Clinical Course

Type	No. of cases	Relapse (%)	Died (%)
Relapsing-remitting	161	41 (25)	13 (8)
Chronic-continuous	60	18 (30)	5 (8)
Acute-fulminating	20	4 (20)	7 (35)
One attack only	19	4 (21)	2 (11)
Unknown	9	4 (44)	0 (0)
Total	269	71 (26)	27 (10)

the relapsing-remitting type. The mortality rate was very high in the acute-fulminating type (35%).

Table 7 presents the macroscopic findings at the time of resection. There were 98 cases (36%) of pseudopolyposis type, 66 cases (25%) of the atrophic type, and 74 cases (28%) of the mixed type, but the difference in macroscopic findings between the relapse rate and mortality rate was not so great.

TABLE 7. Macroscopic Findings at the Time of Resection

Type	No. of cases	Relapse (%)	Died (%)
Pseudopolyposis	98	34 (35)	9 (9)
Atrophic	66	19 (29)	4 (6)
Mixed	74	14 (19)	6 (8)
Unknown	31	4 (13)	8 (26)
Total	269	71 (26)	27 (10)

Table 8 shows the types of operation in these 269 cases. The sphincter-saving type of operation was most common and was performed on 124 cases (46%); it included ileorectal anastomosis, ileoanal anastomosis, ascendoproctostomy, and transversoproctostomy.

Hartmann's technique, that is, colectomy with covering proctostomy, was performed on 42 cases (16%) and had the highest mortality rate. The prognosis of this operation was poor with only 13 cases for coming radical operation. The rectum was resected in 11 cases, and a sphincter-saving operation was done in 3 cases.

TABLE 8. Type of Operation Performed

Type of operation	No. of cases	Died (%)
Sphincter-saving	124	10 (8)
Hartmann	42	9 (21)
Proctocolectomy and ileostomy	54	4 (4)
Proctocolectomy and colostomy	32	1 (3)
Diverting colostomy	13	1 (8)
Diverting ileostomy	1	0 (0)
Ileostomy + mucous fistula	1	0 (0)
Exploratory laparotomy	2	2 (100)
Total	269	27 (10)

Ileostomy and/or colostomy was performed on 143 cases (53%); proctocolectomy with ileostomy on 54 cases (20%) and subtotal proctocolectomy with colostomy on 32 cases (12%).

Next, a study was made on ileorectal anastomosis (IRA), which has become popular recently as a sphincter-saving operation. Table 9 shows the stage, operative mortality, and leakage rate. Among the 58 cases of IRA, the operation was performed in the active stage in 43 cases (74%) and in the remission stage in 15 (26%). There was no significant difference between the two stages in terms of mortality and leakage rates. Operative death was seen in 6 cases (10%), and anastomotic leak was observed in 7 (12%).

TABLE 9. Stage at Ileorectal Anastomosis

Stage	No. of cases	Died (%)	Leak (%)
Active	43	4 (9)	5 (12)
Remission	15	2 (13)	2 (13)
Total	58	6 (10)	7 (12)

Table 10 shows the 58 cases of IRA classified by severity. There were 33 moderate cases (57%) and 19 severe ones (33%). The mortality and leakage rates were high in severe cases at 16% and 21%, respectively.

These 58 cases were divided into two groups (before 1974 and after 1975) and a comparison was made according to the time when the IRA was performed (Table 11). Before 1974, 5 (13%) of 38 cases died. After 1975, however, good results were obtained, with operative death found in only one (5%) of 20 cases. Anastomotic leak was found in 2 (10%) of 20 cases after 1975.

The prognosis of these 58 cases by IRA is illustrated in Fig. 1. Of the 58 cases, 52 cases are alive and 28 cases have had no relapse. The remaining 24 cases have suffered relapse. Of those that relapsed, 18 cases were

TABLE 10. Severity at Ileorectal Anastomosis

Severity	No. of cases	Died (%)	Leak (%)
Mild	5	1 (20)	1 (20)
Moderate	33	2 (6)	2 (6)
Severe	19	3 (16)	4 (21)
Fulminant	1	0 (0)	0 (0)
Total	58	6 (10)	7 (12)

TABLE 11. Operative Mortality and Complication of Ileorectal Anastomosis

	No. of cases	Died (%)	Leak (%)
Before 1974	38	5 (13)	5 (13)
After 1975	20	1 (5)	2 (10)
Total	58	6 (10)	7 (12)

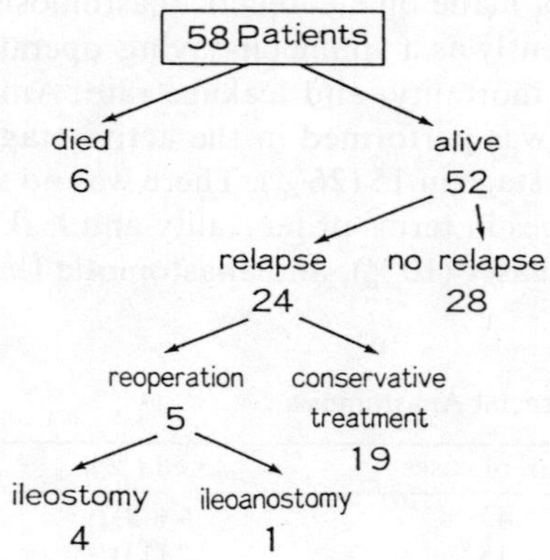

FIG. 1. Patients' prognosis in ileorectal anastomosis.

controlled by conservative therapy, and 5 cases underwent a second operation. Four cases of reoperation were ileostomies, and the other was an ileoanostomy.

To summarize these results, 47 (81%) of 58 patients may be considered examples of success with IRA.

Table 12 shows bowel action after IRA. Most patients did not have more than 10 stools a day; 1–3 stools in 10 cases (23%), 4–6 stools in 15 cases (35%), and 7–9 stools in 15 cases (35%).

Table 13 shows the social status of patients who underwent IRA. Full-time workers accounted for 31 of 44 cases. Light work was done in 5 cases, housework in 5 cases, and only 2 cases were unable to work.

Table 14 shows the operative mortality and leakage of IRA in various

TABLE 12. Bowel Action after Ileorectal Anastomosis

No. of stools/day	Cases (%)
1–3	10 (23)
4–6	15 (35)
7–9	15 (35)
10<	3 (7)
Total	43

TABLE 13. Social Status of Patients Who Underwent Ileorectal Anastomosis

Type	No. of cases (%)
Full-time work	31 (53)
Light work	5 (9)
Housework	6 (10)
Unable to work	2 (4)
Unknown	14 (24)
Total	58

TABLE 14. Operative Mortality and Complications of Ileorectal Anastomosis

	No. of IRA	Mortality (%)	Leak (%)
Aylett (1966)[4]	300	5.7	12.4
Baker (1970)[5]	41	5	14.6
Sprechler and Baden (1971)[6]	48	2	0
Fazio (1975)[7]	157	1.9	1.2
Jones *et al.* (1977)[8]	32	3	3.1
Japan: before 1974	38	13	13
after 1975	20	5	10

foreign countries and Japan.[4–8] The mortality is less than 5% in foreign countries, but was a high 13% before 1974 in Japan. After 1975, however, results improved in Japan, with a mortality of less than 5%. Little significant difference is observed for anastomotic leak, although low rates are given in some reports.

DISCUSSION

In Japan, compared with Western countries, the history of surgical treatment for ulcerative colitis has been short due to a low incidence of ulcerative colitis, a small number of cases, and inadequate follow-up. Therefore, no definite conclusions have been reached yet on surgical treatment.

However, surgical therapeutic results obtained in Japan over the past 10 years are approaching the level of Western countries. At present, there are about 5,000 patients with ulcerative colitis in Japan, and about 10%

of them appear to have received surgical treatment. The questionnaire of the present study conducted mainly by the Research Committee of the Ministry of Health and Welfare used about half the patients operated on in Japan as its subjects.

Operative indications in this disease are cases not responsive to the conservative treatment for severe or fulminating types, and relapsing patients. As absolute indications (emergency operation being indicated), mention can be made of (1) massive hemorrhage, (2) toxic megacolon, (3) severe type, (4) perforation, and (5) acute fulminating type. As relative indications, mention can be made of (1) cases not responding to medical treatment, (2) cases repeating relapse, (3) stenosis of the intestinal tract, and (4) systemic complications.

According to the tabulation for fiscal 1975 by the Research Committee of the Ministry of Health and Welfare,[9] 41 (19%) of 215 cases were categorized as having absolute indications for operation and 173 (81%) as having relative indications. Of the absolute indications for operation, massive hemorrhage occurred most frequently, followed by toxic megacolon and severe type.

The mortality averaged 32% in cases of emergency operation, with 2 cases (12%) of massive hemorrhage, 6 cases (100%) of perforation, one case (14%) of toxic megacolon, 3 cases (38%) of severe type, and one case (33%) of acute fulminating type. The figure is five times higher than that for cases of elective operation. European and American reports have shown it to be about 10 times higher.[10,11]

According to tabulations based on the present questionnaire, surgical operation is performed most often in cases of the active stage, and the mortality increases slightly to 12%; the mortality rates in the severe and acute fulminating types are very high at 17% and 35%, respectively.

For surgical operation to be performed safely and with low mortality, it is important that internists and surgeons cooperate with each other so as not to lose a chance to shift from conservative therapy to surgical treatment.

Proctocolectomy with ileostomy and colectomy with ileorectal anastomosis are available as radical operative methods for this disease. The former is the operative method with the highest radicality since ulcerative colitis is a diffuse disease affecting the entire large intestine. However, this operative method causes problems such as (1) mental stress, (2) development of complications stemming from ileostomy, (3) postoperative sexual dysfunction, and (4) expenditure for appliances for ileostomy. In this respect, the latter is free of the problems associated with ileostomy but has problems such as (1) cancer risk in the remainder of the rectum, (2) relapse, and (3) occurrence of anastomotic leak.

At present, there are pros and cons to each of these operative methods, and the type of operation is selected according to the judgment of the surgeon, and the preoperative state and wishes of the patient.

Table 15 shows the frequency of IRA in various studies.[12–21] Aylett has conducted IRA in 96% of total cases of colectomy.[12] On the other hand, in one hospital IRA was performed in only 10% of total cases, as reported by Adson.[20] Such a difference is the results of differences in surgical judgment.

TABLE 15. Proportion of Patients Undergoing Total Colectomy for Ulcerative Colitis Who Had Ileorectal Anastomosis

	Total colectomies	IRA performed	IRA (%)
Aylett (1974)[12]	461	443	96
Ribet *et al.* (1973)[13]	76	60	79
Vink and Beerstecker (1973)[14]	73	50	68
Ehrenpreis (1966)[15]	45	19	42
Sprechler and Baden (1971)[6]	127	48	38
Yudin (1973)[16]	167	55	33
Muir (1959)[17]	60	19	32
Hughes and Russel (1967)[18]	234	63	27
Mignon *et al.* (1974)[19]	250	28	11
Adson *et al.* (1972)[20]	350	35	10
Veidenheimer *et al.* (1970)[21]	387	36	9.3

In Japan, the sphincter-saving operation was performed in 124 of 269 cases, and IRA in 58 of 124 cases. Accordingly, IRA was performed in 23% of the cases which underwent colectomy. As a recent trend in Japan, the sphincter-saving operation is becoming more widely employed. This surgical procedure was formerly thought to have a high mortality rate and many complications. However, after 1975 the mortality rate declined to 5% and the leakage rate declined to 10%. Thus, recently it has become possible to perform this operation safely.

In conclusion, it appears necessary to make further studies on the surgical treatment of ulcerative colitis, on the basis of the results mentioned above, by increasing the number of cases and by conducting long-term follow-up observations.

REFERENCES

1. Yokota, A., *et al.*: Incidence of idiopathic procto-colitis (IV). In: Proceedings of Inflammatory Bowel Disease Research Committee of the Japanese Ministry of Health and Welfare. p. 239, 1979.
2. Goligher, J. C., *et al.*: Epidemiology. In: Ulcerative Colitis, pp. 47–61. Bailliere Tindall and Cassell, London, 1968.

3. Monk, M., *et al.*: An epidemiological study of ulcerative colitis and regional enteritis among adults in Baltimore. I. Hospital incidence and prevalence, 1960 to 1963. *Gastroenterology*, **53**: 198, 1967.
4. Aylett, S. O.: Three hundred cases of diffuse ulcerative colitis treated by total colectomy and ileorectal anastomosis. *Br. Med. J.*, **1**: 1001, 1966.
5. Baker, W. N. W.: The results of ileorectal anastomosis at St. Mark's hospital from 1953–1968. *Gut*, **11**: 235, 1970.
6. Sprechler, M., *et al.*: Ileorectal anastomosis for ulcerative colitis. *Br. Med. J.*, **1**: 527, 1971.
7. Fazio, V., *et al.*: Ileorectal anastomosis. A stage surgical technique. *Dis. Colon Rectum*, **18**: 107, 1975.
8. Jones, P. F., *et al.*: Colectomy and ileorectal anastomosis for colitis: Report on a personal series, with a critical review. *Br. J. Surg.*, **64**: 615, 1977.
9. Shiratori, T., *et al.*: Questionnaire data on patients who received surgical treatment for ulcerative colitis in Japan. In: Proceedings of Ulcerative Colitis and Crohn's Disease Research Committee of the Japanese Ministry of Health and Welfare. p. 14, 1976.
10. Goligher, J., *et al.*: Ulcerative Colitis. Williams & Wilkins Co., Baltimore, 1968.
11. Emanoel, C. G., *et al.*: Proctocolectomy for ulcerative colitis. *World J. Surg.*, **4**: 195, 1980.
12. Aylett, S. O.: Rectal conservation in surgical treatment of ulcerative colitis. *Arch. Fr. Mal. App. Dig.*, **63**: 585, 1974.
13. Ribet, M., *et al.*: La conservation du rectum dans la rectocolite hemorrhagique. *Chirurgie*, **99**: 474, 1973.
14. Vink, M., *et al.*: A critical evaluation and analysis of total colectomy and ileorectal anastomosis for patients with ulcerative colitis. *Arch. Chir. Neerl.*, **25**: 107, 1973.
15. Ehrenpreis, T.: Surgical treatment of ulcerative colitis in childhood. *Arch. Dis. Child.*, **41**: 137, 1966.
16. Yudin, I. Y.: Some problems of surgical treatment of non-specific ulcerative colitis. *Am. J. Proctol.*, **24**: 403, 1973.
17. Muir, E. G.: Rectal carcinoma seventeen years after ileorectal anastomosis. *Proc. R. Soc. Med.*, **59**: 617, 1966.
18. Hughes, E. S. R. and Russell, I. S.: Ileorectal anastomosis for ulcerative colitis. *Dis. Colon Rectum*, **10**: 35, 1967.
19. Mignon, M., *et al.*: Les indications de la conservation du rectum dans les colectomies pour rectocolite hemorrhagique. *Arch. Fr. Mal. App. Dig.*, **63**: 541, 1974.
20. Adson, M. A., *et al.*: Ileorectostomy for ulcerative disease of the colon. *Arch. Surg.*, **104**: 424, 1972.
21. Veidenheimer, M. C., *et al.*: Ileorectal anastomosis for inflammatory disease of the large bowel. *Am. J. Surg.*, **119**: 375, 1970.

Temporary Colostomy or Ileostomy in the Treatment of Severe Cases of Ulcerative Colitis

Tsuneo Shiratori, Hiroshige Nakano, Naoki Inatsugi, Takasumi Hosoi, Nao Sekiya, Hisao Fujii, and Koji Murakami

INTRODUCTION

The diagnosis and treatment of ulcerative colitis in Japan have improved remarkably with increasing interest in the diseases of the large intestine. Particularly with the accumulation of experience in medical treatment, even cases of severe proctocolitis have come to be well controlled by pharmacotherapy using sulfasalazine and steroid hormones and by nutritional management including intravenous hyperalimentation and elemental diet. However, some types of this disease, e.g., the fulminant type, severe type, and moderate type of the chronic continuous type, are not responding to pharmacotherapy. In such cases, surgical treatment is necessary.

In 1975 an enquête study on cases operated on for ulcerative colitis was conducted in Japan by the Ulcerative Colitis and Crohn's Disease Study Group (headed by Shuji Tsuchiya) of the Ministry of Health and Welfare, and 214 cases were tabulated.[1)]

Table 1 shows the operative indications and mortality in the 41 cases treated by emergency operation among the 214 cases. Cases of massive hemorrhage were the most numerous, followed by cases of severe attack, toxic megacolon, perforation, and sudden deterioration. The mortality was 32%, or 13 out of 214 cases, and the mortality due to perforation was as high as 100%.

Table 2 presents the operative indications and postoperative mortality in cases treated by elective surgery. Cases of frequent relapse and failure of medical treatment accounted for the majority. The mortality was 3%, or 5 cases.

As previously noted, the postoperative mortality in cases of emergency operation is 10 times higher than that in cases of elective surgery. This indicates the great danger involved in emergency operations.

First Department of Surgery, Nara Medical University, Kashihara, Nara, Japan

TABLE 1. Operative Indications and Mortality in Emergency Cases of Ulcerative Colitis[1)]

Indication	No. of cases	No. of deaths	(%)
Massive hemorrhage	17	2	(12)
Perforation	6	6	(100)
Toxic Megacolon	7	1	(14)
Severe attack	8	3	(38)
Sudden deterioration	3	1	(33)
Total	41	13	(32)

TABLE 2. Operative Indications and Mortality in Elective Cases of Ulcerative Colitis[1)]

Indication	No. of cases	No. of deaths	(%)
Frequent relapsing	98	4	(4)
Failure of treatment	60	1	(2)
Systemic complications	1		
Suspected cancer	3		
Obstruction	6		
Fistula formation	0		
Social indications	5		
Total	173	5	(3)

Administration of steroid hormones prior to operation should be mentioned as one of the factors affecting mortality in emergency operations. Table 3 shows the postoperative complications among patients with steroid treatment and those without.

There appear to be more wound dehiscence and perineal sepsis in cases given steroid hormone, 7,000 mg (Predonine) for 3 months or more,

TABLE 3. Postoperative Complications of Steroid-Treated and Nonsteriod-Treated Patients with Ulcerative Colitis

Postoperative complication	Steroid-treated patients (38 cases)			Patients without steroid treatment (29 cases)	Total
	>3 months >Cortisone 7,000 mg (23 cases)		< 3 months <Cortisone 7,000 mg (15 cases)		
	Continued (9 cases)	Discontinued (14 cases)			
Wound dehiscence	1	3	1		5
Perineal sepsis	1	2	1		4
Peritonitis	1		1	1	3
Leakage	4 (1)*	2		2	8 (1)*
Hemorrhage				3	3
Intestinal obstruction				3	3

*( ): No. of deaths.

compared with cases given a lesser dose for a shorter period or those without steroid treatment.

As can be seen from such results, the lessening of mortality in cases of emergency operation and reduction of postoperative complications are problems to be solved in the surgical treatment of this disease.

We have treated severe cases of ulcerative colitis in accordance with the therapeutic criteria illustrated in Fig. 1 and have obtained satisfactory results.[2)] The criteria are as follows: The severe type of ulcerative colitis is initially treated by an intensive intravenous regimen.[3)] The therapeutic effect of this regimen is evaluated within five days. In cases where it has been effective, a decrease in bloody stool and frequency of bowel actions as well as relief of fever and abdominal pain are observed. Cases responsive to this regimen are subsequently subjected either to conservative therapy or to surgical treatment including second-stage operation after withdrawal from steroid therapy.

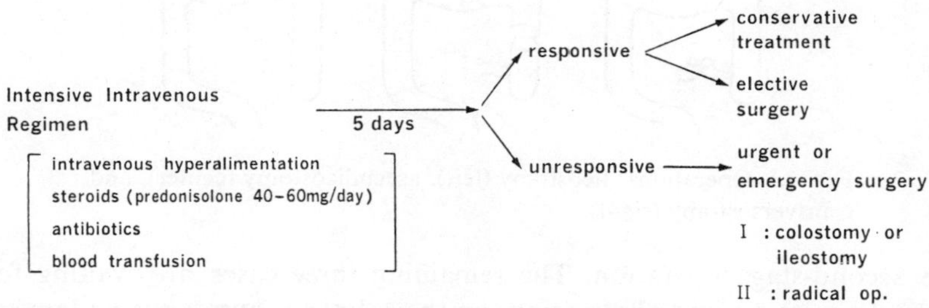

FIG. 1. Therapeutic criteria for severe ulcerative colitis.

In cases in which the regimen is ineffective, emergency or urgent operation is performed. In these cases, radical operation is not performed as the first stage. Ileostomy or right-sided colostomy involving less surgical intervention is performed first, and after confirming improvement in general condition, radical surgery is performed.

RESULTS OF TEMPORARY COLOSTOMY OR ILEOSTOMY

Temporary right-sided colostomy or ileostomy was undertaken in accordance with the therapeutic criteria in 12 cases. Operative indications and prognosis of these 12 cases are shown in Table 4.

Two cases which underwent ileostomy were of the severe attack type, and a sphincter-saving operation was performed as the second-stage operation. Four cases of ascendicostomy were also of the severe attack type, and one of them underwent permanent ileostomy with total colectomy as

TABLE 4. Indications for Colostomy or Ileostomy and Their Outcome

Operation performed*	No. of cases	Indication for operation	No. of cases	Outcome		
				Sphincter-saving operation	Colostomy or ileostomy with resection	Colostomy or ileostomy without resection
Ileostomy	2	Severe attack	2	2	0	0
Ascendicostomy	4	Severe attack	4	0	1	3
Transversostomy	6**	Severe attack	3	4	1	1
		Massive hemorrhage	2			
		Failure ofmedical treatment	1			

*Each operation is illustrated in Fig. 2.
**One: leakage.

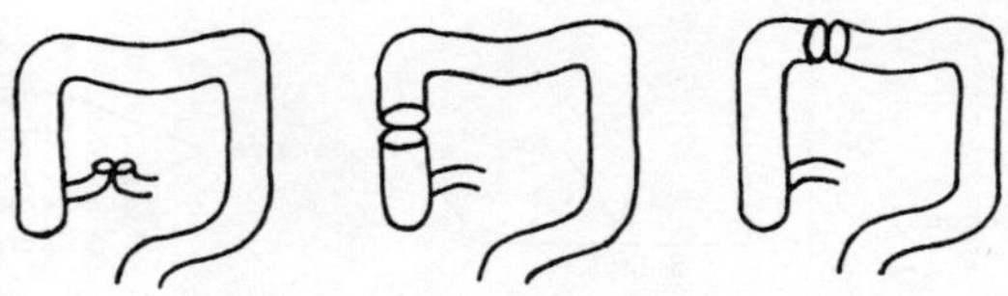

FIG. 2. Operations: ileostomy (left), ascendicostomy (center), and transversostomy (right).

the second-stage operation. The remaining three cases are waiting for radical operation, and observations on their clinical courses are underway.

Of six cases in which transversostomy was undertaken, three cases were operated on for severe attack, two cases for masssive hemorrhage, and one case for failure of the medical treatment.

Five out of these six cases had already undergone radical operation as the second-stage operation, that is, permanent ascendicostomy with resection in one case and sphincter-saving operation in four cases. In the remaining one case, transversostomy is the only operation so far performed and observations on its clinical course are underway.

Figure 3 shows the clinical course of seven cases which have recently undergone colostomy or ileostomy in terms of fever, erythrocyte sedimentation rate, body weight, and serum total protein; a decrease in fever and improvement in the increased erythrocyte sedimentation rate are observed. Further, a marked improvement in general condition is observed along with a marked increase in body weight and serum protein.

Figure 4 illustrates the detailed clinical course of one among these seven cases. The patient is a 36-year-old male. Complaining of 10–20 mucous and blood-streaked stools daily, severe abdominal pain, and fever, he was

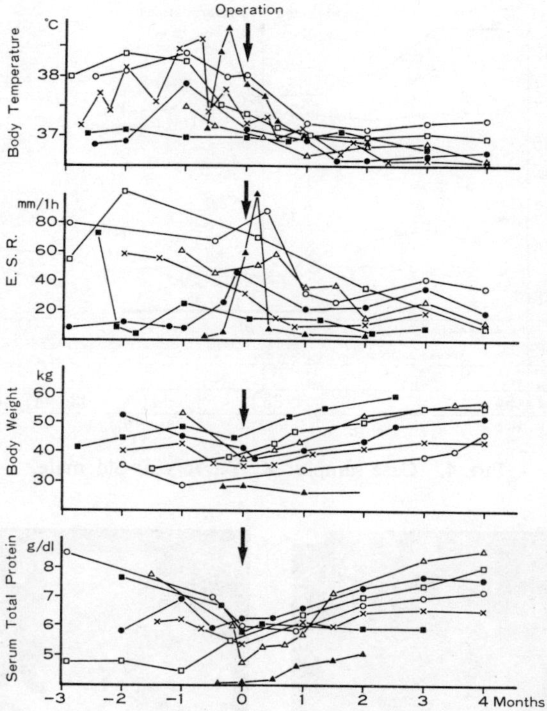

FIG. 3. Clinical course of 7 cases after colostomy or ileostomy.

admitted for emergency treatment. He was immediately put on a fast and started on intravenous hyperalimentation based on the intensive intravenous regimen. His condition did not improve even after administration of Predonine 40 mg/day, antibiotics, and blood transfusion. Furthermore, exacerbation of conditions such as bloody stool, abdominal pain, and loss of body weight were observed even after administration of ACTH 50 U per day. Thus, right-sided transversostomy was undertaken the first month after admission.

Figure 5a shows a barium enema examination just before the operation, and Fig. 5b denotes barium enema examination on the 40th day after operation.

The body weight at the time of operation was 38 kg, a reduction of 16 kg from the normal body weight. On the 40th day of oral ingestion of food, which was started from the first week after operation, however, the body weight had increased by 10 kg to show an evident improvement.

No aggravation was observed even following withdrawal from the

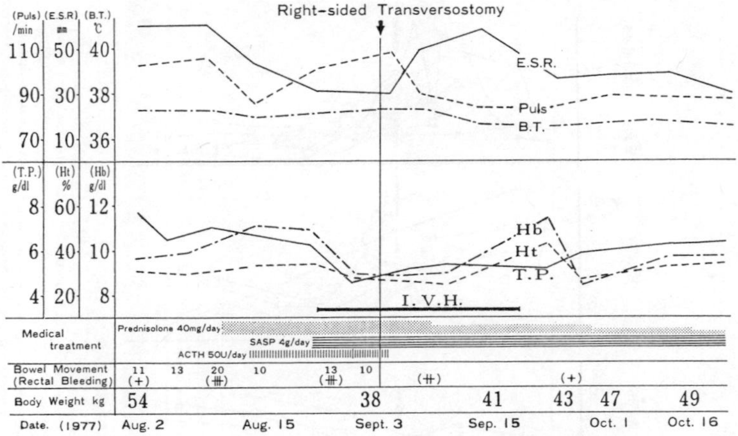

FIG. 4. Case sample: K. Y., 36-year-old male.

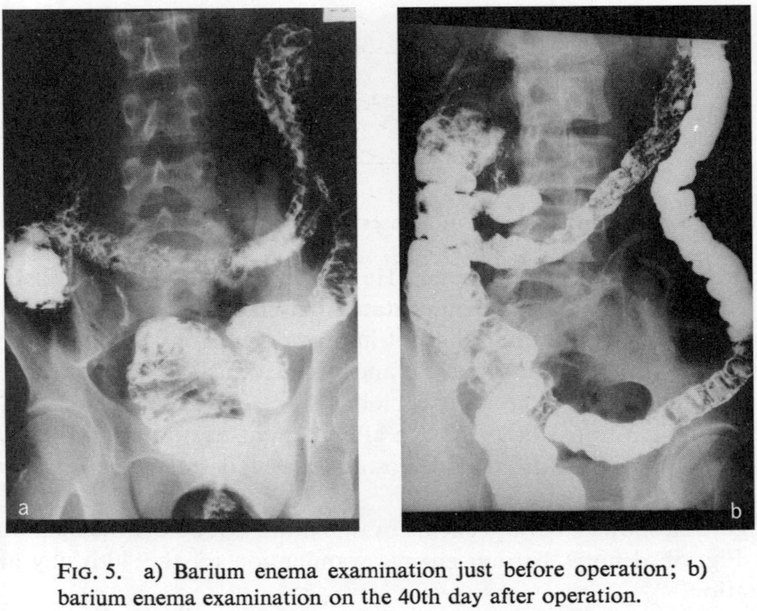

FIG. 5. a) Barium enema examination just before operation; b) barium enema examination on the 40th day after operation.

steroid therapy started after right-sided transversostomy; the steroid therapy was withdrawn completely at the second month and radical operation was performed two months later (Fig. 6). The surgical procedure used makes use of ileal interposition and preserves the slightly affected cecum.

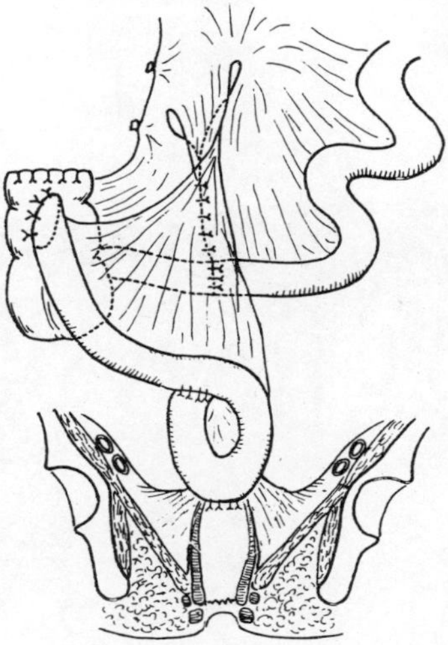

FIG. 6. Scheme of cecum-preserving subtotal proctocolectomy with ileal interposition.

According to macroscopic findings in the isolated specimen, the mucosal inflammation on the oral side was alleviated almost to normal at the site of colostomy, whereas the mucosa on the anal side showed a pattern typical of the active stage with intense redness and edema. Figure 7 illustrates the histology of the isolated specimen, with a) representing the oral side of the colostomy and b) the anal side.

Atrophy of the regenerated epithelium and inflammatory cell infiltration were observed on the oral side, while intense inflammatory cell infiltration, edema of the lamina propria mucosae, and crypt abscess were present to indicate histology of the active stage on the anal side.

Seven cases in which macroscopic and histologic examination was possible showed findings almost identical to those of the case mentioned above.

From these findings, it is surmised that colostomy or ileostomy without resection of the affected area, though not leading to the cure of lesions, will prevent intervention (for instance, physical, chemical, immunological, or bacteriological) by blocking the fecal stream and subsequently bring about improvement in general conditions.

On the basis of such clinical experience, we speculate that both etiologic factors and aggravating factors exist in this disease and that feces are quite likely to be an aggravating factor in the active stage.

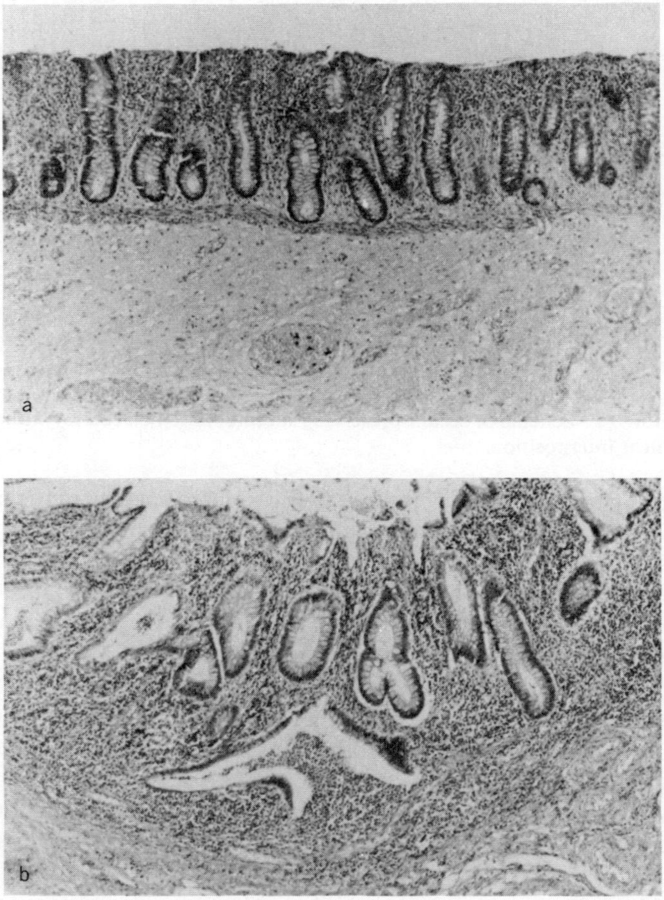

FIG. 7. Histology of the isolated specimen: a) the oral side of colostomy; b) the anal side of colostomy.

INDICATIONS

The following four items may be listed as the operative indications for temporary colostomy or ileostomy in serious ulcerative colitis:

1) Where improvement in general condition with less surgical interven-

tion is desired in the surgical treatment of serious cases, the usefulness of this surgical procedure is high, particularly when consideration is given to the fact that results of radical operation are poor in cases of massive hemorrhage, toxic megacolon, and perforation.

2) Where withdrawal from steroid therapy is difficult in cases placed on a long-term massive administration of steroids, this surgical procedure makes such withdrawal possible.

3) This surgical procedure is effective as a preliminary preparation for performing reconstructive surgery of the anus safely in severe cases.

4) This surgical procedure alone results in such an improvement in general condition as to enable social rehabilitation. Thus, it is indicated where radical operation is made impossible for one reason or another.

DISCUSSION

The decision to operate and the selection of operative procedures are of paramount importance in surgical colitis. Particular attention should be given to the saving of lives of patients with severe disease, massive hemorrhage, and toxic megacolon and to the selecting of an adequate surgical procedure.

According to the result of investigation in 2,071 cases of surgical operation by Goligher *et al*,.[4] the rate of operative death was 3–4% in cases of total colectomy performed as a second-stage operation and 10–70% in cases of total colectomy performed as an emergency operation.

In contrast, the postoperative mortality in cases of ileostomy alone without colectomy is reported to be 19.5% by Goligher *et al.*[4] and 16.1% by Truelove *et al.*[5]

Based on these results, many in Europe and the U.S.A. are of the view that the mortality in cases of emergency operation is affected largely by the timing of the operation rather than by the selection of operative procedure.[4,5] In Japan, the number of cases of emergency operation is small and not enough study has been done yet on the correlation between the timing of operation, operative procedures, and operative death.

We have established therapeutic criteria on the basis of results obtained in Europe and the U.S.A. and our own experience, and conducted treatment according to these criteria to obtain satisfactory results.

According to Goligher,[6] the method to prevent feces from flowing through the affected colon originated from ileostomy performed by Baum (1879) and Schinginger (1881). After that, Follet (1885) and Novaro (1887) also performed cecostomy. These procedures occasionally yielded remarkable results, but the efficacy was temporary in most cases.

Formerly, ileostomy and colostomy were performed in anticipation of radical cure, but failed to produce drastic efficacy. Historically, therefore, these may be known as operative procedures that were forsaken.

From our experience in surgical treatment since 1955, including cases which underwent ileostomy or ascendicostomy without colectomy and showed improvement in general condition and cases under long-term observation which showed no intense recurrence of the disease, we have rated the usefulness of this operative procedure highly and have been performing it in selected cases.

Turnbull *et al.*[7] performed ileostomy and transversostomy for reducing the pressure in 41 cases of toxic megacolon (ulcerative colitis 25 cases, Crohn's disease 16 cases) to obtain excellent results: one operative death, or 2.4%. These results are very interesting since they are similar to ours in that a procedure for reducing pressure was taken and that the fecal stream was prevented from passing through the affected colon; however, comparing the two for evaluation is difficult because of the difference in the subject of study, that is, toxic megacolon in their results and the severe type in ours.

Our experience is derived from a small number of cases, and further studies are needed to determine whether or not our operative procedure is effective for all severe ulcerative colitis cases.

REFERENCES

1. Shiratori. T., *et al.*: A questionnaire data on patients who received the surgical treatment for ulcerative colitis in Japan. In: The Proceedings of Ulcerative Colitis and Crohn's Disease Research Committee of the Japanese Ministry of Health and Welfare. p. 14, 1976.
2. Shiratori, T., *et al.*: Treatment of ulcerative colitis. *Gastroenterological Surgery*, **13**: 2053, 1980.
3. Truelove, S. C.: Intensive intravenous regimen for severe attacks of ulcerative colitis. *Lancet,* **1**: 1067, 1974.
4. Goligher, J. C., Dedombal, F. T., Watts, J. M., *et al.*: Ulcerative Colitis. Williams & Wilkins Co., Baltimore, 1968.
5. Truelove, S. C., Ellis, H., and Webster, C. U.: Place of a double-barrelled ileostomy in ulcerative colitis and Crohn's disease of the colon: A preliminary report. *Br. Med. J.*, **1**: 150–153, 1965.
6. Goligher, J. C.: Ulcerative Colitis. 2nd ed. Bailliere Tindall and Cassell, London, 1968.
7. Turnbull, R. B., Hawk, W. A., and Weakley, F. L.: Surgical treatment of toxic megacolon, ileostomy and colostomy to prepare patients for colectomy. *Am. J. Surg.*, **122**: 325–331, 1971.

The Results of Total Proctocolectomy with Ileostomy for Ulcerative Colitis

Takeshi Sekine, Iwao Sasaki,** and Jin-ichi Kameyama***

Various types of operation for ulcerative colitis have been investigated from the point of view of surgical treatment. In the present study, we scrutinized the results of our total proctocolectomy with ileostomy for the total colitis type of ulcerative colitis and discussed the value of this type of operation for the surgical treatment of ulcerative colitis.

MATERIALS AND METHODS

During the 20 years from 1961 to 1981, we experienced a total of 47 patients undergoing operations for ulcerative colitis at Tohoku University Hospital and Saitama Cancer Center Hospital. In classifying the extent of the disease, total colitis was found in 37 (79%) of the 47 patients (Table 1). They consisted of 16 males and 21 females, with ages ranging between 11 and 54 years with a mean of 30 years. Viewed from the severity of the disease, 21 (57%) of the 37 patients with total colitis were severe, including 4 operative deaths. However, 8 of 9 patients with left-sided colitis and one with proctitis were mild or moderately severe (Table 2).

The indications for operation of the 37 patients with total colitis are shown in Table 3. The indications for urgent or emergency operation were acute fulminating type and massive hemorrhage in 6 (16%) of the 37

TABLE 1. Extent of Disease, 1961–1981

Extent	No. of cases
Total colitis	37 (4) 78.7%
Left-sided colitis	9 19.2%
Proctitis	1 2.1%

( ): Operative death.

*Abdominal Surgery Clinic, Saitama Cancer Center Hospital, Ina, Saitama, Japan
**Department of Surgery, Tohoku University School of Medicine, Sendai, Japan

TABLE 2. Severity of Disease

Extent	Mild	Moderately severe	Severe	Total
Total	7	9	21 [5] (4)	37 [5] (4)
Left-sided colitis	4	4	1	9
Proctitis	1			1

[ ]: Acute fulminating type.
( ): Operative death.

TABLE 3. Indications for Operation: Total Colitis Type

Indication	No. of cases
Urgent or emergency operation	
Acute fulminating type	5* (2)
Massive hemorrhage	1
Elective operation	
Intractability and chronic invalidism (unresponsive to medical treatment)	23 (1)
Systemic complications	
Moon face	4**
Toxic megacolon	2
Steroid diabetes	1 (1)
Fistula-in-ano	1

*Includes one case complicated by toxic megacolon and perforation.
**Includes one case complicated by secondary aldosteronism.
( ): Operative death.

patients. One of the 5 patients of acute fulminating type had evidence of complicating toxic megacolon and perforation. The indications for elective operation were relapsing-remitting type, that is, intractability and chronic invalidism (unresponsive to medical treatment), in the majority of the 37 patients, or as many as 30 (81%). Among them, systemic complications such as moon face, toxic megacolon, and steroid diabetes were observed in 4, 2, and one patient, respectively. Further, preoperative administration of corticosteroids, as shown in Table 4, was performed in 32 (86%) of the 37 patients with total colitis. These 32 patients included 17 (46%) of the 37 patients that received an excessive dosage of corticosteroids for more than 3 months (over 7,000 mg calculated in terms of cortisone), in all likelihood significantly influencing the operative results.

Regarding the operative procedures employed for the 47 patients with ulcerative colitis, artificial anus operation was performed in 33 patients, and sphincter-saving operation in 14 (Table 5). In patients with total colitis, artificial anus operation was often a forced choice in preference to sphincter-saving operation, as demonstrated in the present study with 27 (73%) of the 37 patients. Among these 27 patients with artificial anus

TABLE 4. Systemic Administration of Corticosteroid

Corticosteroid	Total colitis	Left-Sided colitis	Proctitis
Administered	32* [5] (4)	6	1
Not administered	5	3	

*Includes 17 cases with long-term and excessive administration of corticosteriod (more than 3 months over 7,000 mg calculated in terms of cortisone).
[ ]: Acute fulminating type.
( ): Operative death.

TABLE 5. Operative Procedures

Type of operation	Total colitis	Left-Sided colitis and proctitis
Artificial anus operation (33 cases)		
Total proctocolectomy with ileostomy	14 (1)	
Total colectomy with retained rectum and ileostomy	4 (2)	
Subtotal proctocolectomy with colostomy	9	4
Colostomy		1
Abdominoperineal excision		1
Sphincter-saving operation (14 cases)		
Total colectomy with ileorectal anastomosis	9 (1)	
Subtotal colectomy with colorectal anastomosis	1	
Left hemicolectomy	4	

( ): Operative death.

operation, 14 had undergone total proctocolectomy with ileostomy, including 3 with interposition of antiperistaltic ileal segment and 2 with Kock's continent ileostomy. Total colectomy with retained rectum and ileostomy was performed in 4 patients with acute fulminating type with the aim of preventing death in consideration of the general condition.

Follow-up studies, comprised of questionnaires and personal interviews, were done on the 32 patients with various types of operation for ulcerative colitis—the total 47 patients minus 4 operative deaths, 3 follow-up deaths from another disease, and 8 patients failing to respond (Table 6). Of these 32 patients, 26 patients with artificial anus operation were available for the follow-up study. Follow-up periods ranged from 1 to 19 years, with a mean of 8 years. The types of operation were artificial anus operation in 26 patients (total proctocolectomy with ileostomy in 15, subtotal proctocolectomy with colostomy in 11) and sphincter-saving operation in 6 patients (total colectomy with ileorectal anastomosis in 5, subtotal colectomy with colorectal anastomosis in one).

TABLE 6. Follow-Up Study: Questionnaire Review and Personal Interviews (32 Cases)

Type of operation	No. of cases
Artificial anus operation	
Total proctocolectomy with ileostomy	15
Subtotal proctocolectomy with colostomy	11
Sphincter-saving operation	
Total colectomy with ileorectal anastomosis	5
Subtotal colectomy with colorectal anastomosis	1

RESULTS

Operative mortality

As shown in Table 7, operative mortality was identified in 4 (9%) of the 47 patients, all with severe total colitis, showing serious hypoproteinemia and anemia. All the four patients had had long-term and excessive administrations of corticosteroids preoperatively. One of them underwent total proctocolectomy with ileostomy (with interposition of antiperistaltic ileal segment), and two had total colectomy with retained rectum and ileostomy. Particularly in one of the latter cases, uncontrollable rectal bleeding occurred despite the medical treatment. The four patients died of anastomotic leakage, diffuse peritonitis, and wound dehiscence, reminiscent of the time before 1970 when indications for operation as well as medical treatment of total colitis had not thoroughly been investigated. However, no instance of operative death has been identified since 1971.

Recurrence and reoperation

As shown in Fig. 1, 4 (9%) of the 47 cases encountered recurrences and were subjected to reoperations, not including any total proctocolectomy with ileostomy. However, one case with total colectomy with retained rectum and ileostomy frequently encountered recurrence, eventually requiring subsequent rectal excision.

Follow-up results

Frequency of bowel movements. As shown in Table 8, bowel movements were over five times per day in the majority of cases with ileostomy. Instances with bowel movements more than 10 times daily shared a high proportion of 40%, or 6 of 15 cases with ileostomy, contrasted with 18%, or 2 of 11 cases with colostomy. It was notable that the two cases with Kock's continent ileostomy showed a favorable incidence of bowel movements, three times or less per day. The case with interposition of antiperistaltic ileal segment had bowel movements six or seven times per day.

TABLE 7. Operative Mortality

Case No.	Age and sex	Duration of symptom (mos.)	Preoperative complications	Laboratory findings*	Indication	Operative procedures	Postoperative complications
1	14/M	11	Steroid diabetes	RBC: 280 TP: 5.0	Relapsing-remitting type (unresponsive to medical treatment)	Total colectomy with ileorectal anastomosis (inversed 9 type)	Anastomotic leakage, diffuse peritonitis
2	38/F	69	Hypoproteinemia	RBC: 238 TP: 5.2	ditto	Total proctocolectomy with ileostomy (anti-peristaltic segment)	Anastomotic leakage, wound dehiscence
3**	27/F	1	Hypoproteinemia	RBC: 324 TP: 5.2	Acute fulminating type	Total colectomy with retained rectum and ileostomy	Diffuse peritonitis, wound dehiscence
4	44/F	1	Toxic megacolon, hypoproteinemia	RBC: 360 TP: 4.8	ditto	ditto	ditto

*RBC: $\times 10^4/mm^3$, TP: g/dl.

**Onset during pregnancy and exacerbation after abortion.

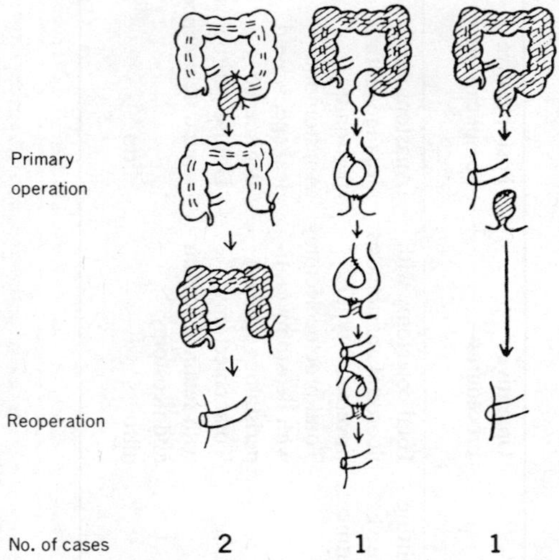

FIG. 1. Recurrence and reoperation. Shaded area represents extent of disease.

TABLE 8. Follow-Up Results: Frequency of Bowel Movements

Bowel motions (No. of stools/day)	Ileostomy (15 cases)			Colostomy (11 cases)		
	<5	5–10	10<	<5	5–10	10<
No. of cases	5 (2)	4 [1]	6 {1}	8	1	2

( ): Kock's continent ileostomy.
[ ]: Interposition of antiperistaltic ileal segment.
{ }: Total colectomy with retained rectum and ileostomy.

Consistency of feces. Table 9 shows the consistency of feces in the cases followed up. With ileostomy, most cases, or 10 of 15 (67%), had loose stool, while watery stool and muddy stool were identified in one and 3 cases, respectively. In the 2 cases with Kock's continent ileostomy, the stool was muddy; the case with interposition of antiperistaltic ileal segment showed loose stool. On the other hand, in 2 (18%) of the 11 cases with colostomy, the stool was formed without any instance of watery or muddy stool. There was no evidence of mucous and bloody stool or steatorrhea in the cases with ileostomy.

Diet control in reference to the influence of food on bowel movements was practiced in about half of the cases with ileostomy.

Marriage, pregnancy, and childbirth. Postoperative marriages were observed in three cases with ileostomy, consisting of two males and one

TABLE 9. Follow-Up Results: Consistency of Feces

	Ileostomy	Colostomy
Watery stool	1	
Muddy stool	3 (2)	
Loose stool	10 [1]	9
Formed stool	1	2

No instance with mucous and bloody stool.
( ): Kock's continent ileostomy.
[ ]: Interposition of antiperistaltic ileal segment.

female (Kock's continent ileostomy), and in one male with colostomy. One female with ileostomy gave birth to a normal baby.

Changes in body weight. As shown in Table 10, in cases with ileostomy, the body weight gained more than 5 kg at the follow-up in 9 (60%) of 15 cases. There was no instance of weight loss.

TABLE 10. Follow-Up Results: Body Weight

Body weight	Ileostomy	Colostomy
Gained	9 (2)	5
Stable	6 [1]	4
Lost		2

( ): Kock's continent ileostomy.
[ ]: Interposition of antiperistaltic ileal segment.

Occupational return. As shown in Table 11, most of the patients had been restored to preoperative condition, competent for working or studying. In cases with ileostomy, the occupational returnees numbered 14 (93%) of 15 cases, with no instance proving unable to work.

TABLE 11. Follow-Up Results: Occupational Return

	Ileostomy	Colostomy
Return to work	14 (2) [1]	9
Change to light work		1
Occasionally able to work	1	1

( ): Kock's continent ileostomy.
[ ]: Interposition of antiperistaltic ileal segment.

Subjective results of operation. As regards the subjective results of operation, 13 (87%) of 15 cases with ileostomy rated it "satisfactory," as opposed to the "unknown" expressed by 2 cases (Table 12). These 2 cases had bowel movements over 10 times per day. However, there was no instance of dissatisfaction being expressed with the operation.

TABLE 12. Follow-Up Results: Subjective Results of Operation

Satisfaction with the operation	Ileostomy	Colostomy
Satisfactory	13 (2) [1]	11
Unknown	2	

No instance expressing dissatisfaction with the operation.
( ): Kock's continent ileostomy.
[ ]: Interposition of antiperistaltic ileal segment.

DISCUSSION

It is generally accepted that of all the patients with ulcerative colitis, 17–48% of them require surgical treatment.[1] Essential in the surgical treatment of ulcerative colitis is to remove as much of the lesion as possible and to preserve the sphincter function of the anus as well as possible. We have made it a rule to select the best type of operation on an individual basis, taking into account the extent and severity of the disease, the patient's age, the inflammatory changes in the rectum, and the postoperative bowel movements.[2–9] Among varying types of operation, total proctocolectomy with ileostomy is the most radical and safe from the point of view of recurrence. However, it involves troublesome postoperative problems such as persistent watery or muddy diarrhea associated with frequent bowel movements and severe excoriation of the skin around the ileostomy.

When total proctocolectomy with ileostomy is performed in an elective operation, we individually choose interposition of antiperistaltic ileal segment 7–8 cm, and Kock's continent ileostomy,[10] which with the device of a nipple valve can control the bowel movements. Certainly the latter may be an elective operation, but in view of the technical difficulties and meticulous care needed in its application, this method should be contraindicated for the aged, severe total colitis cases, and those with long-term and excessive administration of corticosteroids.[8,10] On the other hand, there may be some patients who have general condition so extremely serious that total colectomy with retained rectum and ileostomy (Hartmann's operation) is indicated for the sake of saving their lives. We applied this type of operation to two patients with acute fulminating type. One of the two died of massive hemorrhage from the retained rectum, leaving problems about the indication for this type of operation and the value of retaining the rectum. Also, Flatmark *et al.*[11] reported that out of 63 cases of severe total colitis with this type of operation, 2 were forced to undergo reoperations because of massive hemorrhage with the retained rectum.

With regard to the problem of recurrence, many researchers, including Kon *et al.*[12] and Hamano *et al.*,[13] reported that total colectomy with retained rectum and ileostomy failed to attain favorable remission and that persistent inflammatory changes forced the patient to undergo reoperations with subsequent rectal excision. Binder *et al.*,[14] in 80 patients with urgent or emergency operations out of their total 111 patients undergoing operation, compared the results of total proctocolectomy with those of total colectomy with retained rectum, and found that there was no distinctive difference between the two but that about 80% of the latter cases required reoperations to excise the retained rectum. Based on these findings, they argued that in the surgical treatment of ulcerative colitis with total colitis type, it is safe to perform one-stage total proctocolectomy with ileostomy. According to their valuable advice, what should be emphasized is that the rectum must be retained in as short a length as possible. In our routine, the retained rectum is at a length of about 5–6 cm from the anal verge. In either event, preserving the rectum involves various problems including the risk of developing carcinoma in patients with ulcerative colitis; thus consistent observation and investigation should never be neglected in this regard. Therefore, in view of radical surgery with no recurrence, total proctocolectomy with ileostomy, despite its mental impact on the patient, is nonetheless the most favorable and safest type of operation for ulcerative colitis with total colitis. Based on the follow-up results of 143 cases observed by Waugh *et al.*[15] with "good" or "excellent" comprising as many as 94% of them, along with our favorable follow-up results,[6,16,17] this type of operation is convincingly preferable for the total colitis type of ulcerative colitis with severe inflammatory changes in the rectum.[18,19]

SUMMARY

Eighteen patients with total colitis type of ulcerative colitis were subjected to total proctocolectomy with ileostomy and total colectomy with retained rectum and ileostomy. The results were scrutinized and evaluated from the point of view of surgical treatment.

Total proctocolectomy with ileostomy certainly involves troublesome postoperative problems, such as mental distress and frequent bowel movements, but its virtue in respect of a radical operation with no incidence of recurrence may well justify its evaluation as the most adequate and preferable type of operation for the total colitis type, with severe inflammatory changes in the rectum, of ulcerative colitis.

REFERENCES

1. Goligher, J. C.: Surgery of the Anus, Rectum and Colon. 3rd ed. Bailliere Tindall & Cassell, London, 1975.

2. Maki, T., Shiratori, T., and Machida, T.: An investigation of various types of operation for ulcerative colitis. *Surg. Therapy*, **15**: 42–51, 1966 (in Japanese).
3. Shiratori, T. and Sekine, T.: Surgical treatment of ulcerative colitis, with special reference to the operative results. *Shujutsu*, **24**: 1151–1160, 1970 (in Japanese).
4. Tsukamoto, M. and Sekine, T.: Surgical treatment of ulcerative colitis. *Shujutsu*, **28**: 1101–1109, 1974 (in Japanese).
5. Yamazaki, T. and Tsukamoto, M.: Operative results of ulcerative colitis, with special reference to total colitis type. *Shujutsu*, **31**: 949–956, 1977 (in Japanese).
6. Sekine, T., Yamazaki, T., Kameyama, J., Sasaki, I., Momono, S., Imamura, M., and Sato, T.: Surgical treatment of ulcerative colitis, with special reference to indication, selection of operation and follow-up results. *Jap. J. Gastroent. Surgery*, **12**: 35–40, 1979 (in Japanese).
7. Sekine, T., Imamura, M., Inui, M., Miyakawa, H., Sasaki, I., Kameyama, J., and Sato, T.: Surgical treatment of ulcerative colitis, with special reference to the operative mortality. *Surg. Therapy*, **41**: 127–132, 1979 (in Japanese).
8. Sekine, T., Kameyama, J., Sasaki, I., Imamura, M., Inui, M., and Miyakawa, H.: Surgical treatment of ulcerative colitis, with special reference to Kock's continent ileostomy. *Surg. Therapy*, **45**: 369–375, 1981 (in Japanese).
9. Sekine, T. and Sato, T.: Operative procedure for ulcerative colitis—Panproctocolectomy with permanent ileostomy. *Shujutsu*, **32**: 819–825, 1978 (in Japanese).
10. Kock, N. G.: Continent ileostomy. *Progr. Surg.*, **12**: 180–201, 1973.
11. Flatmark, A., Fretheim, B., and Gjone, E.: Early colectomy in severe ulcerative colitis. *Scand. J. Gastroent.*, **10**: 427–431, 1975.
12. Kon, M., Murakami, T., Sasaki, M., Shishido, Y., Yokoyama, Y., Takano, T., Ito, S., Harada, M., Morita, T., Inamoto, J., Matsuda, K., and Ouchi, K.: Surgical treatment of ulcerative colitis viewed from historical background, with special reference to sphincter-saving operation. *Shujutsu*, **31**: 937–948, 1977 (in Japanese).
13. Hamano, K., Akimoto, S., Omori, N., Yuri, T., Kameoka, S., Nagasaki, K., Sasaki, H., and Yamada, A.: Surgical indication and result of ulcerative colitis. *Jap. J. Gastroent. Surgery*, **12**: 48-53, 1979 (in Japanese).
14. Binder, S. C., Miller, H. H., and Deterling, R. A.: Emergency and urgent operations for ulcerative colitis; the procedure of choice. *Arch. Surg.*, **110**: 284–289, 1975.
15. Waugh, J. M., Peck, D. A., Beahrs, O. H., and Sauer, W. G.: Surgical management of chronic ulcerative colitis. *Arch. Surg.*, **88**: 556–569, 1964.
16. Sekine, T., Sasaki, I., Momono, S., and Sato, T.: An evaluation of total colectomy or subtotal colectomy—With special reference to surgical treatment of ulcerative colitis. *Surg. Therapy*, **31**: 307–315, 1974 (in Japanese).
17. Sasaki, I., Kameyama, J., Imamura, M., Miyakawa, H., Inui, M., Konno, Y., Tsuchiya, T., Naito, H., Narui, H., and Sato, T.: Appraisal of surgical

procedure for ulcerative colitis viewed from follow-up results after operation. *Surg. Therapy*, **46**: 665–672, 1982 (in Japanese).

18. Meyers, R. T. and Hightower, F.: Critical follow-up of surgically treated ulcerative colitis. *Ann. Surg.*, **167**: 920–925, 1968.
19. Roy, P. H., Sauer, W. G., Beahrs, O. H., and Farrow, G. M.: Experience with ileostomies. Evaluation of long-term rehabilitation in 497 patients. *Amer. J. Surg.*, **119**: 77–86, 1970.

Total Colectomy and Ileorectal Anastomosis for Surgical Treatment of Ulcerative Colitis with Special Reference to the Two-Stage Procedure

Tetsuichiro Muto, Junjiro Kamiya, Toshio Sawada, and Kenichi Sugihara

Although the generally accepted surgical treatment for ulcerative colitis is proctocolectomy with permanent ileostomy, the alternative procedure of total colectomy with ileorectal anastomosis has been championed by Aylett[1] and more recently by others.[2–4] We have been trying, as much as possible, to perform sphincter-saving operations for ulcerative colitis over the past several years. The purpose of this paper is to present our limited experience of the sphincter-saving operation for ulcerative colitis with special reference to the two-stage procedure and its results.

PATIENTS AND SURGICAL PROCEDURES

A total of 28 patients with ulcerative colitis were operated on at University of Tokyo Hospital and affiliated hospitals from 1963 through 1981. All patients had total active colitis. Between 1963 and 1969 proctocolectomy was performed in 60% of cases, whereas it was never performed after 1976 (Table 1).

TABLE 1. Type of Operation

	Proctocolectomy	Sphincter-saving operation	Total
1963–1969	6	4*	10
1970–1975	2	4	6
1976–1981	0	12*	12

*One case failed.

Among 28 operated cases, sphincter-saving operations of various types were attempted or performed in 20 (71%) with an annual increase of the proportion of ileorectal anastomosis (IRA). All 20 patients who received

Department of Surgery, Faculty of Medicine, University of Tokyo, Tokyo, Japan sphincter-saving operation had had mild or moderate active disease of the rectum. Out of 20 patients with IRA, one-stage operation was performed in 9 and two-stage operation in 11 (Table 2), the proportion of two-stage operations increasing over the past several years. All patients receiving two-stage operation has been on steroids for many years and showed evident clinical signs of steroid side effects, such as moon face and osteoporosis, at the time of surgery; some patients showed marked adrenal suppression when examined.

TABLE 2. Type of Sphincter-Saving Operation

	One-stage	Two-stage	Total
1967–1975	6	2	8
1976–1981	3	9	12

Two-stage IRA was performed in order to prevent anastomotic leakage in patients with moderate to severe steroid side effects. The types of sphincter-saving operation performed are illustrated in Fig. 1. In two patients, the two-stage sphincter-saving operation was attempted but failed. In another two patients diverting colostomy with subsequent colectomy and IRA was performed, and the outcome was quite satisfactory. In one patient, colectomy with ileostomy and mucous fistula was performed, followed by subsequent sigmoidectomy and IRA.

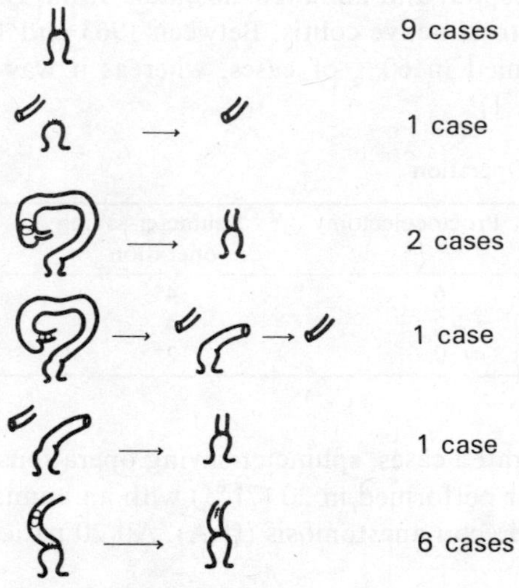

FIG. 1. Illustration of sphincter-saving operations performed.

After having tried various types of two-stage sphincter-saving operations for ulcerative colitis, we found that inflammation of the retained diseased colon did not improve even after the first operation diverted the fecal stream. On the contrary, colonic mucosa sometimes showed much more severe inflammation which made patients ill. Therefore, we thought that the entire diseased colon should be removed in the initial operation, and for this purpose, colectomy with IRA and diverting ileostomy to cover the anastomosis was performed recently in six patients. In five patients, covering loop ileostomy was closed 7 to 11 months after the first operation, and one patient is now waiting for the ileostomy closure. The end-to-end procedure is the usual type of anastomosis employed, although EEA stapler anastomosis has been recently used successfully.

RESULTS

The outcome of one-stage and two-stage sphincter-saving operations for chronic ulcerative colitis is illustrated in Tables 3 and 4. Of the nine patients receiving one-stage sphincter-saving operation, eight enjoyed good health and normal life and one was lost to follow-up (Table 3). Although some patients had to be treated for recurrent proctitis of the retained rectum, no subsequent rectal excision was necessary. There was only one anastomotic leakage and no operative deaths in this group of patients. In the treatment of proctitis of the retained rectum, steroid suppository was most effective.

Among the 11 patients receiving two-stage sphincter-saving operation, one patient with colectomy and Hartmann's procedure died of malnutrition 3 years and 5 months after having her retained rectum excised. In another patient, loop-ileostomy did not improve retained colonic inflammation and several months later colectomy with mucus fistula and

TABLE 3. Outcome of One-Stage Sphincter-Saving Operation

Age & sex	Type of operation	Rectal disease at operation	Outcome after operation	
1. K. F., 34m	Colectomy + ileo-proctostomy	mild	13 yrs 7 mos	healthy
2. H. N., 19m	do	mild	13 yrs 5 mos	healthy
3. H. K., 28m	do	moderate	12 yrs	healthy
4. S. I., 25m	do	mild	10 yrs	healthy
5. Y. I., 19m	do	mild	7 yrs	healthy
6. Y. K., 31m	do	mild	6 yrs	lost to follow-up
7. H. M., 32m	do	moderate	4 yrs 8 mos	healthy
8. F. M., 46f	do	inactive	4 yrs	healthy
9. H. S., 43m	do	mild	3 yrs 10 mos	healthy

TABLE 4. Outcome of Two-Stage Sphincter-Saving Operation

Age & sex	Type of operation	Interval between 1st & 2nd op.	Rectal disease at 1st op.	Outcome after 2nd operation	
1. K. M., 15f	Colectomy + ileoproctostomy + ileostomy → ileostomy closure	7 mos	inactive	2 yrs 7 mos	healthy
2. K. I., 45m	do	9 mos	moderate	1 yr	healthy
3. Y. A., 63f	do	10 mos	moderate	1 yr	healthy
4. N. Y., 31m	do	11 mos	moderate	5 mos	healthy
5. H. K., 32m	do	9 mos	mild	6 mos	diarrhea
6. N. K., 44m	Colectomy + ileoproctostomy + ileostomy	—	mild	—	healthy
7. M. O., 46m	Colectomy + mucous fistula + ileostomy → sigmoidectomy + ileoproctostomy	1 yr	mild–moderate	1 yr 5 mos	healthy
8. K. K., 24f	Ascendicostomy → colectomy + ileoproctostomy	1 yr 2 mos	mild	6 yrs	healthy
9. H. T., 31m	Transverse colostomy → colectomy + ileoproctostomy	1 yr	mild	1 yr 10 mos	healthy
10. S. K., 48m	Loop ileostomy → colectomy + mucus fistula → proctosigmoidectomy + ileostomy	—	moderate	—	healthy
11. A. I., 23f	Colectomy + ileostomy+ Hartmann op. → rectal excision	11 mos	severe	3 yrs 5 mos	died

ileostomy was performed for colonic perforation. However, the retained sigmoid and rectum had to be excised because of narrowing of the lumen and continuous inflammation. Apart from these two cases, the eight remaining patients receiving two-stage sphincter-saving operation enjoyed good health and normal life up to six years after the second operation (Table 4). There was neither anastomotic leakage nor operative death, and no retained rectum was excised after completion of ileorectal anastomosis. All patients showing recurrent proctitis of the retained rectum were successfully treated by steroid suppository and oral salazopyrin. There was no carcinoma detected in up to 13 years follow-up after IRA.

DISCUSSION

Sphincter-saving operation for ulcerative colitis is desirable provided that it can be safely completed and the reoperation rate for the retained rectum is low. As patients suffering from ulcerative colitis are generally young, it is reasonable that they prefer normal bowel action through their preserved anus to abnormal action through permanent ileostomy. The psychological impact on these young patients of having permanent ileostomy is also to be considered.[5] Some patients even fail to go to the doctor to receive proper treatment for ulcerative colitis for fear of being persuaded to undergo permanent ileostomy. In considering these emotional reactions of patients towards ileostomy we have been trying to perform sphincter-saving operations for ulcerative colitis whenever possible, and the relative proportion of this procedure has been increasing over the past several years.

One of the reasons for the recent increased number of IRA is assumed to be a marked decrease in the number of severe case, probably due to early diagnosis and proper treatment of the disease. Recent indications for surgical treatment of ulcerative colitis in our clinic have been longstanding continuous disease together with steroid administration. Although the patients are not severely ill, they cannot enjoy a normal life with continuous mild disease and occasional moderate to severe relapse. Because oral steroids of up to 20–30 mg/day have been given continuously for months or even years, they usually showed marked clinical symptoms of steroid side effects.

Performing IRA for these patients in one stage seems to be too risky because anastomotic leakage may occur easily, and may be fatal if it does. Therefore, we have adopted the two-stage sphincter-saving operation as the safest procedure. After having tried various types of procedures, we have found colectomy with IRA and covering loop ileostomy and subsequent ileostomy closure to be the best one, provided rectal inflammation is not severe. Aylett[1] has advocated the same procedure for his large IRA series, and we have followed his use of IRA in patients with ulcerative colitis suffering from the side effects of long-term steroid administration. In cases that rectal inflammation is severe, colectomy with mucous fistula and subsequent IRA is the operation of choice if a sphincter-saving operation is attempted. Simple ileostomy or colostomy may improve patients' general health because they can start eating. However, we abandoned this procedure as the retained colon sometimes showed severe attacks of inflammation despite the diverted fecal stream, and patients became very sick; consequently steroid withdrawal had to be postponed.

The disadvantage of the two-stage sphincter-saving operation is the long interval between the first and the second operations. It took seven months to more than one year for ileostomy closure after the initial operation. This interval was necessary for gradual steroid withdrawal and complete recovery of the adrenal function, which was checked before the second operation. Initially, we treated retained rectal inflammation by steroid suppository until complete healing. However, rectal inflammation was usually rather resistant to the suppository treatment and it took several months for complete healing. However, we found that inflammation of the retained rectum would become milder or even heal after ileostomy closure; thus it was not always necessary to wait for complete healing of the diverted rectal inflammation.

It seems that the fecal stream, probably bacterial flora, may have some favorable effect on mucosal inflammation in ulcerative colitis. Interestingly enough, metronidazole enema in the diverted inflamed rectum was very effective in some patients whose retained rectums were resistant to a high dose of steroid suppository treatment, suggesting that anaerobic bacteria have a role in maintaining mucosal inflammation.

By using EEA stapler, IRA became much safer and increasing experience indicates that the time interval between the first and second operations can be minimized in the future. On the other hand, it must be kept in mind that the patients receiving two-stage operations must have been operated on earlier, and thus the one-stage sphincter-saving operation will be performed more frequently. Loop ileostomy could be closed even under local anesthesia, and no leakage was encountered.

Recurrent inflammation of the preserved rectum after completing IRA is another problem of the sphincter-saving operation for ulcerative colitis. Local treatment by steroid suppository together with oral salazopyrin is our treatment of choice, as it is for ordinary idiopathic proctitis. The grade of inflammation is usually mild or moderate, but if untreated, may become severe. In one patient, inflammation of the retained rectum was so severe that he had to be hospitalized and treated by systemic steroids. All patients except three required steroid suppository treatment for recurrent inflammation of the retained rectum, but no rectal excision was necessary. In order to prevent subsequent rectal excision after the sphincter-saving operation, close follow-up and early treatment for the recurrent disease of the retained rectum is absolutely necessary, the same policy being emphasized by others.[3] Recurrent inflammation of the retained rectum tends to become less frequent postoperatively after time passes. At present no carcinoma has been found in the preserved rectum, but further close follow-up is necessary in the long-term schedule. Out of 69 collected cases of the sphincter-saving operation in Japan, there were 7 cases (10.1%) of rectal excision and no carcinoma was found in the retained rectum, giving excellent results as compared to those in Western countries.

All patients but one are enjoying a normal life and are satisfied with the results of their surgical treatment. The other patient is now suffering from intractable diarrhea, for which he is under intensive treatment.

From our limited experience it has become clear that sphincter-saving operations are feasible for selected patients with ulcerative colitis, and the outcome after surgery has been satisfactory without operative death or subsequent rectal excision.

SUMMARY

Our experience in the surgical treatment for ulcerative colitis was presented with special reference to the sphincter-saving operation. Two-stage ileorectal anastomosis was the safest and most satisfactory procedure in patients receiving long-term steroid treatment with side effects. The outcome after sugery was quite satisfactory, both in one-stage and two-stage sphincter-saving operations. There were no operative deaths or subsequent rectal excision. Although many patients required treatment for recurrent inflammation of the retained rectum, it was controllable by steroid suppository.

REFERENCES

1. Aylett, S. O.: Three hundred cases of diffuse ulcerative colitis treated by total colectomy and ileo-rectal anastomosis. *Brit. Med. J.*, **1**: 1001–1005, 1966.
2. Baker, W. N. W.: The results of ileorectal anastomosis at St. Mark's Hospital from 1953 to 1968. *Gut*, **11**: 235–239, 1970.
3. Khubachandani, I. T., Trimpi, H. D., Sheets, J. A., Stasik, J. J., and Kleckner, F. S.: Ileorectal anastomosis for ulcerative colitis and Crohn's colitis. *Am. J. Surg.*, **135**: 751–756, 1978.
4. Farnell, M. B., Van Heerden, J. A., Beart, R. W., Jr., and Weiland, L. H.:

Rectal preservation in nonspecific inflammatory disease of the colon. *Ann. Surg.*, **192**: 249–253, 1979.

5. Jones, P. F., Bevan, P. G., and Hawley, P. R.: Ileostomy or ileorectal anastomosis for ulcerative colitis? *Brit. Med. J.*, **1**: 1459–1463, 1978.

The Results of Total Colectomy with Ileoproctostomy Preserving the Whole Rectum in Ulcerative Colitis

Hiroshi Takemura, Tsuneo Fukushima, and Shuji Tsuchiya

There are many conflicting arguments as to whether or not ileorectal anastomosis is the operation of choice for ulcerative colitis. In this series, total colectomy with ileoproctostomy sparing all the rectum distal to the rectosigmoid junction was performed on 20 patients who were followed up during medical therapy and who underwent periodic postoperative examinations. This paper presents the postoperative results of our series and discusses the indications and methods for ileorectal anastomosis.

MATERIALS AND METHODS

In a consecutive series of 25 patients with ulcerative colitis operated on since 1974, 20 patients underwent ileorectal anastomosis. The age of the patients ranged from 17 to 53 years (mean age 28.4 years) (Table 1). Three out of the 20 patients were operated on urgently or semi-urgently (Table 2). On the basis of histology of the rectum before operation, 11 out of the 20 patients were classified as severe (grade 5) or moderate (grade 4), having

TABLE 1. Age and Sex Distributions of the 20 Operated Patients

Age	No. of patients		Total
	Male	Female	
Less than 10	0	0	0
10–19	1	1	2
20–29	9	3	12
30–39	2	0	2
40–49	1	1	2
50–59	1	1	2
Total	14	6	20

Second Surgical Department, Yokohama City University School of Medicine, Yokohama, Japan

TABLE 2. Urgency of Operation in 20 Ileoproctostomies

Urgent	1	3(15%)
Semi-urgent	2	
Elective	17	

ulcer or crypt abscess; and the other 9 as grade 3 or 2, having mild inflammation (Table 3). Four patients who had deteriorated rapidly with or without associated toxic megacolon underwent decompression colostomy and diverting ileostomy as a first-stage procedure, followed by ileoproctostomy at the second stage (Table 4). In 8 patients, temporary ileostomy or appendicostomy was constructed for the sake of protection of the anastomotic site, especially in the patients with severe inflammation and in a poor nutritional state (Table 5). Without exception, ileorectal anastomosis was performed at the level of the rectosigmoid junction or sacral promontory preserving the whole rectum. Anastomosis was done in end-to-end fashion on 13 patients and in side-to-end fashion on 7 patients.

As postoperative medical treatment, salicylazosulfapyridine (2.0–3.0 g/day) and prednisolone (5–20 mg/day) were administered orally or rectally until rectal inflammation regressed. As continuing medical treatment, postoperative studies were undertaken every two weeks by symptomatology, endoscopy, and biopsy. Particularly, the number of daily stools and pas-

TABLE 3. Histological Grading of Rectal Inflammation at the Time of Ileoproctostomy

Grading (Matts)	No. of patients	
5 (ulcer)	7	11 (55%)
4 (crypt abscess)	4	
3	2	
2	7	

TABLE 4. Number of Primary and Secondary Ileoproctostomy

Ileoproctostomy	No. of patients
Primary	16
Secondary*	4 (20%)

* Decompression colostomy and diverting ileostomy preceded ileoproctostomy.

TABLE 5. Ileoproctostomy with or without Covering Ileostomy

Ileoproctostomy	No. of patients	
With covering ileostomy	6	8 (40%)
With covering appendicostomy	2	
Without covering ileostomy	12	

sage of muco-bloody stools were checked every time because they are simple relevant indices for postoperative evaluation. Endoscopic examination was usually done by anoscope, occasionally by sigmoidoscopy or fiberoptic colonoscopy. The findings of endoscopy were classified into four gradings and those of biopsy into six gradings, according to Matts.

RESULTS

The postoperative results were evaluated mainly on occurrence of anastomotic leakage, changes in retained rectal inflammation and function, and development of rectal dysplasia and carcinoma.

Incidence of anastomotic insufficiency. Minor anastomotic leakage occurred in two patients. Covering ileostomy had been carried out on them and leakage closed eventually. There has been no operative mortality so far.

Changes of retained rectal inflammation. In most of the operated patients, inflammation of the spared rectum was proved, by biopsy, to be medically controllable within a few years (Table 6). But, in the case of a 25-year-old male, intensive medical care had been ineffective and excision of the rectum with permanent ileostomy was undertaken 1 year and 10 months after the first operation. Failure of the operation was 5% in our series.

TABLE 6. Changes of Postoperative Grading of Rectal Inflammation

Grading \ Year of operation	0	1	2	3	4	5	6	7	8
5	7	0	0	0	0	1	0	0	0
4	4	6	4	3	1	0	0	0	0
3	2	6	9	2	6	3	3	3	1
2	7	5	3	4	2	1	1	1	1

Postoperative bowel movements and laboratory examinations. At every postoperative year, each patient was evaluated as to whether or not he or she was in good condition in terms of rectal function and general status (Fig. 1). Many patients were in poor condition one year after operation but improved as time passed. All patients but one returned to their previous lives and occupations less than one year postoperatively.

Development of rectal dysplasia and carcinoma. Neither rectal dysplasia nor carcinoma has been recognized so far.

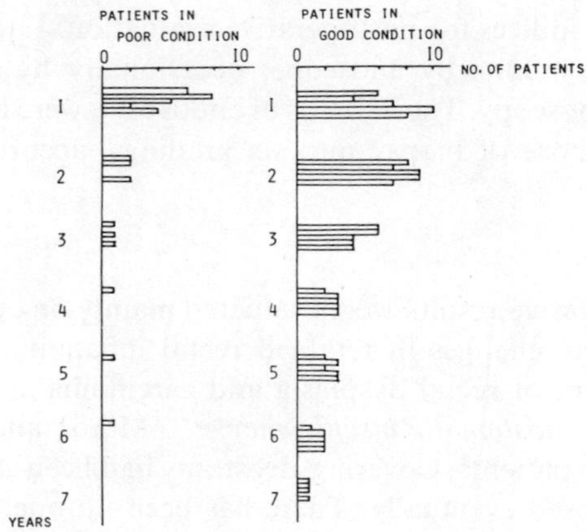

INDICES	POOR CONDITION	GOOD CONDITION
FREQUENCY OF DAILY STOOLS	> 6 TIMES/DAY	< 5 TIMES/DAY
HEMOGLOBIN CONCENTRATION	< 12.0GM/DL	> 12.0 GM/DL
SERUM ALBUMIN CONCENTRATION	< 4.2 GM/DL	> 4.2 GM/DL
$ALPHA_2$ GLOBULIN CON.	> 9.7 GM/DL	< 9.7 GM/DL
PLATELET COUNTS	> 32×10^4/ML	< 32×10^4/ ML

FIG. 1. Postoperative frequency of stools and laboratory examinations.

DISCUSSION

Many surgeons have preferred proctocolectomy with ileostomy to total colectomy with ileoproctostomy, recognizing the risk for development of cancer and operative failure due to anastomotic leakage, persistence of inflammation, and anorectal dysfunction.

In order to lessen the occurrence of anastomotic leakage and anorectal dysfunction, the rectum was retained distal to the rectosigmoid junction and anastomosed easily and safely in the abdominal cavity, not in the pelvic cavity. It was not only very effective in preventing the failure of anastomosis, but also preserved good anorectal function. Anastomotic leakage was likely to occur in patients with severely diseased rectum having crypt abscess and ulceration, and covering ileostomy is preferable for these patients (Table 7). Covering ileostomy was ineffective in preventing anastomotic leakage itself, but was certainly effective in preventing the spread of intrapelvic inflammation. Minor leakage occurred in 10% of our series, but covering ileostomy had been carried out on them and leakage closed without surgical intervention.

Postoperative medical treatment of retained rectal inflammation was important in maintaining good anorectal function. In most of our series,

TABLE 7. Grading of Rectal Inflammation at Time of Ileoproctostomy, Covering Ileostomy and Anastomotic Insufficiency

Grading of inflammation	No. of patients	Anastomotic insufficiency	
5	7 (3)	1 (1)	2(10%)
4	4 (2)	1 (1)	
3	2 (0)	0	
2	7 (3)	0	

( ): No. of patients with covering ileostomy or appendicostomy.

inflammation of the spared rectum gradually regressed by medical therapy within a few years, regardless of preoperative severity of inflammation. There was no reason to abandon ileoproctostomy because of rectal inflammation. A 21-year-old female case with toxic megacolon underwent total colectomy with ileoproctostomy in a second-stage operation and recovered uneventfully. From the outcome of follow-up studies, it was concluded that postoperative medical therapy should be indicated without exception for the first year and is desirable for the second year. After the third year, it should be maintained only in necessary cases.

CONCLUSION

Total colectomy with ileoproctostomy preserving all the rectum distal to rectosigmoid junction should be the first choice of operation in almost all operative candidates affected by ulcerative colitis. Continuous postoperative medical treatment and examinations at regular intervals should be provided.

Sphincter-Saving Operation for Ulcerative Colitis

——Results in Twenty-Six Patients

Naoki Inatsugi, Tsuneo Shiratori, Hiroshige Nakano, Takasumi Hosoi, Hisao Fujii, Nao Sekiya, and Koji Murakami

For the purpose of attaining radicality, proctocolectomy with ileostomy is a very useful operative method in ulcerative colitis. On the other hand, an operative method which avoids colostomy or ileostomy and employs a sphincter-saving operation when possible is to be favored because this disease usually develops in the young and is a benign disease. In Japan, the frequency of sphincter-saving operations has increased gradually, although the number of cases operated on for this disease is small when compared with Europe and the U.S.A.

Sphincter-saving operations (SSO) have been performed in 26 cases, and the therapeutic results of this operative method will be reported in this paper.

MATERIALS AND METHODS

We encountered 50 cases of ulcerative colitis from 1955 to 1982. As shown in Table 1, the frequency of SSO performed at Nara Medical University has gradually increased to a rate of 80%, or 16 of 20 cases from 1973 to 1982; at Tohoku University the figure was about 33%, or 10 of 30 cases from 1955 to 1972.

TABLE 1. Surgical Procedures Performed for Ulcerative Colitis

	Proctocolectomy with sphincter-saving operation	Proctocolectomy with colostomy or ileostomy	Total
1955–1972 (Tohoku Univ.)	10 (33%)	20 (67%)	30
1973–1982 (Nara Med. Univ.)	16 (80%)	4 (20%)	20
Total	26 (52%)	24 (48%)	50

First Department of Surgery, Nara Medical University, Kashihara, Nara, Japan

The sex-age distribution is presented in Table 2. There were 13 male and 13 famale patients. By age at operation, 12 patients were in their teens or 20s, accounting for about half of the total.

TABLE 2. Sex-Age Distribution of the 26 Patients Undergoing Sphincter-Saving Operation

Sex:	Male	13
	Female	13
Age:	10 yr–	8
	20 yr–	4
	30 yr–	7
	40 yr–	4
	50 yr–	2
	60 yr–	0
	70 yr–	1

The operative indications are shown in Table 3. Emergency or urgent operations were performed in 8 cases, or 31% of the total, and elective operations in 18 cases, or 69%.

TABLE 3. Operative Indications

Emergency or urgent cases		Elective cases	
Massive hemorrhage	1	Frequent relapsing	12
Perforation with toxic megacolon	1	Failure of medical treatment	5
Toxic megacolon	1	Social indication	1
Severe attack	5		
Total	8 (31%)	Total	18 (69%)

As indications for emergency or urgent operation, five cases were ranked as severe attack, followed by one case each of massive hemorrhage, perforation with toxic megacolon, and toxic megacolon.

Of the elective operations, 12 cases were ranked as frequent relapsing, followed by failure of medical treatment (5 cases) and social indication (one case).

For severe ulcerative colitis, treatment was done on the basis of the therapeutic criteria illustrated in Fig. 1. As a first step, severe cases are treated on the basis of an intensive intravenous regimen. Whether or not this regimen is effective is then tested. If it is effective, conservative therapy or elective surgery is performed. If it proves ineffective, urgent surgery is performed within a week. In such a case, a radical operation is not performed at once, but ileostomy or right-sided colostomy is performed as a first-stage operation in order to leave the involved colon intact. This brings about improvement in most cases. Then after successful withdrawal

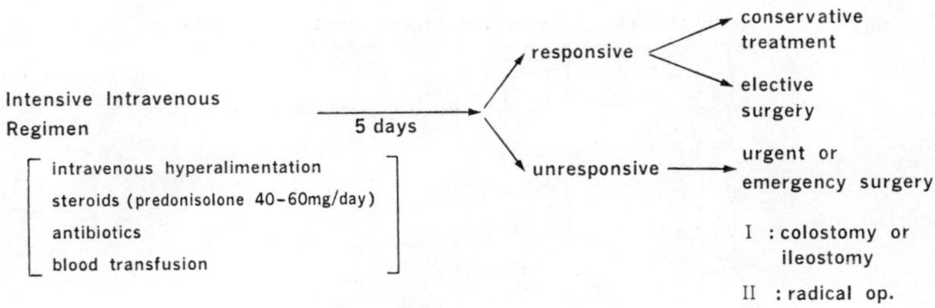

FIG. 1. Therapeutic criteria for severe ulcerative colitis.

from steroid therapy, the radical operation is performed safely as a second-stage operation.

In eight patients of emergency or urgent operation, SSO was performed as a multi-stage operation extending over two or three stages. Of these eight patients, in one patient with massive hemorrhage and in five patients of severe attack, treatment was made on the basis of our therapeutic criteria; the remaining two patients underwent their initial operation in another hospital.

The initial operation included colectomy and ileostomy in two cases, right-sided colostomy in five cases, and ileostomy with colonic mucous fistula in one case.

To determine the best surgical procedure among several selective procedures, the presence of fistula or stenosis in the rectum and anal canal was first examined. When the anal sphincter mechanism was defective, permanent ileostomy or colostomy was performed; if the right-sided colonic lesion was mild, ascendicostomy was performed to preserve the ileocecal valve. If the anal sphincter mechanism was good, SSO was performed even when the involved rectum was in active stage. In this case, if the right-sided colonic lesion was mild, the colon was partially preserved; if the lesion was severely affected, the colon was totally removed for anastomosis with the rectum.

The range of preservation of the rectum should be as follows: the peritoneal reflection and the site of anastomosis is usually placed 4–7 cm to the oral side from the anal verge so that the postoperative bowel action will be maintained and relapsing-recurrence will be held to a minimum.

Figure 2 illustrates the location of disease and method of reconstruction of 26 cases with SSO. Descendoproctostomy was performed on one case of proctitis, and transversoproctostomy was performed on three cases of left-sided proctocolitis. In these four cases operation was made at the early stage, whereas the remaining 22 cases were in the remission stage at operation.

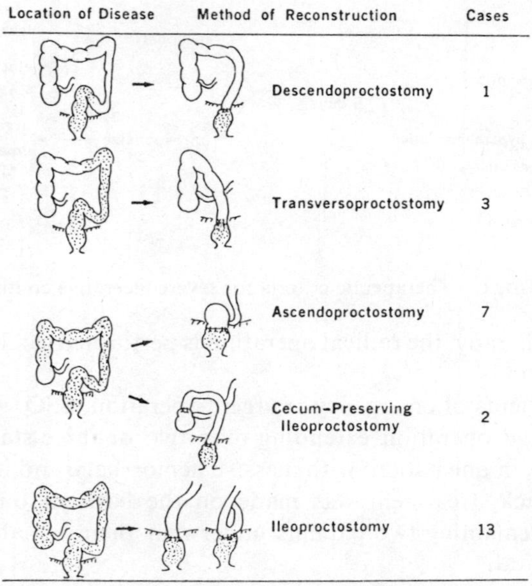

FIG. 2. Relationship of location of disease and operation.

Of nine cases in which the right-sided colonic lesion was mild, ascendicostomy was performed in seven cases, and cecum-preserving ileoproctostomy in two cases.

In the 13 cases in which the right-sided colonic lesion was severely affected, ileoproctostomy increased.

RESULTS

Postoperative follow-up study was done for 3 months to 26 years, averaging 8 years. Table 4 shows postoperative complications divided into early and late phases. As early complications, leakage occurred in 7 cases, followed by one case each of abscess and wound dehiscence. As late complications, there was intestinal obstruction in 3 cases; gallstone in 2 cases; and one case each of meningitis, urinary calculus, and hepatitis. In cases of this disease with SSO, attention should be paid to anastomotic leakage in the early phase and intestinal obstruction in the late phase.

Death was found in one case each of anastomotic leak and postoperative intestinal obstruction. As described above, anastomotic leak is considered a major problem as an early complication in cases of this disease with SSO.

Table 5 shows the treatment for 7 cases of anastomotic leak. Anastomotic

TABLE 4. Complications

		No. of cases
Early phase:	Leakage	7 (1)
	Abscess	1
	Wound dehiscence	1
Late phase:	Intestinal obstruction	3 (1)
	Gallstone	2
	Meningitis	1
	Urinary calculus	1
	Hepatitis	1

( ): died.

TABLE 5. Treatment for Anastomotic Leak

Ascendoproctostomy: 1/7 →	Drainage: 1	
Ileoproctostomy: 6/13 →	Conservative Treatment: 1	
	Ileostomy: 5 →	Temporary: 3
		Permanent: 2 (1)

( ): died.

leak occurred in one patient among 7 with ascendoproctostomy and in 6 of 13 patients with ileoproctostomy. The former patient was cured by a drainage operation. Of the latter six patients, one patient was cured by conservative treatment, three patients by temporary ileostomy, and two patients were not cured. The two uncured patients were subjected to reoperation and permanent ileostomy.

As one measure to prevent anastomotic leak, we have recently performed autosuture using EEA on three cases and obtained satisfactory results.

In Fig. 3 the prognosis of patients with SSO is shown. Postoperative death was found in one (3.8%) among 26 patients. The death occurred among the patients with elective operation. Postoperative death was not found in any of the patients with emergency or urgent operation. This may be an indication of the safety of the multi-stage operation.

Of 25 patients (excluding the patient who died), 23 patients had complete SSO and 2 patients had SSO with covering ileostomy. Excluding the patient who had permanent ileostomy for anastomotic leak, 22 patients (96%) may be recognized as examples of success with this surgical procedure.

Table 6 shows the number of postoperative relapses in 21 out of the 22 patients (excluding the patient who died because of intestinal obstruction in the fourth year after operation). A clinically definite relapse was observed in 2 out of 7 cases with ascendoproctostomy and 2 out of 11 cases with ileoproctostomy. The site of relapse in these cases was the rectum. The

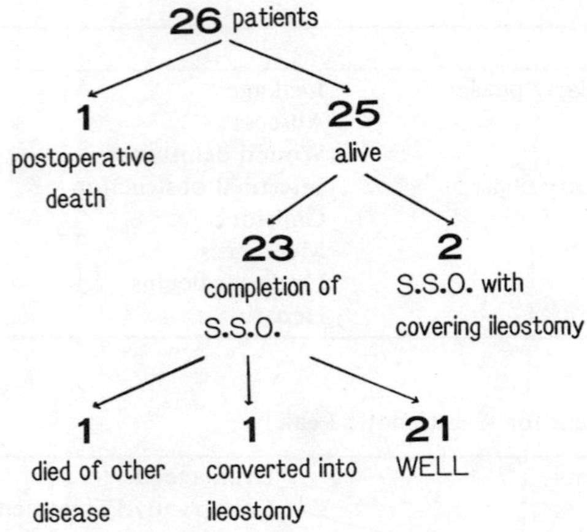

FIG. 3. Patients' prognosis following sphincter-saving operation.

TABLE 6. Postoperative Relapse

Operative method	Relapse	Therapy
Descendoproctostomy (1)	0	—
Transversoproctostomy (2)	0	—
Ascendoproctostomy (7)	2	SASP
Ileoproctostomy (11)	2	SASP, steroid (supp.)

relapse was mild in all cases and was cured by oral administration of Salazopyrin or by steroid suppository. In no case was reoperation necessitated by the relapse.

Table 7 shows bowel function after surgery. There was a tendency for bowel action to decrease in frequency, especially when the colon was preserved. The frequency of bowel actions was rather high in ileoproctostomy, with 4–9 stools a day seen in 9 cases. Viewed in terms of the postoperative clinical course, cases with 7–9 stools daily were found up to 6

TABLE 7. Bowel Actions after Operation

Bowel actions per day	Operative procedure			
	Descendoproctostomy (1)	Transversoproctostomy (2)	Ascendoproctostomy (3)	Ileoproctostomy (11)
1–3	1	2	2	1
4–6			3	5
7–9			2	4
10<				1

months after operation. After that, however, the bowel action improved, with the frequency decreased to 4–6 stools daily.

As a follow-up after surgery, endoscopy and biopsy were performed once a year as a rule. In our experience, no case has resulted in dysplasia and no cancer risk has appeared in the preserved colon or rectum.

DISCUSSION

Proctocolectomy with ileostomy and total colectomy with ileorectal anastomosis are mainly employed as radical operations in the surgical treatment of ulcerative colitis. However, as disadvantages of permanent ileostomy and proctocolectomy, Khubchandani *et al.*[1] have mentioned the following: 1) psychological unacceptability, 2) stomal complications needing subsequent surgical revisions, 3) sexual dysfunction, 4) expenditure for appliances, and 5) unhealed perineal wounds in some patients. On the other hand, the following must be mentioned as disadvantages of ileorectal anastomosis by those favoring total proctocolectomy: 1) retention of rectal segment with potential risk for development of cancer, 2) possible recrudescence of inflammatory disease necessitating subsequent major operation, 3) leakage after anastomosis, and 4) frequent bowel movements. Thus, there are these two surgical procedures, and the operative methods chosen depend on the preoperative state of the patient, the wish of the patient, and the recommendation of the surgeon.

Aylett[2] has been the most enthusiastic proponent of ileorectal anastomosis. In 1974 he performed ileorectal anastomosis in 443 (96%) of 461 cases of this disease. He reported that this operative method proved successful in 90% of them. According to Jones *et al.*,[3] other surgeons have performed ileorectal anastomosis in 30–40% of cases with colectomy. Prior to 1972, we performed the sphincter-saving operation in 26 cases, 52% of the 50 cases operated. From 1972 onward, however, the sphincter-saving operation has been performed in 16 (80%) of 20 cases.

In the sphincter-saving operation, we performed ileorectal anastomosis and coloproctostomy (inclusive of cecum-preserving colectomy with ileal interposition) in 13 cases. Coloproctostomy was performed where right-sided colonic lesion was absent or mild. None of these cases suffered from relapsing or recurrence in the preserved colon, and bowel function after operation was good.

Roediger *et al.*[4] also performed subtotal colectomy, preserving 10–20 cm of the ascending colon distal to the ileocecal valve, a mucosal proctectomy and subsequently a coloanal anastomosis in 6 cases in which right-sided colonic lesion was absent or mild. The results seem to be satisfactory.

Aylett[2] has proposed that the sphincter-saving operation can be employed for cases without stenosis or fistula of the rectum regardless of the severity of rectal inflammation. Our results agree with his view and we propose the use of this operative method. In contrast, Ehrenpreis[5] and Nixon *et al.*[6] proposed that this operative method should be limited to cases where the rectal lesion is mild to moderate.

In the resection of the rectum, Aylett[2] and Jones *et al.*[3] excise it in the vicinity of the promontrium, while Watts *et al.*[7] excise it near the peritoneal reflection. We have stressed the need to preserve a small part of the rectum since preserving a large part of it results in high incidence of relapsing or recurrence and high dependence on postoperative therapies. We made it a point to set the resection line below the peritoneal reflection and performed resection along that line in all of our 26 cases.

The operative mortality in ileorectal anastomosis is given as about 3% in many reports.[3] In our experience, too, a similar trend was found with a postoperative mortality of one, or 4%, in the 26 cases of the sphincter-saving operation.

Of the postoperative complications, anastomotic leak is the major problem, and its incidence is reported to be 3–20%.[3] In our study, the incidence was slightly higher, being 7 of 26 cases, or 27%. This was probably due to the difficulty of the anastomosis and to the severity of inflammation in the mucous membrane of the rectum preserved because the leak often occurred at a low level: 2–3 cm from the dentate line on the anastomosed side. Recently, therefore, we have performed anastomosis using EEA to obtain better results.

In terms of bowel function after operation, 22 of 23 cases in our study showed good bowel action, with less than 6 stools a day, in contrast to Jones' results[3] for ileorectal anastomosis. In our results, too, 10 or more soft stools a day are seen immediately after operation, but decrease to 3–5 stools a day, and several months further after operation, enabling patients to enjoy a much more comfortable life than ileostomy.

Cancer risk in the preserved colon–rectum was reported to be 12 of 461 cases (2.6%) by Aylett,[2] 2 out of 41 cases (5%) by Dennis *et al.*,[8] and 2 out of 67 cases (3%) by Richie.[9] The incidence of cancer risk is expected to become higher in the future with long-term follow-up observation. In our cases, none showed dysplasia or carcinoma, but a follow-up study is needed.

Relapsing and recurrence after operation are liable to develop early after operation, but cease to occur with the progress of the clinical course. Should relapsing or recurrence develop, it is easy to treat and can be controlled well by oral administration of Salazopyrin or with steroid hormone suppository. In our cases, only a small portion of the rectum is preserved, so there seems little relapsing or recurrence of the rectal lesion.

SUMMARY

1) Where no stenosis of the recto-anal region is observed, the sphincter-saving operation can be performed even if the rectal lesion is in active stage.

2) The sphincter-saving operation can be performed safely by the multi-stage operative method even in cases indicated for emergency or urgent operation.

3) The incidence of relapsing or recurrence is low even when a part of the cecum–ascending colon is preserved in cases in which the right-sided colonic lesion is mild.

4) The dependence on pharmacotherapy after operation is reduced by setting the range of sphincter-saving operation below the peritoneal reflection.

5) The incidence of anastomotic leak is high as a postoperative complication. Measures to prevent it are important. Autosuture is useful in this capacity.

6) Bowel function after operation does not interfere with social rehabilitation.

7) Careful consideration should be given to cancer risk of the preserved colon–rectum. Roentgenographic, endoscopic, and histologic examinations are needed once a year.

REFERENCES

1. Khubchandani, I. T., Trimpi, H. D., Sheets, J. A., Stasik, J. J., and Kleckner, F. S.: Ileorectal anastomosis for ulcerative and Crohn's colitis. *Am. J. Surg.*, **135**: 751–756, 1978.
2. Aylett, S. O.: Rectal conservation in surgical treatment of ulcerative colitis. *Arch. Fr. Mal. App. Dig.*, **63**: 585–587, 1974.
3. Jones, P. F., Munro, A., and Ewen, S. W. B.: Colectomy and ileorectal anastomosis for colitis: Report on a personal series, with a critical review. *Br. J. Surg.*, **64**: 615–623, 1977.
4. Roediger, W. E. W., Pihl, E., and Hughes, S. E.: Preserving the ascending colon as an alternative surgical option in ulcerative colitis. *Surg. Gynecol. Obstet.*, **154**: 348–350, 1982.
5. Ehrenpreis, T.: Surgical treatment of ulcerative colitis in childhood. *Arch. Dis. Child.*, **41**: 137–142, 1966.
6. Nixon, H. H.: Ileorectal anastomosis for inflammatory bowel disease in children. *Arch. Fr. Mal. App. Dig.*, **63**: 590–591, 1974.
7. Watts, J. and Hughes, E. S. R.: Ileorectal anastomosis for ulcerative colitis. In: Advance Abstracts of the Fourth World Congress of Gastroenterology (ed. P. Riis), p. 229. Copenhagen, 1970.
8. Dennis, D. and Karlson, K. E.: Surgical measures as supplements to the

management of idiopathic ulcerative colitis, cancer, cirrhosis and arthritis as frequent complication. *Surgery*, **32**: 892–912, 1952.
9. Ritchie, J. K.: Further results of surgery for inflammatory bowel disease—A further survey of one hospital region. *Br. Med. J.*, **1**: 264–268, 1974.

Total Colectomy and Ileorectal Anastomosis for Ulcerative Colitis

Mitsuru Konn, Mutsuo Sasaki, Takayuki Morita, Tetsuyuki Murakami, Shinobu Karoji, and Keiichi Ono

INTRODUCTION

The etiology of ulcerative colitis has not yet been established. In terms of its surgical treatment, the operative indications are complex and many factors are involved because this disease sits on the borderline of medicine and surgery, as do other benign diseases such as gastric ulcer. When it comes to the selection of an operative procedure, the complexity increases because one must consider various factors such as social rehabilitation and postoperative defecating dysfunction, besides those involved in the disease itself such as severity of disease, extent of lesion, general condition, and even postoperative complications on an individual basis.

Because of the nature of this disease, a better case can perhaps be made for total colectomy than for extensive resection of colon. The former procedure is thought to be an ideal one from the viewpoint of cure since there is no recurrence. However, permanent abdominal ileostomy, which is unavoidable in this procedure, causes the patient both mental and physical distress and is undoubtedly a great deterrent to his or her returning to social activity.

Hence, looking hard for better procedures, surgeons as well as patients wish to use anal sphincter-saving operations whenever possible. However, since follow-up reviews of anal sphincter-saving operations have disclosed some recurrences, there is still a need for further study of indication requirements. This paper describes the indication requirements of ulcerative colitis for total colectomy and resection of the upper rectum with ileorectostomy, and pertinent recurrent cases.

Second Department of Surgery, Hirosaki University School of Medicine, Hirosaki, Japan

SUBJECTS AND METHODS

The number of primary operative cases of ulcerative colitis in our clinic from March 1954 through the end of December 1981 was 29. There were 23 males aged 14 to 65 (mean 32 years) and 6 females aged 33 to 56 (mean 43 years), the overall average age being 34 (14 to 65) (Table 1). Anal sphincter-saving operations were tried throughout the period based on our operation protocol. However, since our series covered the long period of 27 years, any discussion without attention to the advancing medical background of diagnosis and treatment in assessing results of the procedure will cause some confusion. Hence, the entire period of time was divided into two parts: early (1954–1965) and recent (1966–1981). In the latter period, with the aid of colonoscope it was possible to observe the entire bowel mucosa and diagnose the affected site with more certainty; furthermore, in combination with intraoperative biopsy, the pathohistological criteria of diagnosis could be established. There were 13 cases with primary operation in the former period and 16 in the latter. Seven of 13 cases in the early period and 7 of 16 cases in the recent period underwent anal sphincter-saving operation. All cases with Hartmann's operation were excluded in this series (Table 2).

TABLE 1. Characteristics of Primary Operated Cases with CUC (1954–1981)

Sex	No. of pts.	Age (yr)	Average age (yr)
Male	23	14–65	32 } 34
Female	6	33–56	43 }

TABLE 2. Historical Studies on Operative Procedures

Operative procedures	No. of pts.		
	1954–1965	1966–1981	Total
Ileostomy or colostomy	6 (2)*	9	15
One-stage sphincter-saving method	7	7 (3)**	14

*Operative death.
**Reoperated with ileostomy.

RESULTS

Cases with anal sphincter-saving operation were 7 each in the early and recent periods, totalling 14. In the early period, because of attempts to minimize operative intervention by resecting the lesion site and saving the anus, operative procedures varied widely, and it is not an exaggeration to say that they differed with each different case. Nevertheless, meticulous procedures were used. In the recent period, advances in various aspects of medicine, particularly attempts at saving the intact part of the intestinal tract by the use of intraoperative histological diagnosis, led to total resection of the large bowel with ileoanal anastomosis, total colectomy and resection of the upper rectum with ileorectostomy, and total colectomy and resection of rectum with cecoanal anastomosis (Table 3).

TABLE 3. Surgical Procedures of Sphincter-Saving Operation for CUC

1954–1965		1966–1981		
Left hemicolectomy	2	Subtotal colectomy and resection of rectum	1	
Transversorectostomy	1 (1)	Cecoanal anastomosis		1
Ascendicorectostomy	1	Total colectomy and resection of rectum	1	
Subtotal colectomy	5	Ileoanal anastomosis		1 (1)
Ascendicosigmoidostomy	1 (1)	Total colectomy and partial resection of rectum	5	
Cecosigmoidostomy	1			
Cecorectostomy	1	Ileorectostomy		5 (2)
Ileosigmoidostomy	2 (1*)			

( ): Recurrent case.
*Operative death after second operation.

Criteria for intraoperative histological diagnosis were established by rapid frozen sectioning of whole layers of the cut end of the resected intestinal tract at operation, and the suspected cases with slightly inflammatory changes were indicated for resection. The criteria reasonably indicated for resection included ulcer formation grossly appreciable as mucosal changes, presence of crypt abscess, vascular congestion, and highly inflammatory cell infiltration. In addition, presence of cryptitis, or crypt cell changes observed at the early stage of cryptitis showing infiltration of a small number of inflammatory cells into the interspace of crypt cells, picnosis of crypt cells, and their vacuole degeneration to a minimal degree were all accepted as criteria in the resecting of the intestinal tract for potential sources of recurrence (Figs. la–c).

Early Cases

Seven out of 13 cases with primary operation in the early period underwent anal sphincter-saving operation, and the remaining 6 received either ileostomy or colostomy. One was an operative death after the second operation.

As shown in Table 4, the modality of anal sphincter-saving operations consisted of left hemicolectomy in 2 cases; transversorectostomy in one and ascendicorectostomy in one (recurred 1 year and 7 months later). Subtotal colectomy was performed in 5 cases; ascendicosigmoidostomy in one (recurred 1 year and 5 months after operation), cecosigmoidostomy in

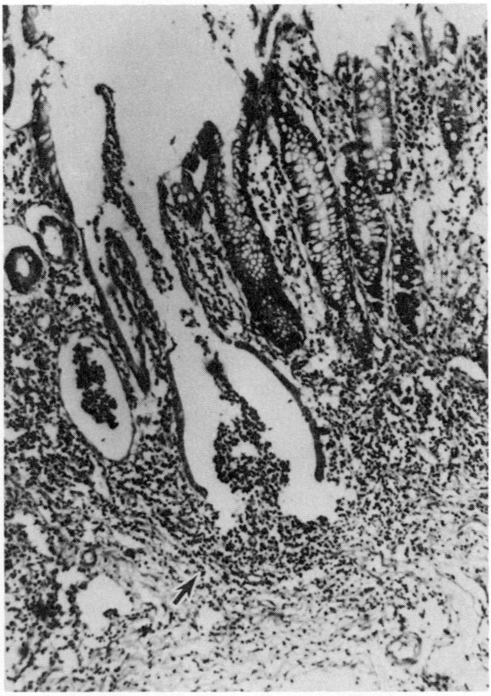

FIG. 1a. Crypt abscess.

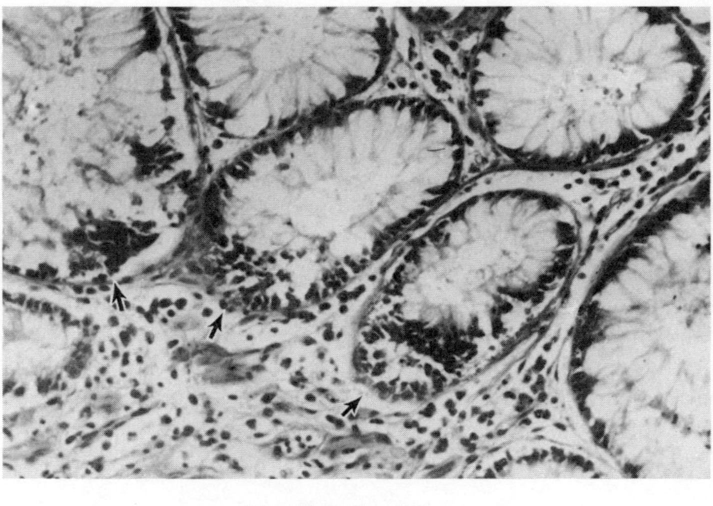

FIG. 1b. Cryptitis.

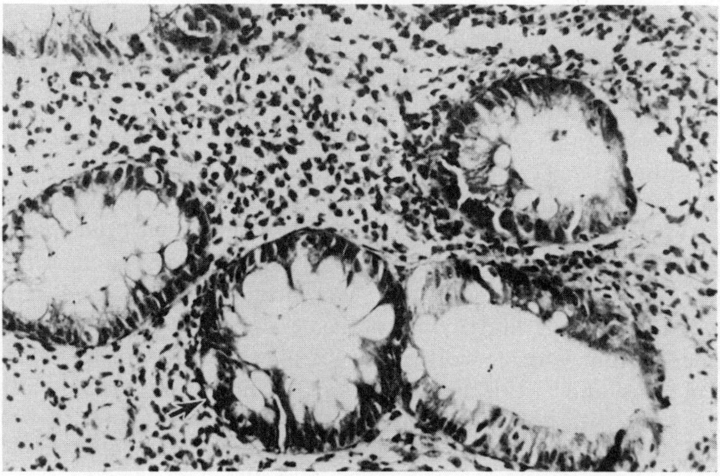

FIG. 1c. Early stage of cryptitis.

TABLE 4. Surgical Procedures of Sphincter-Saving Operation for CUC in Early Cases

Operation performed	1954–1965
Left hemicolectomy	2
Transversorectostomy	1 (1)
Ascendicorectostomy	1
Subtotal colectomy	5
Ascendicosigmoidostomy	1 (1)
Cecosigmoidostomy	1
Cecorectostomy	1
Ileosigmoidostomy	2 (1)*

( ): Recurrent case.
*Operative death after second operation.

one, cecorectostomy in one, and ileosigmoidostomy in 2 (one of which developed recurrence that ended in death 12 months after operation). Recurrence took place in 3 of 7 cases and reoperation had to be performed. A 27-year-old male patient who underwent ileosigmoidostomy died of acute suppurative panperitonitis due to perforation of the remaining rectum. Our unfortunate experience with this case prompted us to establish intraoperative histological diagnostic criteria for determining the extent of resection.

Recent Cases

In the recent period, with the development of the endoscope, the extent of the affected area could be more clearly diagnosed; moreover, review of the recurrent cases in the early period suggested that macroscopic findings of the lesion were inadequate alone and that histological examination was necessary. This led to our policy that procedures for the remaining intestinal tract should be decided only after intraoperative histological diagnosis. As a result, even in anal sphincter-saving operations, the procedure of leaving the rectum or part of the cecum was employed in performing subtotal colectomy or total colectomy in some cases.

Seven cases with anal sphincter-saving operation consisted of one with subtotal colectomy and resection of the upper rectum with cecoanal anastomosis, one with total colectomy and resection of the rectum with ileoanal anastomosis (recurred 6 years after operation and required abdominal ileostomy), and 5 with total colectomy and partial resection of the upper rectum with ileorectostomy (2 of which developed recurrence after 6 months, and 7 years and 4 months after operation) (Table 5). In one out of 5 cases with ileorectostomy, anastomosis was made at an obvious inflammatory site with no histological diagnostic criteria applied. Our method of ileorectostomy is to anastomose the ileal loop to the rectal remnant at the peritoneal reflection level (Fig. 2). Five cases with ileorectostomy are shown in Table 6 (4 males and one female aged 20 to 56, average age 29.4). Their disease activity was mild in one, moderate in 2, and severe in 2 cases. Steroids were administered in a total dose of from

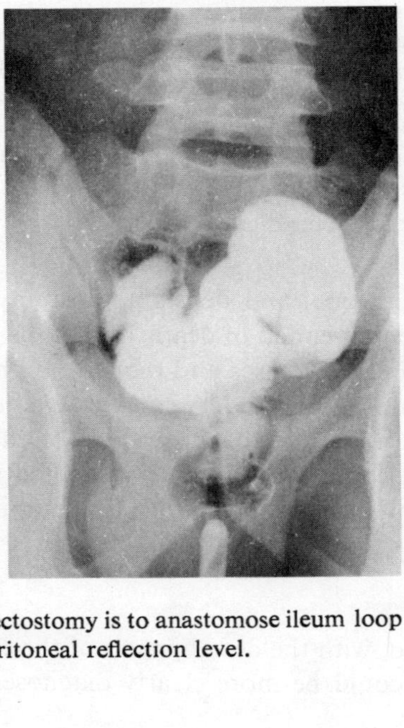

FIG. 2. Ileorectostomy is to anastomose ileum loop to rectal remnant at the peritoneal reflection level.

TABLE 5. Surgical Procedures of Sphincter-Saving Operation for CUC in Recent Cases

Operation performed	1966–1981	
Subtotal colectomy and resection of rectum	1	
Cecoanal anastomosis		1
Total colectomy and resection of rectum	1	
Ileoanal anastomosis		1 (1)
Total colectomy and partial resection of rectum	5	
Ileorectostomy		5 (2)

( ): Recurrent case.

TABLE 6. Long-Term Results of Ileorectostomy Performed in Recent Cases

No.	Case No.	Name	Age and sex	Onset to operation	Amount of steroid (mg)	Disease activity	Result
1	19	K. T.	27M	1 yr 3 mos	1,765	Mild	Good
2	20	K. O.	21M	9 mos	3,900	Moderate	Recurrent*
3	23	N. K.	56F	1 yr	——	Moderate	Good
4	25	Y. K.	23M	2 yrs	15,592	Severe	Recurrent**
5	35	H. H.	20M	3 mos	1,780	Severe	Good

*Recurrent 6 mos later.
**Recurrent 7 yrs later.

1,765 to 15,592 mg. Recurrence developed in two patients and they were forced to undergo permanent abdominal ileostomy. These two cases are discussed below.

a) Case No. 20 (K. O., 21-year-old male). The diseased colon was of the entire type, with the main lesion in the descending and ascending colon. Cortisone was administered in a total dose of 6,400 mg. Total colectomy and resection of the upper rectum with ileorectostomy was performed, and the absence of lesion in the remaining rectal stump was confirmed at surgery by frozen section examination of whole layers of the resected tract. However, uncontrollable massive bleeding occurred 6 months after operation, and the ileal loop, the residual rectum, and the anus were resected and abdominal ileostomy had to be performed (Fig. 3).

Specimens obtained at surgery showed obvious backwash ileitis, and the inflammatory appearance of ulceration was also observed in the resected rectum. Partial epithelial regeneration was noted (Figs. 4a and 4b).

The patient was married 8 years after the reoperation at the age of 28 and became the father of a boy one and a half years later. Although somewhat annoyed by management of the ileostomy, he is engaged in gardening as an occupation and leads a happy life.

b) Case No. 25 (Y. K., 23-year-old male). This case is that of the entire colitis type with the main lesion involving the entire large bowel. As preoperative steroid therapy, 38,270 mg of cortisone was administered before

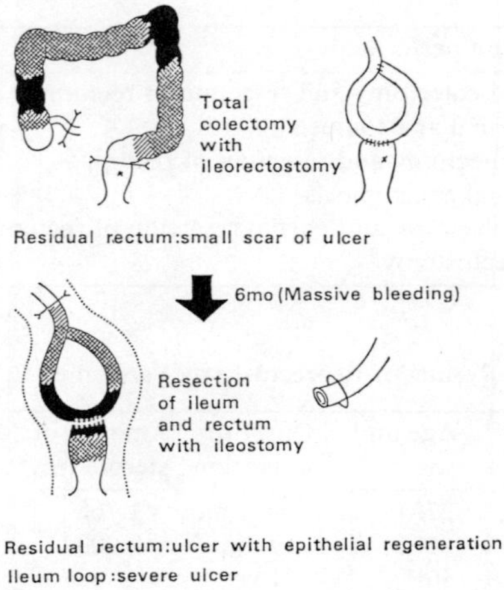

FIG. 3. Clinical course of case No. 20 (K. O., 21-year-old male).

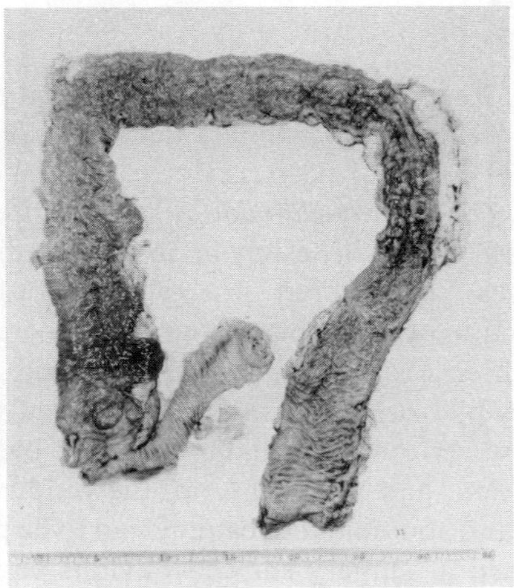

FIG. 4a. Removed specimen of case No. 20 at first operation (total colectomy and resection of upper rectum).

operation. Total colectomy and resection of the upper rectum with ileorectostomy were performed. Absence of lesion at the remaining rectal stump was confirmed by the frozen section technique as with case 20. The postoperative clinical course was fair until 5 years after operation, when he had to undergo partial nephrectomy due to right nephrolithiasis which

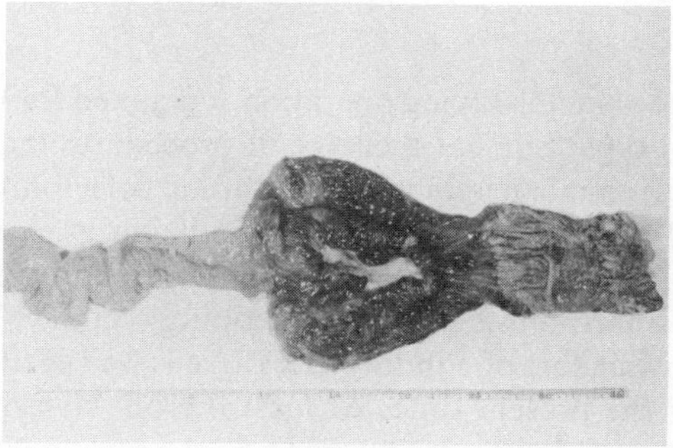

FIG. 4b. Removed specimen of case No. 20 at second operation (resection of ileum loop and residual rectum).

had been recognized since the first operation. Later, the patient began to complain of mucous and bloody stool with subsequent erosion at the anus. Severe ulcer and anal fistula were noted in the rectal remnant 7 years and 4 months after primary operation and were followed by high fever and anal bleeding. Revision of operation with permanent abdominal ileostomy was required (second operation, performed at Department of Surgery, Shinshu University) (Fig. 5).

The patient was married 2 years after the second operation, when he was 33 years old. Now, he is enjoying a happy life as a wage worker.

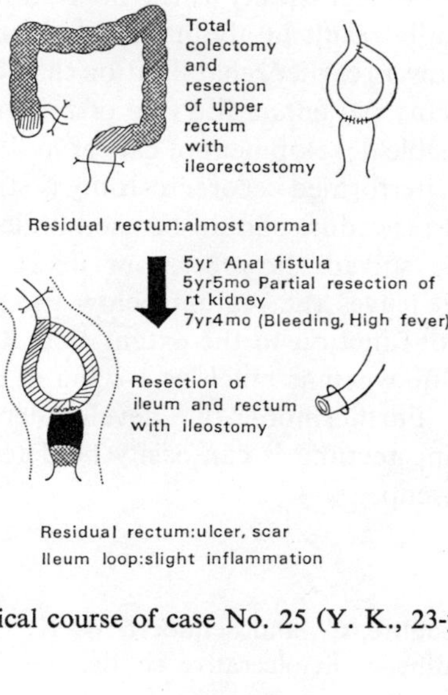

FIG. 5. Clinical course of case No. 25 (Y. K., 23-year-old male).

DISCUSSION

When an anal sphincter-saving operation is planned for ulcerative colitis (the entire colon type) one has a choice of procedures including: 1) total colectomy with ileoanal anastomosis, 2) subtotal colectomy and removal of the lower rectal mucosa through which the ileum is passed for ileoanal anastomosis,[1,2] 3) ileorectostomy with the remaining lower rectum,[3] and 4) cecoanal anastomosis with the remaining cecum.[4] What procedure is indicated for what sort of conditions? There is no specific procedure accepted by all at the present time. At least the one described in 2) above (removing all intestinal mucosa) seems to be the most encouraging in anal sphincter-saving operations from the viewpoint of recurrence. However, as far as social rehabilitation is concerned, the delay in returning to a normal pattern of life due to postoperative stool dysfunction should be considered, although this is not so severe as seen with the procedure in 1).

Whenever no lesion was demonstrated in the remaining rectum by intraoperative histological diagnosis, we have made it a rule since 1966 to perform ileorectostomy as the anal sphincter-saving operation which is believed to be the shortest path to social rehabilitation. We had only four patients to whom this operative procedure was applied (there was one case that received this procedure with obvious lesion in the rectal remnant). Among the four patients, two developed recurrence, and eventually had to have abdominal ileostomy.

We rather argue for ileorectostomy as the operation of first choice even though it may eventually result in abdominal ileostomy. This is because our procedure may allow an earlier rehabilitation than other procedures do, and may also offer many patients a life free of recurrence, although one must consider the possible development of cancer in the remaining rectum. A patient in whom we performed cecorectostomy is still doing well 8 years after operation. What procedure should be used under what conditions is still a problem to be solved; however, our ileorectostomy method is noteworthy because it leaves the rectum below the peritoneal reflection level. It preserves stool function to the extent that it does not give embarrassment in daily life when as much as 1–2 cm of rectum and the anal canal are preserved. Furthermore, the development of recurrence or cancer in the remaining rectum[5,6] can easily be detected by only digital examination and anoscope.

REFERENCES

1. Martin, L. W., LeCoultre, C., and Schubert, W. K.: Total colectomy with preservation of continence in ulcerative colitis. *Ann. Surg.*, **186**: 477–480, 1977.

2. Utsunomiya, J., Iwama, T., Imajo, M., Matsuo S., Sawai, S., Yaegashi, K., and Hirayama, R.: Total colectomy, mucosal proctectomy, and ileoanal anastomosis. *Dis. Col. & Rect.*, **23**: 459–466, 1980.
3. Aylett, S. O.: Ulcerative colitis treated by total colectomy and ileorectal anastomosis: A ten-year review. *Proc. Soc. Med.*, **56**: 183–190, 1963.
4. Hughes, E. S. R. and Bennett, R. C.: Caecal pull-through operation for distal ulcerative colitis; A preliminary report. *N. Z. J. Surg.*, **42**: 26–30, 1972.
5. Grundfest, S. F., Fazio, V., Weiss, R. A., Jagelman, D., Lavery, I., Weakley, F. L., and Turnbull, R. B.: The risk of cancer following colectomy and ileorectal anastomosis for extensive mucosal ulcerative colitis. *Ann. Surg.*, **193**: 9–14, 1981.
6. Kurtz, L. M., Flint, G. W., Platt, N., and Wise, L.: Carcinoma in the retained rectum after colectomy for ulcerative colitis. *Dis. Col. & Rect.*, **23**: 346–350, 1980.

Ileoanostomy Surgery

Joji Utsunomiya, Takeo Iwama, Kanji Yaegashi, and Renzo Hirayama*

In surgery for adenomatosis coli (AC) and total ulcerative colitis (UC), there is a controversy between two principles: 1) the primary total removal of the large bowel and 2) its subtotal removal followed by additional conservative treatment on the retained rectum.

In AC, total colectomy with ileorectal anastomosis followed by fulguration is the most popular practice. The risk of advanced cancer in the retained rectum was reported as 13% and 42%, 10 and 42 years after colectomy at the Mayo Clinic,[1] whereas at St. Mark's Hospital, the risk was only 2.1% during 10 years after surgery and under strict surveillance of the retained rectum.[2] In practice, as Parks *et al.*[3] indicated, many surgeons may admit the difficulty in giving lifetime guarantee on the retained rectum to colectomized patients. In our Polyposis Center, the central register of polyposis in Japan, we have observed an increasing number of AC patients with a retained rectum who are not under adequate surveillance.

Results of the rectum-preserving operation for ulcerative colitis (Aylett operation) in the U.S.A. have been dismal, with more than three fourths of the patients having required subsequent proctectomy even when the rectum was diverted with a mucous fistula,[4] and with 54% failure in children.[5] The cumulative risk of cancer in the retained rectum in colitis is 6% at 20 years.[6] The remarkable increase in colorectal cancer seen in Japan in recent years indicates Japanese UC patients will probably not be an exception to the increased risk of cancer of the rectum.

Surgery of abdominal ileostomy has recently made significant achievements in stoma care and in improved surgical techniques, as seen in Kock's continent stoma. The patient requiring an abdominal ileostomy is usually young and their disease is benign. Thus a better quality of post-

Second Department of Surgery and Polyposis Center, Tokyo Medical and Dental University, Tokyo, Japan

*Present address: Second Department of Surgery, Hyogo College of Medicine, Nishinomiya, Hyogo, Japan

operative life has been ever more demanded, as it has in other surgical fields.

The total removal of the diseased large bowel mucosa with preservation of natural anal continence is an ideal solution to this problem. Operative procedures aimed at this goal have been called total colectomy, rectal mucosectomy (or mucosal proctectomy), and ileoanal anastomosis, or more simply ileoanostomy or anal ileostomy. The first clinical trial of ileoanostomy was made by Nissen[7] in 1932 in a boy with AC who had undergone an anastomosis between the ileum and the anus through a sacral incision, but without success. In 1947, Ravitch and Sabiston[8,9] initiated a surgical study on ileoanostomy. After a series of animal experiments, they reported their clinical experience in performing ileoanostomy through the method of an endoanal pull-through anastomosis with rectal mucosectomy in two UC patients. They were reported to have performed the operation on 11 additional cases by 1951.[10] Devine and Webb,[11] independently, performed ileoanostomy by an original technique in two AC cases. (According to a recent letter to us from Dr. Webb, they performed this operation in four cases all together. Two did very well indeed, but two failed and had to have an ileostomy. The main problem was severe sepsis around the anus.)

Best,[10] in 1952, summarized the clinical results of ileoanostomy performed by the above authors including his own cases. He found that satisfactory results were about 59%. Finally, he concluded that he had difficulty in convincing himself that "facing the issues (many complications and technical difficulties) was not worth the sweat and tears of both patient and surgeon," and commented that further improvements in technique to limit the complications would be the answer to a wider acceptance of this procedure. Thus, the ileoanostomy did not acquire a position in surgery for AC[12] or for UC.[13,14] The studies, however, were continued: in construction of an ileal reservoir,[15] in use of a diverting ileostomy,[16] in trials to replace the rectal mucosa,[17,18] and in sporadic clinical experiences.[19,20] Since the beginning of the 1970s, ileoanostomy surgery has rekindled the interest of surgeons, stimulated by clinical successes in AC by Safaie-Shirazi and Soper[21] and in UC by Martine *et al.*[22] Encouraging results have been further reported by Ferrai and Fonkalsrud,[23] by Parks and Nicholls,[3,24] by Peck,[25] by Telander *et al.*,[26,27] and by Johnston *et al.*[28] In the World Congress of Colo-Proctology in 1982, ileoanostomy became one of the major topics.

As a result of our study of surgery on AC, in 1977 we decided to initiate a series of clinical projects using our original method (Fig. 1) with a J-shaped reservoir after animal experimental studies had been performed. The encouraging preliminary results were reported in 1980.[29] Analysis has recently been completed on 45 cases, including 34 AC and 11 UC

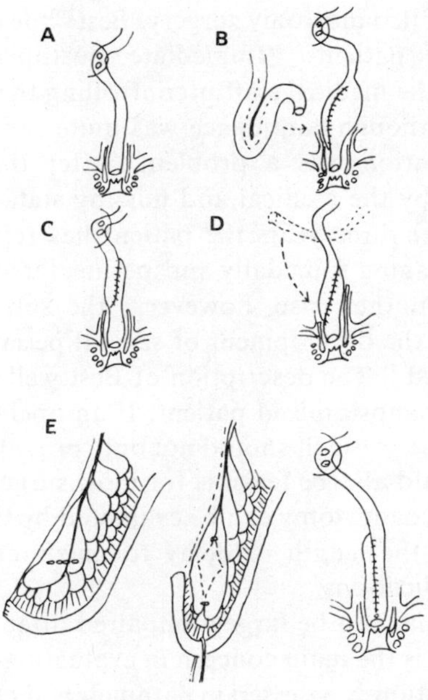

FIG. 1. Type of ileal reservoir. A: non-pouch method (Martine *et al.*, Telander *et al.*, Utsunomiya *et al.*), B: S-pouch method (Parks and Nicholls), C: H-pouch method (Fonkalsrud, Utsunomiya *et al.*), D: secondary H-pouch method (Peck), E: J-pouch method (Utsunomiya *et al.*).

patients, who underwent ileoanostomy by various technical modalities concerning types of ileal reservoir, extent of rectal mucosectomy, and so on. The clinical and functional results have also been studied in 33 patients who underwent closure of a loop-ileostomy and have been observed for an average of 19 months.[30)]

In this paper, we discuss the current specific problems of ileoanostomy and possible tactics for their solution by reviewing our own experience as well as information obtained from the literature.

SPECIFIC PROBLEMS OF ILEOANOSTOMY

Based on reported information and our own experiences, three major problems remain to be solved before practical procedures can be established: 1) how to obtain optimal bowel function, 2) how to reduce the frequency of complications, and 3) how to improve the technical difficulties involved in this procedure.

Bowel function and rehabilitation

In the early era of ileoanostomy surgery, Best[10] described his experience in a postoperative patient: "Immediate postoperative period taxed resourcefullness of the medical staff in controlling the urgency of stool and loose movement, although continence was quite satisfactory. Discomfort from perianal irritation was a problem. After three weeks of rather constant attending by the medical and nursing staffs, these problems lessened and now after three years the patient has reported having proper control, stools averaging four daily and perineal irritation occurring only occasionally." In another case, however, "the suture line did not heal smoothly and after the development of several perianal fistulae, an ileostomy was established." The description of Best well indicates the specific problems of the ileoanostomized patient. If an operative method is to be accepted for continuous use, it should not only provide high-quality life for the patient but should also be feasible for most surgeons. The quality of a patient's life after ileoanostomy can be evaluated by the degree of recovery of bowel function, the length of delay to maximum recovery, and the frequency of complications.

Bowel function that can be largely impaired after total removal of the large bowel mucosa is the main concern in evaluating the clinical results of ileoanostomy. Function is assessed in parameters including daily stool frequency (DSF); fecal leakage (degree of "incontinence"); and ability to discriminate air, liquid, or solid bowel content. In cases with reservoirs, need to use catheterization and time required to evacuate for each urge are placed under consideration. To evaluate the degree of patient satisfaction, DSF and fecal leak are the major parameters generally used, as seen in Peck's criteria (Table 1). DSF of six times or less, which Peck defined as excellent patient satisfaction, might be reasonable. Lillehei and Wangensteen[31] defined the colectomized patient with a DSF of six or more as having poor clinical bowel function.

Frequent stooling, as much as 10 times or more per day, was seen

TABLE 1. Clinical Value for Ileoanostomized Patient (Modified from Peck)

	Stooling frequency (per day)	Fecal leakage	Anal sensation
Excellent (fair)	6 or less	None	+
Good (poor)	7–10	Once at night	±
Fair (poor)	11 or more	At night and 2 or fewer per day	−
Failure (poor)	Incontinence	Incontinence	Incontinence

( ) indicates the criteria for colectomized patients by Lillehei and Wangensteen.

immediately after the diverting ileostomy was closed to let the bowel content pass through the natural anus; but within 6 months it rapidly decreased by adaptation, and after this period it continued to decrease although quite slowly (Fig. 2). It is apparently important to fix the timing of clinical assessment in the period following early adaptation. The interval required for adaptation is another parameter for evaluating the procedure.

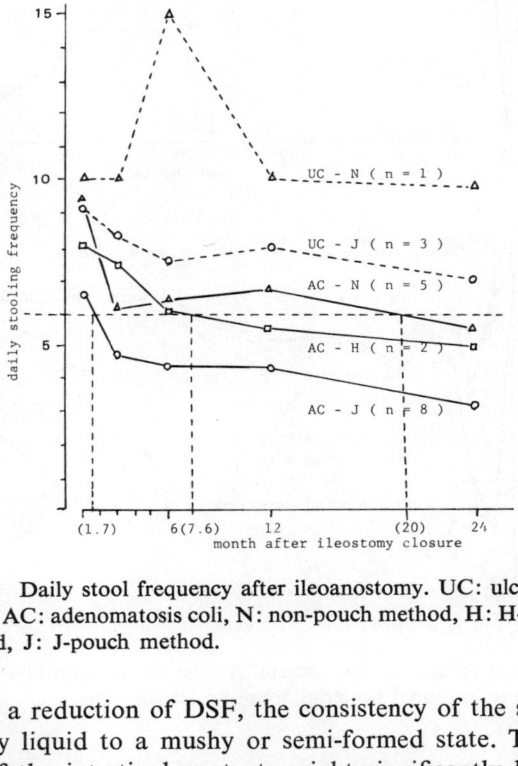

FIG. 2. Daily stool frequency after ileoanostomy. UC: ulcerative colitis, AC: adenomatosis coli, N: non-pouch method, H: H-pouch method, J: J-pouch method.

Along with a reduction of DSF, the consistency of the stool changed from a watery liquid to a mushy or semi-formed state. This increased consistency of the intestinal contents might significantly help the fecal continence. Imajo's study[32] of our patients revealed that the water content of the stool decreased from 85% to 75% and its viscosity increased within 8 weeks after the ileostomy closure. This change was found to correlate with the prolongation of the ileal transit time and with the characteristic change seen in the aerobic-dominant bacterial pattern of the ileostomy excreta to an anaerobic-dominant pattern similar to feces in the colon (Fig. 3).

Liquid stool leaks in almost all cases immediately after ileostomy

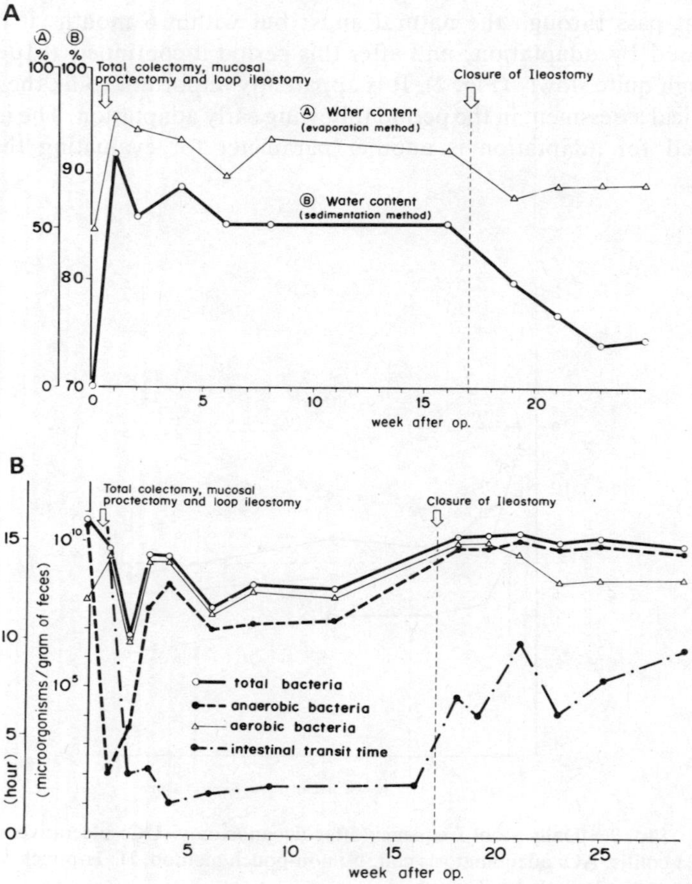

FIG. 3. Changes in ileal excreta. A: change in water content, B: change in intestinal bacterial flora and transit time.

closure, but it subsides with time, as DSF reduces, and if the patient should still leak after the sixth month, he or she should be considered to have abnormal fecal leakage or fecal "incontinence," which implies a persisting partial disturbance in control of the ileal content. This may be a phenomenon specific to the ileoanostomized patient. When the minimum fecal leakage occurs exclusively during sleep, the patient can be entirely normally active (a slight leak or "good" clinical result by Peck). When the stool leaks occasionally during day and night, the perianal skin is excoriated and causes the patient discomfort. The patient could tolerate this condition with a small pad or medication and be active (a moderate leakage or "fair" clinical result). Occasionally an unconscious fecal discharge could occur that makes the patient so dismal as to give up his or her ileoanostomy, and the surgery is evaluated as "failure." From 33–60% of ileoanostomized patients experience fecal leakage depending on the type of procedure (Table 2). Our J-pouch procedure yields the minimum morbidity of leakage compared with other procedures.

TABLE 2. Clinical Results of Ileoanostomy

	"Success" rate	"Excellent" rate	Leakage rate
Ravitch, Wangensteen, Devine, Best (1952)	17/29 (58.6%)	—	
Parks *et al.* (1980) S-pouch	20/21 (95.2%)	10/21* (47.6%)	52.4%
Peck (1980) H-pouch	23/25 (92.0%)	10/25 (40.0%)	60.0%
Telander *et al.* (1980) Non-pouch	20/24 (83.3%)	6/24 (25.0%)	54.2%
Utsunomiya *et al.* (1981)			
J-pouch	21**/26 (80.8%)	16/26 (61.5%)	33.3%
Non-pouch and H-pouch	7/9 (77.8%)	4/9 (44.4%)	44.4%

*Indicates number of cases of spontaneous evacuation.
**Not including the cases with re-established ileostomy to be closed.

The success rate of ileoanostomy has been found to be apparently improved in recent series of cases reported since 1980, and has shown a result of above 80%, compared with less than 60%, as described by Best in 1951 (Table 2). Looking at quality of life, however, patients enjoying excellent satisfaction are seen in less than half of the cases in most reports. This fact clearly indicates there is a need to improve the procedure to provide the patients with a better life after surgery.

Complications

A substantial number of various postoperative complications have been reported, even in the recent literature, with rates of 40%,[3] 50%,[28] 72.4%,[25] and 62.2%.[30] This again presents one of the reasons for the controversy surrounding ileoanostomy. The most frequent and specific complication is pelvic sepsis. The denuded rectum is less resistant to infection, and so-called "cuff abscess" is apt to occur between the cuff and transposed ileum. This destroys the muscular structure of the anorectal region, produces a stricture around the anastomosis, and finally results in incontinence. Diverting ileostomy, strict bowel preparation, and effective drainage work in the cuff are the essential tactics for preventing this sequela, but they are not able to eradicate it. An important recent finding is the less frequent occurrence of sepsis in the shorter rectal cuff (Table 3).

Bowel obstruction itself is not specific to this procedure, but it tends to occur with a higher frequency than in other major laparotomies, as seen in 11% of our series,[30] 12.3%,[3] 27%,[25] and 16%.[27] Hemorrhage inside or outside of the pouch was reported in 6.7% of our series, one or 4.7% of Parks', and one or 3.4% of Peck's series. Peritoneal fistulae were occasionally seen in 4.4% of our series, two or 9.5% of Parks', and one or 4.1% of Peck's. We have experienced loop ileostomy-related sequelae in 8.9% of cases. The one operative death that was recorded in our series was a 62-year-old female with UC who had a severe stress ulcer after surgery.

TABLE 3. Incidence of Pelvic Sepsis

Level of proximal margin of the cuff	Incidence
Supra-peritoneal (the long cuff method)	
Utsunomiya *et al.*	11/39 (28.2%)
Peck *et al.*	10/38 (30.3%)
Fonkalsrud *et al.*	1/5 (20.0%)
Peritoneal reflection	
Johnston *et al.*	2/22 (9.1%)
Parks *et al.** (?)	3/21 (14.3%)
Subperitoneal (the short cuff method)	
Telander *et al.*	0/24
Utsunomiya *et al.*	0/4

*May be including both long and short cuff cases.

Four patients with a J-pouch experienced late complications, persisting or transitional, anemia, diarrhea, and lower abdominal distension. Biopsy of the ileal mucosa revealed chronic ileitis. Reservoir ileitis or pouchitis, already known in Kock's pouch, is a late complication of ileoanostomy with a pouch, as Parks has already reported. The metabolic disorders relating to Vit B12 absorption, bile acid cycle, and other nutritional components should be studied for a longer period of time. The fate of the adapted ileum is another question. Theoretically, the colonized ileum may have an increased susceptibility for neoplastic transformation in the AC patient, and in the UC patient, flashback ileitis may occur if any amount of the rectal mucosa should be left behind. Disturbance of sexual function has not yet been recorded, but specific attention is essential to totally avoid this sequela, for the patient is usually young.

Technical difficulty and complexity

The entire course of ileoanostomy surgery requires a long duration of time: usually more than seven hours based on our experience and other reports. This eventually results in a large blood loss (2,000 ml on the average in our experience) and predisposes the patient to a higher frequency of postoperative complication. Extensive mucosectomy in the rectum is mainly responsible for the problem. This procedure does not produce consistent results, even when done by an experienced surgeon, in UC cases because of the technical difficulty of stripping the inflamed mucosa leaving the lowest rectal muscle layer intact.

After surgery, a great effort must be made to cope with the various complications. Modern ileoanostomy surgery has made significant progress in the extensive use of antibiotics, in improved nutritional support by an intravenous hyperalimentation or by elemental diet, in sophisticated stoma care, in machine suture techniques, and so on. Nevertheless, surgeons must sometimes feel in sympathy with Best's comment.

Next we will discuss the technical problems with an eye to finding solutions to these problems.

ILEOANOSTOMY TECHNIQUES

The ileoanostomy is a composite of several surgical techniques, some of which are specific and controversial.

Rectal mucosectomy

Rectal mucosal resection is the core of the operation and is technically the most difficult procedure. The questions are how much of and which part of the rectal mucosa should be removed without disturbing the bowel function and how to remove it completely without damaging the lowest part of the rectal muscular structure and the internal sphincter.

The proximal limit of the mucosectomy or the length of the rectal muscular cuff is one of the most controversial parts of this procedure (Fig. 4). Ravitch liberated the rectum down to the muscular pelvic diaphragm and left only a short stump of the rectum 5–8 cm in length in the pelvis ("the short cuff method"). Devine and Webb felt the necessity of preserving a significant amount of the rectal muscular layer with the intrinsic nerve plexus and the connection with the sacral segment of the spinal cord, based on the study made by Denny Brown and Riberton,[33] and performed the mucosectomy starting at the level of the rectosigmoidal junction ("the long cuff method"). This concept has been followed by many surgeons such as von Esparre,[19] Reifferscheid,[20] Safaie-Shirazi *et al.*,[21] Wolfstein *et al.*,[34] Emmerman,[35] Peck,[25] and Utsunomiya *et al.*[29] Soave[36] inde-

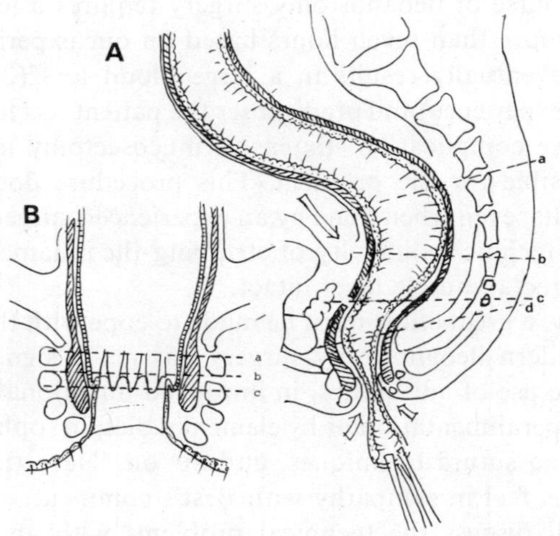

FIG. 4. Rectal mucosectomy. A: length of cuff. a: long cuff method, b: intermediate cuff method, c: short cuff method, d: ultra-short cuff method; B: level of distal mucosectomy. a: high mucosectomy, b: intermediate mucosectomy, c: low mucosectomy.

pendently devised an abdominal endorectal mucosectomy for use in coloanal anastomosis. In the procedures by Martin *et al.*, Parks and Nichols, and Telander *et al.*, the endorectal mucosectomy began just at or below the peritoneal reflection.

The long cuff method has been found to have two disadvantages: 1) producing a higher frequency of cuff abscess, as discussed before, and 2) requiring a longer operation time. Parks[37] already indicated that neither the mucosa nor the muscle wall of the rectum plays a part in the maintenance of continence, based on his experience with endoanal coloanostomy, and has applied this theory to his recent ileoanostomy. Telander *et al.*[27] modified their method of the long cuff to the short cuff, in order to simplify the technique, with good results. They carried out the pelvic dissection of the rectum in a manner similar to Swenson's (for avoiding sexual disturbance) down to the levator and left a distal rectal cuff of about 8 cm. Recently, we[30] have found excellent bowel function in two AC cases associated with rectal cancer who underwent ileoanostomy with the rectal wall above the levator muscle and the mucosa of the anal canal excised (the ultra-short cuff) and with a standard pelvic dissection performed. Based on our experience, we have modified our technique such that endorectal mucosectomy is totally made from the anus at a distance of 7–8 cm in a prone jack-knife position followed by the rest of the procedure at the Lloyd-Davis position (Fig. 4).

The distal limits of mucosectomy

Devine and Webb left a small part of the rectal mucosa above the dentate line as a censor area because they thought it was essential for discriminating the solid or fluid nature of the bowel content. This principle was followed by Martine *et al.*, Safaie-Shirazi *et al.*, and many surgeons. Our experience has shown that cancer occurred in some instances just above the dentate line in AC patients, and histological examination revealed many micro-foci of adenomas involving the transitional epithelium near the dentate line. If the area is not removed, the risk of cancer remains, and the patient must be placed on a regular check-up schedule as is practiced for patients retaining their entire rectum. Such an operation should be called subtotal mucosectomy to distinguish it from the total mucosectomy, which entirely removes the risk of cancer from the rectum.

Subtotal mucosectomy definitely reduces the advantages of ileoanostomy over low ileorectostomy, which can be much more easily performed. Peck, Parks *et al.*, and Telander also conceived the importance of total removal of the rectal mucosa and suggested that the rectal mucosa be incised at the dentate line (Parks, Telander) or the level of the crypt of Morgagni (Peck). On the other hand, it is well appreciated that extensive excision of the transitional anal mucosa can result in incontinence, as seen in the patients who underwent Whitehead's operation. We have performed three types of distal mucosectomy which differ in regard to the level at which they initiate (Fig. 4). The low distal mucosectomy in which the incision is made at the line of the crypt of Morgagni showed a slight disturbance of continence, with soiling at night in two out of five cases. Therefore, we think that the incision should be made at the top of the pecten or a few millimeters above it.

Rectal mucosectomy has been carried out in different ways by different surgeons. The principal requirements of the mucosectomy are avoidance of injury to the underlying muscular structure at the lowest part of the rectum and anal canal, and avoidance of leaving any mucosal fragment on the surface of the muscular cuff which will eventually cause delayed cuff abscess. We were able to find some technical principles to be followed in order to perform mucosectomy successfully. First of all, the field must be kept dry at all times using a succor and bipolar coagulating forceps. This requires the coordinated action of the operator and assistants. Second, the muscle layer must always be everted so it can be detached from the mucosal layer by using pusher or scissors. We have previously used an anoabdominal approach, as other surgeons such as Martine, Parks, and

Peck have done. Johnston started mucosectomy first from the anus and then completed it from the abdomen at lithotomy position ("the supine-anoabdominal approach"). For the short cuff method by Telander, the mucosectomy was performed on the rectal segment that had already been cut from the abdominal approach and everted out from the anus. Parks removed about 8 cm of rectal mucosa by a perineal approach at lithotomy position, while he divided the mucosa in three strips. Matsuo[38] studied our cases and revealed that the maximum anal canal pressure at rest can predict the fecal functional outcome after surgery (Fig. 5). This finding led us to conclude that most important technique for obtaining good fecal continence is to preserve the lowest part of the rectal muscular structure and the internal sphincter as completely as possible. In order to conduct this important phase of the operation with better exposure of the surgical field and with less physical strain on the surgeon, we decided to start the distal mucosectomy at the beginning of the operation with the patient placed at a prone jack-knife position ("the prone anoabdominal approach"). This technique was especially useful for UC cases. The details of the technique are described separately.[30]

Construction of an ileal reservoir

Frequent stoolings and occasional fecal leakage in the ileoanostomized patient is thought to be caused by a limited capacity and by frequent peri-

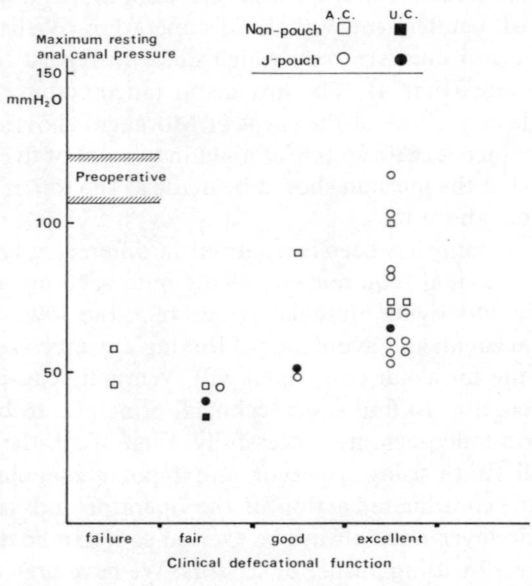

FIG. 5. Maximum anal canal pressure at rest and clinical result.

stalsis of the ileum. Martine *et al.*[22] and Telander *et al.*[26] reported satisfactory results in pediatric patients treated by ileoanostomy without reservoir. It was said that Martine's patients required heavy medication with anti-diarrheal agents and a prolonged period of rehabilitation.[39] To provide some storage capacity for feces and lessen the severity of post-ileoanostomy diarrhea, ileal reservoirs of different types have been constructed since the first experimental trial was made by Valiente and Bacon in 1955. Koch's study had promoted clinical use of an ileal pouch in ileoanostomy.[24,40] At present, there are four types of ileal pouch that are being used in clinical practice. The S-shaped or triplicated pouch by Parks,[24] which is similar to the idea of Valiente; the isoperistaltic double loop or H-shaped pouch, primarily (Fonkalsrud[41]) and secondarily (Peck[25]) constructed; and the J-shaped pouch or antiperistaltic double loop (Utsunomiya) (Fig. 1). Peck had first started his study with the idea of rectal mucosal replacement to eliminate ileal peristalsis and preserve rectal muscular function, but after having found shrinkage of the grafted rectum, he created a reservoir by a long side-to-side anastomosis at the second laparotomy. We first constructed a J-shaped reservoir in an AC patient in June 1978, with our original idea to place the reservoir at the lowest portion of the pelvis directly connected to the anus in order for it to be smoothly evacuated. The other advantages of the J-pouch are simplicity of construction and a low risk of reservoir necrosis (the pouch has a bilateral blood supply). So far we have performed the J-pouch in 33 cases and compared its clinical results with other methods. Daily stooling frequency of the J-pouch (median 4.5) is apparently less than those without reservoir (6.0 in our series and 7.0 in Telander's series) and those with Peck's pouch (5.5) (Fig. 6). Parks' pouch shows less frequent stooling (4.0) than ours, but a half of his patients were required to evacuate the reservoir contents using self-catheterization. Telander's idea to simply dilatate a straight ileal loop using a specially made intestinal balloon in order to accelerate the ileal dilatation has not yet been assessed in terms of its clinical results. In evaluating the adaptation time, patients with the J-pouch have a DSF of 6 times or less with a much shorter delay period (1 7 months) than cases with the H-pouch (7.5 months) or without pouch (20 months) (Fig. 2).

Other attempts to preserve the ileal content, such as the ileal myotomy or grafting of antimesenteric ileal segment, have not been widely accepted.

Ileoanal anastomosis

Primary clean healing of an ileoanal anastomosis is essential for obtaining good continence. Therefore, anastomotic technique and drainage work are of considerable importance for avoiding early or late pelvic infection.

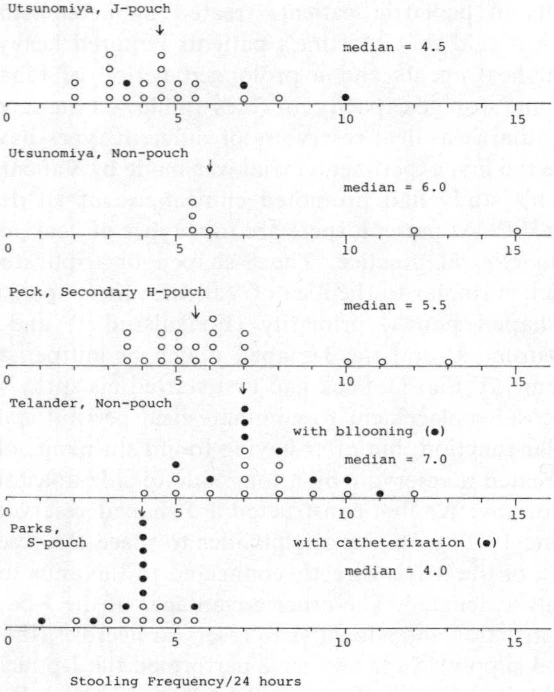

FIG. 6. Median daily frequency of stooling in different procedures.

Ravitch used three-layer anastomosis: an ileal serosa–rectal muscle, an ileal serosa–external sphincter, and an ileal wall–anal skin using catgut. This was modified by Best to a secondary pulled-through anastomosis. These anastomoses were too low based on our present knowledge. Many surgeons have followed Devine's method of suturing above the dentate line. Park's contribution[37)] on the transanal anastomotic technique greatly facilitated this technique. By his method, each interrupted suture incorporates the mucosa of the mid-anal canal, a deep bite of the internal sphincter, and the full thickness of the ileal wall using (000) Dexon. Our suture is quite similar to Parks' in principle, but is different in that our anastomosis is carried out in a side-to-end fashion. According to our experience, a side-to-end anastomosis can be performed more easily and more cleanly than those of an end-to-end fashion because the size of the anastomotic opening in the ileal wall can be adequately adjusted to the size of the anal canal. The vertical mattress technique was useful in adapting the mucosal layers. We never use silk or catgut because the former can cause persistent infection and the latter is absorbed too soon. We always use (000) Dexon, as do other surgeons, and feel that the use of Dexon may be one of the major achievements in ileoanostomy surgery. An EEA stapler can be employed in the high anastomosis (at the level of the anorectal junction), but cannot be used in the low anastomosis just above the dentate line because the rectal muscle could be cut together with the mucosa.

Effective drainage work is essential to remove the fluid and blood accumulated within the muscular cuff which will eventually cause cuff abscess. Transanastomotic Penrose drainage has not been used by us because it leaves a slit at the anastomosis that could cause infection into the cuff. Transperitoneal drainage is most commonly used by Safaie-Shirazi, Parks *et al.*, Telander *et al.*, and by us. Until recently, transabdominal drain has been our routine procedure. However, analysis revealed that the transabdominal drain alone was not effective in preventing pelvic sepsis and that the combined use with the transperineal drain was more effective. The most effective drainage of the cuff can be obtained by reducing the dead space within the cuff (the short cuff method).

Diverting ileostomy

Routine use of diverting ileostomy advocated by Schneider[16)] and Martine *et al.*[22)] was one of the most significant contributions to the prevention and treatment of pelvic sepsis. A loop ileostomy by the Turnbull method[42)] (Martine *et al.*, Parks *et al.*, Utsunomiya *et al.*) and an endo-ileostomy (Peck, Johnston *et al.*) have been reported. We experienced both and found that the latter was easier and functioned just as well. Complications such as stoma recession or prolapse were seen in 3 out of 44 performances, and one intestinal obstruction and one anastomotic leakage occurred in 33 closures. The frequency of complications has been reduced in recent series. Turnbull's principle of stoma siting has given patients increased activity during the waiting period before closure, which may occasionally require a year or more. A loop ileostomy is usually closed in six to eight weeks (Parks *et al.*, Telander *et al.*) or in three months at least (Utsumoniya *et al.*). The average waiting time of our 33 patients who had an ileostomy closed was 207 days. Before a decision regarding ileostomy closure is made, a clean healing at the anastomosis must be confirmed both by endoscopic and barium enema examination. We assumed that a small fistula left unhealed was the cause of pelvic sepsis that occurred after the ileostomy closure in our two cases. The closure is better delayed until the time when the maximum anal pressure at rest recovers to above 50 cm/H_2O. A sphincter that had not recovered sufficiently would produce perianal irritation that would further reduce sphincteric function. The site of loop ileostomy varied from 20 cm to 60 cm from the end in our series. All the cases with a loop ileostomy have enjoyed normal activity for up to three years at the most under regular consultation with a stomatherapist. The volume of ileal excreta decreased rapidly after establishment of a loop ileostomy and stabilized at the sixth month at an average volume of 687 ml in 13 cases with a terminal ileal diversion of 50–60 cm, 1.56 times the average volume of ileal excreta from a terminal endoileostomy (439 ml/4 cases).[32] Metabolic disturbance has not been observed in the cases with a retained loop ileostomy.

INDICATIONS

A successful ileoanostomy can only be achieved through the skill and experience of the surgeon in all the components of this complex surgery which have been discussed above. With this condition fulfilled, candidates for ileoanostomy are all the cases of AC for which rectum-preserving surgery is indicated; UC patients who have an indication for colectomy or proctocolectomy can be included, if the internal sphincter is healthy. Patients with AC or UC that are older than approximately 55 years had better be excluded from selection because their anal sphincteric function could probably not recover sufficiently after surgery, and the advantage of avoiding an abdominal ileostomy is less than in those of younger age. We propose a new surgical policy for UC in order to avoid ileostomy. Our procedure could be performed primarily during the remission stage as elective surgery (Fig. 7). A cecorectal anastomosis is advisable if the rectum-preserving operation is indicated because it preserves the ileocolic vessels which would be advantageous in a later construction of the J-shaped reservoir. Total colonic diversion, or primary or secondary rectal diversion with a suprapubic mucous fistula, is initially indicated for the cases with fulminating or severe colitis, followed by ileoanostomy using our method after the patient's general condition and rectal lesion are improved.

CONCLUSION

Total removal of the large bowel mucosa with preservation of anal continence to avoid an abdominal ileostomy is an ideal surgical procedure for AC and UC. It has been one of the major questions left unsolved in gastrointestinal surgery. Ileoanostomy, which had been once disregarded as a practical procedure, has recently rekindled the interest of surgeons due to the encouraging results reported by several institutes since 1980. Analysis of these reports, including our own, has shown an apparent improvement in clinical results if compared with the results of 30 years ago, but

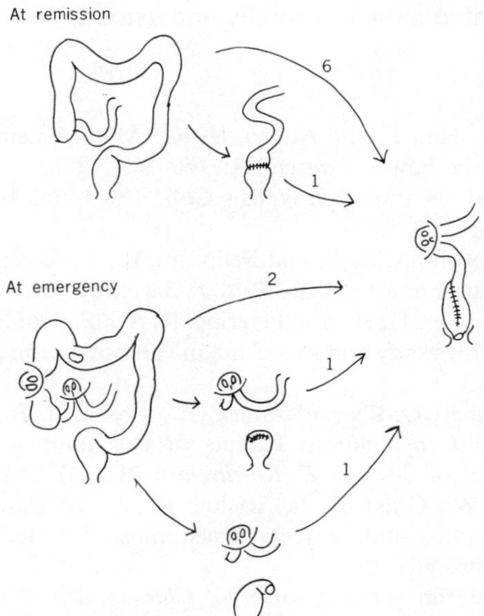

FIG. 7. Indication of ileoanostomy for ulcerative colitis.

has also revealed that there are many problems to be solved before the procedure can be really appreciated for routine use.

The major specific problems are how to obtain optional bowel function after surgery, how to reduce the high frequency of diverse complications, especially of pelvic sepsis, and how to make the technique feasible for practical use. One of the answers can be found in the procedure: the prone anoabdominal short rectal mucosectomy and ileoanal anastomosis with a J-pouch, covered by a temporal loop ileostomy.

Ileoanostomy is "reconstitutional surgery," aimed both at the reduction of potential risk of malignancy and at relative improvement in the quality of patients' lives. The life of the ileoanostomized patient is undoubtedly much more satisfactory than that of an abdominal ileostomy patient, and the cost and time needed for this sophisticated surgery must be paid. To achieve this basic requirement, surgeons must master the surgical disciplines involved in every component of this technically complex operation before he or she decides to practice it. With this condition fulfilled, the ileoanostomy can be justified for the patient, preferably of younger age, with AC or UC who is a candidate for the rectum-preserving operation.

Ileoanostomy surgery will be studied continuously until the final outcome of the operated patient is totally understood.

REFERENCES

1. Moertel, C. G., Hill, J., and Adson, H. R.: Management of multiple polyposis of the large bowel. *Cancer*, **28**: 160–169, 1971.
2. Bussey, H. J. R.: Familial Polyposis Coli. The Johns Hopkins University Press, Baltimore, 1975.
3. Parks, A. G., Nicholls, R. J., and Belliveau, P.: Proctocolectomy with ileal reservoir and anal anastomosis. *Brit. J. Surg.*, **67**: 533–538, 1980.
4. Binder, S. C., Miller, H. H., and Petering, R. A.: Fate of the retained rectum after subtotal colectomy and ileorectal anastomosis. *Am. J. Surg.*, **131**: 201, 1976.
5. Naas, R., Gruner, O.-PN., Flatmark, A., Fretheim, B., and Gjone, E.: Ulcerative colitis in children: Results of colectomy in 38 patients with childhood onset of disease. *Z. Kincllrchir.*, **21**: 237–244, 1977.
6. Baker, W. N. W., Glass, R. E., Richie, K., *et al.*: Cancer of the rectum following colectomy and ileorectal anastomosis for ulcerative colitis. *Brit. J. Surg.*, **65**: 862–868, 1978.
7. Nissen, R.: "Berlin surgical society." *Chirung*, **15**: 888, 1933.
8. Ravitch, M. M. and Sabison, D. C.: Anal ileostomy with preservation of the sphincter: A proposed operation in patients requiring total colectomy for benign lesions. *Surg. Gynec. Obstet.*, **84**: 1095–1099, 1947.
9. Ravitch, M. M.: Anal ileostomy with sphincter preservation in patients requiring total colectomy for benign condition. *Surgery*, **24**: 170–187, 1948.
10. Best, R. R.: Evaluations of ileoproctostomy to avoid ileostomy in various colonic lesions. *JAMA*, **150**: 637–642, 1952.
11. Devine, J. and Webb, R.: Resection of the rectal mucosa, colectomy and anal ileostomy with normal continence. *Surg. Gynec. Obstet.*, **92**: 437–442, 1951.
12. Lockhart-Mummery, H. E., Dukes, C. E., and Bussey, H. J. R.: The surgical treatment of familial polyposis of the colon. *Brit. J. Surg.*, **43**: 476–481, 1956.
13. Goligher, J. C.: The functional result, after sphincter-saving resection of the rectum. *Ann. Roy. Coll. Surg.*, **8**: 421, 1951.
14. Goligher, J. C. and Hughes, E. S. R.: Sensitivity of the rectum and colon: Its role in the mechanism of anal continence. *Lancet*, **1**: 543–547, 1951.
15. Valiente, M. A. and Bacon, H. E.: Construction of pouch using "Pantaloon" technique for pull-through of ileum following total colectomy. *Am. J. Surg.*, **90**: 742–750, 1955.
16. Schneider, S.: Anal ileostomy. Experience with new three-stage procedure. *Arch. Surg.*, **70**: 539–574, 1955.
17. Peck, D. A. and Hallenbeck, G. S.: Fecal continence in the dog after replacement of rectal mucosa with ileal mucosa. *S. G. O.*, **119**: 1312–1320, 1964.

18. Glotzer, D. J.: Preservation of continence after mucosal graft in the rectum and its feasibility in man. *Am. J. Surg.*, **117**: 403–409, 1969.
19. von Esparre, W.: Weitere Erfahrungen mit der chiruigischen Behandlung der *colitis ulcerosa. Z. Kinderchir.*, Suppl. **5**: 84–90, 1967.
20. Reifferscheid, M.: Kontinenzhaltende radikale Exstirpation prämaligner und maligner Adenoma des Rectosigmoids. *Aktuelle Chir.*, **6**: 295–302, 1971.
21. Safaie-Shirazi, S. and Soper, R. T.: Endorectal pull-through procedure in the surgical treatment of familial polyposis coli. *J. Pediat. Surg.*, **8**: 711–715, 1973.
22. Martine, L. W., Le Caultre, C., and Sehubert, W. K.: Total colectomy and mucosal proctectomy with preservation of continence in ulcerative colitis. *Ann. Surg.*, **186**: 477–479, 1977.
23. Ferrai, B. T. and Fonkalsrud, E. W.: Endorectal ileal pull-through operation with ileal reservoir after total colectomy. *Am. J. Surg.*, **136**: 113–120, 1978.
24. Parks, A. G. and Nicholls, R. J.: Proctocolectomy without ileostomy for ulcerative colitis. *Brit. Med. J.*, **2**: 85–88, 1978.
25. Peck, D. A.: Rectal mucosal replacement. *Ann. Surg.*, **191**: 294–303, 1980.
26. Telander, R. J. and Perrault, J.: Total colectomy with rectal mucosectomy and ileoanal anastomosis for chronic ulcerative colitis in children and young adults. *Mayo Clinic Proc.*, **55**: 420–425, 1980.
27. Telander L. and Perrault, J.: Colectomy with rectal mucosectomy and ileoanal anastomosis in young patients: Its use for ulcerative colitis and familial polyposis. *Arch. Surg.*, **116**: 623–629, 1981.
28. Johnston, D., Williams, N. S., Neal, D. E., and Axon, A. T.: The value of preserving the anal sphincter in operations for ulcerative colitis and polyposis: A review of 22 mucosal proctectomies. *Brit. J. Surg.*, **68**: 874–878, 1981.
29. Utsunomiya, J., Iwama, T., Imajo, M., Matsuo, S., Sawai, S., Yaegashi, K., and Hirayama, R.: Total colectomy, mucosal proctectomy, and ileoanal anastomosis. *Dis. Colon Rect.*, **23**: 459–465, 1980.
30. Utsunomiya, J., Iwama, T., Imajo, M., Sawai, S., Okamura, T., Yaegashi, K., and Hirayama, R.: Result of the ileoanostomy on adenomatosis coli and ulcerative colitis. Submitted for publication.
31. Lillehei, R. C. and Wangensteen, O. H.: Bowel function after colectomy for cancer, polyps, and diverticulitis. *JAMA*, **159**: 163–170, 1955.
32. Imajo, M.: Study of the small bowel transit time and physiochemical characteristics of the ileal excreta in abdominal and anal ileostomy. *J. Jap. Surg. Soci.*, **82**, **6**: 874–878, 1981 (Japanese text with English abstract).
33. Denny Brown, D. and Robertson, E. A.: An investigation of the nervous control of defecation. *Brain*, **58**: 256–259, 1935.
34. Wolfstein, I. H., Dreznik, A. J., and Avigaid, S.: Total colectomy and anal ileostomy in multiple polyposis coli. *Arch. Surg.*, **113**: 1101–1106, 1978.
35. Emmerman, H.: Endstaindiges Ileostoma oder kontinenzhaltende Proktomukosektomie nach Kolektomie wegen Adenomatose. *Zbl. Chir.*, **99**: 1139–1143, 1974.
36. Soave, F.: Hirshprung's disease: A new surgical technique. *Arch. Dis. Child.*, **39**: 116–124, 1964.

37. Parks, A. G.: Transanal technique in low rectal anastomosis. *Proc. R. Soc. Med.*, **65**: 975–976, 1972.
38. Matsuo, S.: Anorectal function after total colectomy, mucosal proctectomy and ileoanal anastomosis. *J. Jap. Surg. Soci.*, **82**: 1366–1376, 1981 (Japanese text with English abstract).
39. Goligher, J. C.: The quest for continence in the surgical treatment of ulcerative colitis. *Advance in Surgery*, **14**: 53–84, 1980.
40. Kon, M.: How to treat polyposis coli. *Rinsho-ge-ka*, **31**: 758-711, 1976 (in Japanese).
41. Fonkalsrud, E. W., Ament, M. E., and Byne, W. J.: Clinical experience with total colectomy and euclorectal mucosal resection for inflammatory bowel disease. *Gastroenterology*, **77**: 156–160, 1979.
42. Turnbull, R. G., Jr., Hawk, W. A., and Weakley, F. L.: The surgical treatment of toxic megacolon. Ileostomy and colostomy to prepare patient for colectomy. *Am. J. Surg.*, **122**: 325–331, 1971.

Metabolic Disorders after Total Colectomy

Tsuneo Fukushima, Naoki Ishiguro, Hiroshi Takemura, and Shuji Tsuchiya

After total colectomy, colonic inflammatory lesion is eradicated; however, subsequent metabolic disorders are known to be induced. This paper presents post-total colectomy complications seen in our department.

UROLITHIASIS

In 32 patients with inflammatory bowel disease who received total or proctocolectomy, 4 patients developed urolithiasis. Two of them were affected by ulcerative colitis, and the remaining two were affected by Crohn's disease. The mean period between the operation and initial urinary symptoms was 3.8 years. Ileostomy was more liable to complicate urolithiasis compared to ileoproctostomy, since incidence of urolithiasis in ileostomy was 50% (3 out of 6) but no urolithiasis was seen in 20 cases of total colectomy with ileoproctostomy. One patient (S.O., 30-year-old female) developed renal stones three times in a 9-year follow-up period and another patient (Y.A., 40-year-old male) developed renal stones twice in an 8-year follow-up period. The other two patients had one episode only.

Stones of ileostomy were composed of uric acid and Ca oxalate. Urinary organic acids and electrolytes were measured in patients with urolithiasis after total colectomy (Table 1). Urinary oxalate concentration was markedly increased but uric acid was not increased. Urinary Ca/Mg ratio was increased.

After total colectomy, in addition to decreased urinary output, other lithogenic factors such as low urinary pH, increased oxalate, and increased urinary Ca/Mg ratio facilitate renal stone formation.

Second Department of Surgery, Yokohama City University, Yokohama, Japan

TABLE 1. Urinary Organic Acid and Electrolytes in Urolithiasis after Large Bowel Resection

Patient	Age and sex	Oxalate (mg/dl)	Uric acid (mg/dl)	pH	Na (mEq/*l*)	K (mEq/*l*)	Cl (mEq/*l*)	Ca (mg/dl)	Mg (mg/dl)	Ca/Mg ratio
Y. A.	45/M	7.4		5.0	165	50	236	21	8.0	2.6
S. O.	30/F	9.1	34	5.0	233	72	301	18	3.5	5.3
T. I.	31/M	27.4	128		33	106	1	32	1.8	18.2
K. D.	45/F		16	6.0	111	12	100	6	1.6	3.7
Mean ± SD		14.6 ±11.1	59 ±60		135 ±85	60 ±39	159 ±134	19 ±11	3.7 ±3.0	7.5 ±7.2
Control value ± SD		2.8	51 ±24	5–7	173 ±41	33 ±16	187 ±46	20 ±10	9.7 ±4.8	2.2 ±0.2

CHOLELITHIASIS

Three patients developed cholelithiasis after total colectomy and two of them were proved to have cholesterol stones. Cholesterol stone formation was suggested to be due to a decreased bile acid pool and subsequent increase in lithogenicity of the bile.

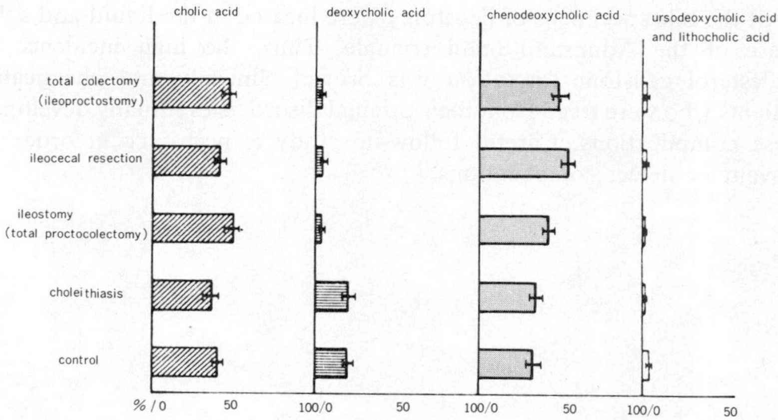

FIG. 1. Bile acid composition in each group. A decrease of deoxycholic acid was noted after ileostomy, ileocecal resection, and total colectomy.

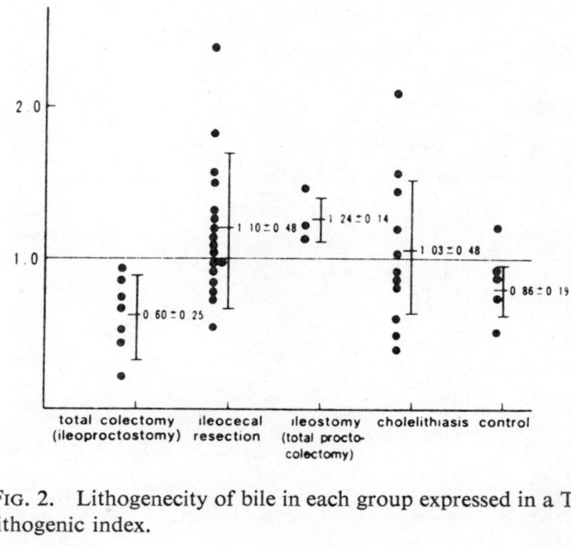

FIG. 2. Lithogenecity of bile in each group expressed in a Thomas lithogenic index.

Bile acid composition was compared in various types of bowel operation (Fig. 1). Percentage of deoxycholic acid was decreased and choenodeoxycholic acid was increased.

The lithogenic index was calculated from the molar ratio of bile acid, cholesterol, and phospholipid in bile. That of ileostomy was 1.24 ± 0.14, higher than that of ileocecal resection, ileoproctostomy, and cholithiasis (Fig. 2).

All the bile specimens of ileostomy were located in the liquid and solid phase of the Admirand-Small triangle. Thus, the high incidence of cholesterol gallstone formation was proved clinically and chemically. Patients who were freed from their original disorders eventually developed these complications. Careful follow-up study is necessary in order to prevent or detect complications.

Ileostomy: Continent or Incontinent?

Keith A. Kelly

SUMMARY

The Brooke ileostomy remains today the safest and most trouble-free procedure for patients requiring proctocolectomy. However, the patients have a stoma, which is incontinent, and they must wear an appliance continuously day and night to collect the fecal output. A pre-stomal, valved ileal pouch (Kock pouch) offers the patients control over their fecal discharge. However, such patients still have a stoma and require intubations. Moreover, some experience valvular malfunction and diarrhea, both of which require continued medical attention and sometimes reoperation. Straight endorectal ileal–anal anastomosis avoids the stoma and the intubations and maintains the transanal route of fecal flow. However, the patients have more bowel movements/day than healthy controls and are sometimes incontinent, especially at night. The ileal pouch–anal anastomosis decreases the frequency of stooling and improves the continence, but it, too, does not lead to a perfect result. Two newer techniques, the use of a stomal obstructing device and electrical pacing, may find application in the future.

Patients with a conventional Brooke ileostomy are completely incontinent of gas and stool and must wear an ileostomy appliance both day and night to collect the effluent from their intestinal tract.[1] These appliances are unsightly, uncomfortable, and odoriferous. Disturbing noises may appear when gas or stool discharges into them. There is the ever-present danger of leakage and subsequent soiling of the clothes. Moreover, the appliances are expensive. In the United States, the estimated cost of maintaining an appliance and its supplies approximates $300.00/year. In addition, ileostomates with an appliance have a number of social, psychological, and sexual disadvantages. The patients have an impaired

Roberts Professor and Head, Section of Gastroenterologic and General Surgery, Mayo Clinic and Mayo Foundation, Rochester, Minnesota, U.S.A.

image of their body and its functions and are reluctant to engage fully in the many activities of a normal, healthy person. The appliances hinder their work, their social interchange with other individuals, and may impair their sexual relations with others. Thus, for a number of reasons, an alternative to an incontinent Brooke ileostomy and its appliance would be desirable.

Our work at Mayo has taken several directions in an attempt to avoid a Brooke ileostomy in patients who require excision of their large intestine. Over the past decade, we have used the pre-stomal, continent ileal pouch (Kock pouch), the straight endorectal ileal–anal anastomosis, and the ileal pouch–anal anastomosis. In addition, we are currently exploring the use of an ileostomy stomal occluding device and electrical pacing as means of achieving fecal continence. In this paper, I will discuss our experience with these various approaches.

THE CONTINENT ILEAL POUCH

General description

The continent ileal pouch or Kock pouch is made from 45 cm of terminal ileum. It consists of three parts: the pouch itself; a valve to keep the pouch from leaking; and an efferent ileal limb leading from the valve to the skin (Fig. 1).[2] The efferent limb ends in a stoma which is made flush with the cutaneous surface at the ileostomy site in the right lower quadrant. The intestinal content travels down the intestine to the pouch, where it remains until the pouch is emptied. The patient empties the pouch by passing a catheter through the stoma and efferent limb, through the valve, and into the reservoir. The ileal content then drains through the catheter directly into the toilet bowl or another suitable receptacle. The catheter is then removed and an occlusive gauze dressing placed over the stoma to protect the clothing from the mucus discharged by the exposed ileal epithelium. When the pouch and valve are working properly, there is no discharge of gas or intestinal content in between intubations. In this way, the patient has complete control over the discharge from the intestinal tract.

Upon initial construction, the pouch will accept only 150 ml of content. However, with the weeks and months passing after the operation, the pouch gradually dilates, and at three months, the pouch holds approximately 500 ml of content. The pouch occupies a position in the right lower abdominal quadrant and pelvis just beneath the stoma at a site formerly occupied by the cecum and sigmoid colon. While the pouch itself dilates, the ileum proximal to the pouch usually retains a normal caliber.

The daily routine of the patients is simple. The patients can eat a regular diet, with the one proviso that they must masticate their food thoroughly.

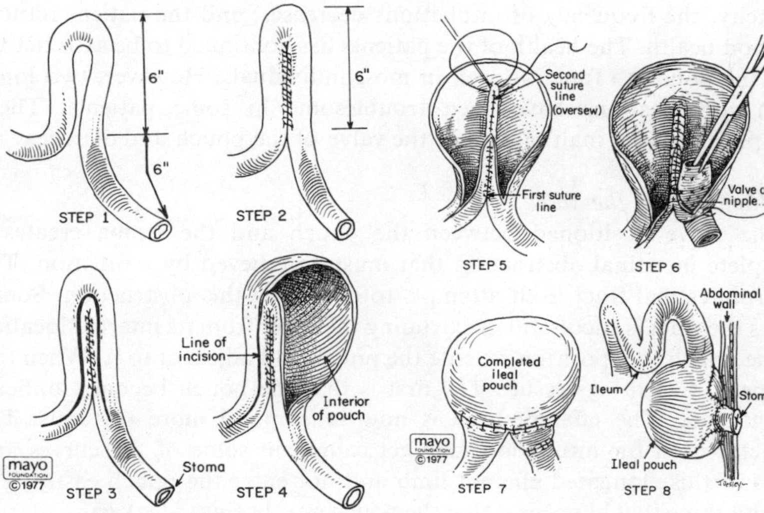

FIG. 1. The continent ileal pouch (Kock pouch) ileostomy. Initial steps (left). Final steps (right). (From *The Ileal Pouch Procedure*, Mayo Clinic and Mayo Foundation, © 1977.)

This applies especially to food containing indigestible fibers, such as raw celery, cabbage, apple skins, orange sections, nuts, and mushrooms. The patients require no medication and usually intubate their pouch 3–4 times/day, but not at night. They may engage in any and all activities with the possible exception of excessively strenuous lifting, which may tend to prolapse their valve. There is no restriction on sexual activities or pregnancies. We have had a number of patients who have delivered full-term pregnancies without disturbing the function of their pouch.

Clinical results

We have constructed continent ileal pouches in about 450 patients at Mayo during the period 1971 through 1982.[3–5] There have been no operative mortalities or mortalities within the first postoperative month. The mean postoperative hospital stay has been about 17 days. In the early days of the operation, among our first 25 patients, only about half had achieved continence at discharge from the hospital. However, in the last 400 patients, nearly all (98%) were continent at discharge. By continent, I mean the patient had complete control over fecal discharge and wore no lieostomy appliance.

In the weeks and months that follow the construction of the pouch, the patients gradually adapt to their new situation. The pouch increases in capacity, the frequency of intubations decreases, and the patient returns to good health. The health of the patients has continued to be satisfactory and the pouch to function well in most individuals. However, two long-term complications have been troublesome in some patients. These complications are malfunction of the valve of the pouch and diarrhea.

Malfunction of the valve

The valve positioned between the pouch and the stoma creates a complete intestinal obstruction that must be relieved by intubation. The gastrointestinal tract itself attempts to overcome this obstruction. Sometimes the tract is successful in extruding the valve from its internal location in the pouch to a position outside the pouch and adjacent to it. When this happens, two things result. The first is that the pouch becomes difficult to intubate. The efferent limb is now longer and more tortuous. The catheter used for intubation may get caught in some of the curves and folds of this elongated efferent limb and not enter the pouch easily. The second thing that happens is that the pouch now begins to leak gas and fecal content. We found in a careful study of our patients that the frequency of valve slippage was greater in males than in females, was greater in patients over 40 years of age than in those less than 40 years of age, and was greater in those having a conversion from a conventional Brooke ileostomy to a continent ileal pouch than in those who had the continent ileal pouch constructed at the time of their proctocolectomy.[4)] In our initial group of patients the incidence of valve slippage in the first postoperative year was approximately 40%.

Because of the large incidence in the need for valve revision, we adopted some technical changes in our more recent patients in an attempt to decrease the need for revision of the valve.[5)] The ileum was thoroughly scarified and its serosa denuded prior to making the intussusception to form the valve. Fat in the ileal mesentery adjacent to the site of intussusception was carefully denuded and excised. The valve was made at least 5 cm in length and was anchored in place with and through nonabsorbable sutures or stainless steel staples. The efferent ileal limb was sutured to the pouch at the site of its exit from the pouch. Nonabsorbable sutures were used. The pouch itself was sewn to the anterior abdominal wall just at the site of exit of the efferent limb from the pouch. The efferent limb connecting the valve and pouch to the cutaneous surface was made as straight and as short as possible to allow the easiest possible intubation. In addition, the pouch was catheterized in the operating room and the catheter left in place for a period of one month after the operation to allow good healing to take place before the pouch and valve were distended by intestinal content.

With these changes, the probability of having a valve revision was decreased markedly. In the early series, 40% of patients required a revision by one year after operation; while in the second series, in which the technical revisions were undertaken, the need for revision had decreased to 20%. Nonetheless, while we have improved the need for revision by our technical modifications, we have not eliminated the need for revision. The technical aspects of valve construction still need attention.

Diarrhea

Diarrhea remains another problem that requires attention in patients with the continent ileal pouch. In health, individuals normally excrete approximately 125 ml of fecal discharge. This quantity increases about five-fold in patients with Brooke ileostomy, to approximately 625 ml. Our patients with the continent ileal pouch fall into two groups.[6] In the first group, about 90% of our patients, the same fecal volume is excreted as among patients with Brooke ileostomy. However, in the second group, approximately 10% of our patients, the output is in excess of 1 liter/day and the excreta contains an increased quantity of fat, nitrogen, vitamin B12, sodium, and potassium.

The cause of the increased output and the malabsorption is obscure. Schjønsby *et al.* have found increased numbers of anaerobic bacteria in the ileostomy effluent of such patients.[7] They treated the patients with lincomycin, an antibiotic that impairs the growth of anaerobic bacteria in the gastrointestinal tract. With the treatment, malabsorption was improved in their patients. We looked at possible causes of diarrhea in our patients. Lactase deficiency or partial intestinal mechanical obstruction explained the increased output in some patients. In other patients no specific cause was identified, but a nonspecific "pouchitis" was sometimes found. The nonspecific pouchitis was characterized by blunting of the villi of the pouch mucosa and by chronic inflammation with erythema, erosions, and ulcerations of the mucosa. However, the appearance of pouchitis was inconsistent in patients with increased output, sometimes being present and sometimes not. Moreover, we were unable to correlate the number or severity of the anatomic, pathologic changes with symptoms or increased output. Thus, morphology is not of help in identifying those patients who have or will have increased fecal output from those who will not and does not explain fully the development of the symptoms when they do appear.

We were, however, able to identify a consistent abnormality in the bacteriology of the gastrointestinal tract in those patients with an ileal pouch and increased output.[8] Patients with ileal pouch and diarrhea had increased numbers of both aerobic and anaerobic bacteria in their jejunal luminal content compared with Brooke ileostomy patients and ileal pouch patients without diarrhea. In contrast, the number of bacteria/g stool in the ileal effluent was nearly identical in the three groups. That the anaerobic bacteria in the jejunal lumen were responsible for the malabsorption is suggested by the fact that when we treated the patients with metronidazole, an antibiotic directed specifically against the anaerobic bacteria, the patients' symptoms improved. Moreover, the improvement in symptoms was accompanied by a decrease in the number of anaerobic organisms in the jejunal content. Thus, the diarrheal syndrome seen in patients with continent ileal pouches may be caused in part by an overgrowth of anaerobic bacteria in the upper gut of the patients. The bacterial overgrowth, either by virtue of the toxic products produced by the bacteria or other factors, impairs digestion and absorption in the small bowel and results in increased output and malabsorption. The overgrowth can be treated by anti-bacterial agents directed against the anaerobic organisms and the treatment is usually successful. However, several courses of treatment may be required.

Conclusions

We concluded that the continent ileal pouch has a great advantage over the Brooke ileostomy; the pouch patients have control over their fecal discharge. Nonetheless, the patients remain with a stoma and require intubations 3–4 times/day to empty their pouch. Moreover, the two nagging problems of valve malfunction, occurring in about 15% of patients, and diarrhea severe enough to require treatment, occurring in about 5% of the patients, remain as lingering and troublesome problems. Thus, another solution to the problem of providing continence after proctocolectomy would be well received.

STRAIGHT ILEAL–ANAL ANASTOMOSIS

In 1979, we began to explore the use of colectomy, mucosal proctectomy, and endorectal ileal–anal anastomosis as a means of providing continence for patients after proctocolectomy (Fig. 2). The major advantages of this approach are that the operation removes all of the diseased mucosa found in chronic ulcerative colitis and familial polyposis, and yet it preserves the anal sphincters and the normal route of fecal flow. An ileostomy is avoided once the operative sequence is completed. Moreover, the pelvic nerves are undisturbed because the distal rectal and perineal portion of

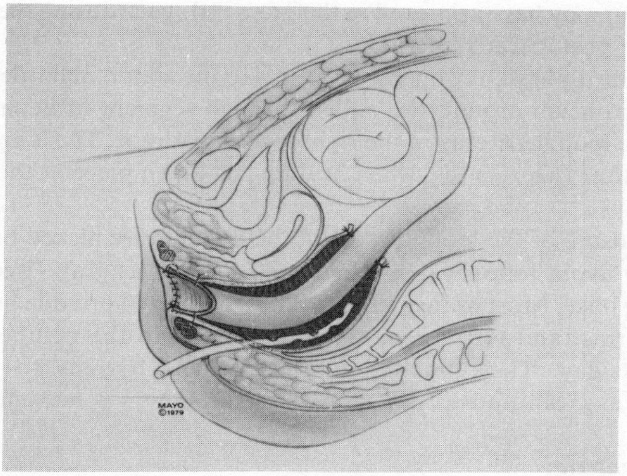

FIG. 2. Endorectal straight, ileal–anal anastomosis. (Reprinted with permission from Telander, R. L. and Perrault, J.[9])

the operation are done endorectally. The chance of injuring the nerves to the genitalia or to the urinary apparatus is minimized. Lastly, because the operation is done endorectally, no perineal wound results. Such wounds are sometimes difficult to heal.

Operative technique

The operation is done in three phases.[9] The first phase, an abdominal phase, is performed with the patients in the lithotomy position. A midline abdominal incision is made and a thorough inspection of the abdominal contents is undertaken to establish the diagnosis and presence of any ancillary diseases. The large intestine is then thoroughly mobilized and the cecum, colon, and proximal rectum excised.

In the second, or perineal phase, the operator, with the patient remaining in the lithotomy position, everts the distal rectum onto the perineal surface by pulling the rectum inside out through the anal canal. Using the cautery, the distal rectal mucosa is then stripped from the dentate line in an oral direction up to a point 7 cm proximal to the dentate line. The distal rectum is then transected at this point completing the stripping procedure. The terminal ileum is then advanced endorectally through the distal rectal muscular cuff and sewn to the dentate line from the perineal side. Two medium-sized round silastic catheters are placed through perineal stab wounds into the plane between the ileum and the rectal muscular cuff and advanced into the presacral space. These drains are used in the postoperative period to remove blood, serum, or intestinal content that may have appeared in the presacral space during the operation and in the postoperative period.

In the third phase, the operator returns to the abdominal side, closes the pelvic peritoneum around the pulled-through segment of ileum and then performs a loop ileostomy in the right lower quadrant. The loop ileostomy is closed after two months, when healing has taken place at the ileal–anal anastomosis.

After closure of the loop ileostomy, the patients are placed on a regular diet. They avoid foods with a laxative effect such as grape juice, prunes, and prune juice. Most of the patients take psyllium to provide bulk in their intestinal tract and loperamide to slow transit and the number of bowel movements/day. They practice careful perineal hygiene to keep their perineum as clean and as dry as possible after bowel movements.

Clinical material

We performed this operation on 50 patients between the years 1979 through 1981, among whom there were 25 males and 25 females.[10] The mean age of the patients was 29 years. Among the 50 patients were 41 with ulcerative colitis, 7 with familial polyposis, and 2 with Crohn's disease. (We would not advise the operation for Crohn's disease today.) Six of the 50 patients had had prior colectomy and ileorectostomy.

Clinical results

Among the 50 patients, there was no mortality and a mean hospital stay of 14 days. Six of the 50 developed an anastomotic leak which required excision of the ileal–anal anastomosis. The remainder healed the anastomosis without difficulty. After closing the loop ileostomy, the mean fecal output was 600 g/day, a figure that does not differ significantly from patients with Brooke ileostomy or from those with Kock pouch. Among 30 patients followed for at least six months, the degree of continence during the day was excellent; 40% of patients had no leakage at all and 40% had only minor leakage. However, the continence at night was not as good, with approximately 20% of the patients having nocturnal leakage that at times soiled the bedclothes and pajamas.

The mean number of stools passed/24 hr was 8, of which 6 were passed during the day and 2 at night. However, the range of stools passed/day was as low as 3 stools/24 hr in one patient to as high as 20 stools/24 hr in another patient. Needless to say, the patient that had 20 stools/24 hr had a marked degree of perineal soreness and excoriation. Continued and active therapy with perineal creams and salves was required. Nine patients with frequent stools needed conversion to a permanent ileostomy.

Among the first 50 patients, then, there were 16 who required excision of the ileal–anal anastomosis: 6 with anastomotic problems, 9 who had frequent stools, and one who developed recurrent Crohn's disease. All 16 were converted from an ileal–anal anastomosis to an ileostomy. Four patients still had the ileostomy present at the time of our review, leaving 30 with the ileal–anal anastomosis intact for long-term evaluation. Among 39 patients who had their ileostomy closed, 30 preferred the ileal–anal anastomosis, but 9 preferred the ileostomy.

Certain disadvantages to the straight ileal–anal anastomosis emerged. Some of the patients have an excessive number of stools/day, and some leak stool, especially at night. Frequent stooling and leakage results in perineal skin excoriation. Moreover, almost all of the patients required the chronic use of psyllium and loperamide to combat diarrhea.

We wondered what aspect of the operation allowed some patients to have an acceptable result following ileal–anal anastomosis, while other patients had a poor result. We studied a spectrum of our patients with physiologic tests to help us answer this question.

Physiologic studies

Anal sphincter function. Anorectal manometry was performed using a specially designed glass probe that had an external diameter of 11 mm and through which were drilled four channels that allowed measurement of intraluminal pressure using a perfused catheter system.[11)] When this probe is passed into the anal canal of a normal, healthy person and withdrawn in 1-cm steps from the rectum to the anus, the intraluminal pressure profile across the sphincter can be measured. The length of the anal sphincter is between 4 and 5 cm in most healthy controls. The pressure in the anal sphincter gradually increases as the probe is withdrawn from the point 4 to 5 cm proximal to the anal verge up to the point 1 to 2 cm from the anal verge, where the pressure is about 80 to 90 mmHg. We performed such measurements in patients with ileal–anal anastomosis and found that their resting anal sphincter pressure had a profile very similar to that of the controls. Thus, the operation preserved resting anal sphincter pressure in the patients.

In a second test of anal sphincteric function, the probe was placed in the area of maximum anal sphincter pressure at rest. The patient was then asked to squeeze voluntarily his anal sphincter for 3 min, and a pressure profile of the squeeze pressure against time was obtained. With the onset of squeezing, the pressure at the anal sphincter usually increases to about twice that of the resting pressure and then gradually declines toward the control even though continual squeezing is maintained. With continual squeezing an increase in sphincteric tone can be maintained at a level approximately

50% greater than the resting pressure. With relaxation of the squeeze, the pressure then returns to control. In the patients with the ileal–anal pull-through operation, the ability to squeeze, increase the pressure, and maintain the pressure over the 3-min period was similar to that in the controls. No impairment in squeeze pressure was identified.

Rectal–anal inhibitory reflex. Attention was then focused on the measurement of the rectal–anal inhibitory reflex. In this test, the bowel is distended with a 20-ml bolus of air at a point 12 cm from the anal verge, while pressure in the anal sphincter 3 cm from the anal verge is being measured concurrently. When the rectum is distended in health, a prompt decrease in proximal anal sphincter pressure of about 40 cmH_2O occurs. The pressure then gradually returns towards the control over a 2-min period. This response can be demonstrated repeatedly. However, after endorectal ileal–anal anastomosis, the rectal–anal inhibitory reflex is either abolished or greatly impaired. In fact, in some of our patients, instead of a decrease in proximal anal sphincter pressure, an increase in pressure was found. The physiologic significance of this abnormality is unclear.

Distal bowel motor pattern. We also examined the motility of the bowel at a point 10 cm from the anal verge. In health, the basal intraluminal pressure within the rectum 10 cm proximal to the anal verge during fasting is about 5 cmH_2O. Superimposed upon this resting pressure are phasic changes in pressure of small amplitude and short duration. The amplitude of the changes is about 10 to 20 cmH_2O and the duration approximately 10 to 20 sec. In contrast, after ileal–anal anastomosis, while the resting pressure remains low, phasic changes in pressure of much greater amplitude and much longer duration are found in the neo-rectum. After ileal–anal anastomosis, the changes in pressure frequently have amplitudes of 100 cmH_2O and often last as long as 30 sec. We believe that these large increases in intraluminal pressure after ileal–anal anastomosis may contribute to the frequency of stooling and the incontinence that some patients experience after the operation.

Pressure–volume relationships. Using another rectal probe with a diameter of 8 mm and with a soft latex balloon attached to its tip, we measured the pressure–volume relationships of the bowel 12 cm from the anal verge in the patients with ileal–anal anastomosis and compared these to the same relationships found in healthy controls. In controls, little increase in pressure occurs as the volume of rectal distension is increased up to 160 ml. At this point, the pressure within the rectal canal has only risen about 10 cmH_2O. However, after ileal–anal anastomosis, a much greater increase in pressure is found with the same volume of distension, so that with 160 ml, the pressure in the neo-rectum is closer to 25 cmH_2O. We calculated the compliance of the bowel as being the reciprocal of the slope of the line depicting the change in volume against the change in pressure. In controls, the compliance of the bowel is approximately 17 ml/cmH_2O. In contrast, after ileal–anal anastomosis, the compliance is much less, being approximately 6 ml/cmH_2O. We also found that the healthy rectum can easily tolerate a volume of approximately 400 ml. However, the maximal capacity of the neo-rectum after ileal–anal anastomosis is much reduced, with the neo-rectum only able to accommodate about 250 ml of H_2O.

We studied the association between the capacity of the neo-rectum and the number of stools per day. In patients with a large neo-rectal capacity, the number of stools/day was far less than in those with a smaller rectal capacity. In fact, an indirect linear correlation was noted between the number of stools/day and the rectal capacity.

The study of our initial patients, thus, identified some strengths and weaknesses of the straight ileal–anal anastomosis. Although the anal sphincters and the voluntary anal squeeze were preserved, the rectal–anal inhibitory reflex was impaired and the rectal capacity markedly reduced. The significance of the abolition of the rectal inhibitory reflex is obscure. However, the reduction of rectal compliance was indirectly correlated with the frequency of bowel movements. Moreover, the greater the frequency of bowel movements, the more the incontinence, the more the perineal soiling, and the greater the need for medications.

Conclusions

The straight ileal–anal anastomosis has an advantage over various types of ileostomy in that the normal transanal route of fecal flow is maintained and a stoma is avoided. However, our initial results indicated that if this operation were eventually to be widely applied, a means of increasing neo-rectal capacity, decreasing the number of stools/day, increasing continence, reducing perineal soiling, and reducing the need for perineal and systemic medications would be required. We wonder if these objectives would be achieved with an ileal pouch–anal anastomosis.

ILEAL POUCH–ANAL ANASTOMOSIS

Operative technique

Beginning in 1981, we began to explore the concept of ileal pouch–anal anastomosis as an alternative to straight ileal–anal anastomosis following proctocolectomy.[12] The hypothesis was that construction of a terminal ileal reservoir would increase ileal capacity, decrease stooling, and improve continence after ileal–anal anastomosis. We constructed an ileal pouch from the terminal 25 cm of ileum by fashioning the terminal ileum into the shape of a J or U. The approach was similar to that used by Utsunomiya and colleagues.[13] The anterior and posterior walls of the newly constructed pouch were formed using two layers of continuous 2–0 chromic catgut. The bottom or crotch of the J was then brought down endorectally to the dentate line, just as in the straight ileal–anal anastomosis, and the bottom of the pouch itself sutured to the dentate line in the anal canal. We chose the J-shaped pouch rather than the S-shaped pouch with an efferent limb because we reasoned that sewing the J-pouch itself to the dentate line would allow the patients to empty the pouch spontaneously and voluntarily. In other words, the patients ought not to have to intubate to empty the pouch.

Clinical material

We employed the ileal pouch–anal anastomosis in a subsequent series of 74 patients. We compared the results from this series to those of the first series of 50 patients with straight ileal–anal anastomosis. The mean age and the range in age as well as the ratio of males to females were similar in both groups. Moreover, the incidence of the diseases for which the operation was performed (chronic ulcerative colitis, familial polyposis, and Crohn's disease) was nearly identical in both groups, with the exception that none of the patients in the second series had Crohn's disease.

Clinical results

No deaths occurred in either series of patients. The incidence of leak and sepsis was similar in both groups, with nine patients having leak or sepsis in the first series and eight patients having it in the second series. However, there were nine patients with excessive stools in the straight ileal–anal group as opposed to none in the ileal pouch–anal group. One patient had recurrent Crohn's disease in the first group, whereas there was none in the second. The early results showed that among the 50 patients in the first series, 16 were considered failures and had to have their ileal–anal anastomosis taken down, whereas only one patient was a failure in the second series. This patient had the ileal pouch–anal anastomosis taken down because of leak and sepsis.

Long-term follow-up was done on the two groups of patients. We were able to trace 30 patients in the first series and 33 patients in the second series. The mean follow-up was longer in the first group (18 months) than in the second group (6 months). All patients were able to defecate voluntarily at all times. In both groups, the number of stools/day improved with time. In the straight ileal–anal anastomosis group, the patients experienced 20 bowel movements/day at the first month, whereas after 18 months, the number of bowel movements had decreased to 9/day. In contrast, among the ileal pouch–anal patients, only 11 bowel movements were evacuated each day by one month, and the number had decreased to 7 movements/day by six months. The difference between the ileal pouch patients and the straight ileal–anal anastomosis patients was significant both at one month and at six or more months. The patients with ileal pouch–anal anastomosis also required less medication than those with the straight anastomosis. At 18 months, 85% of the patients with the straight anastomosis were still using psyllium and loperamide, whereas at six months only 40% of the pouch patients were using this medication.

The degree of continence was better in the patients with ileal pouch–anal anastomosis than in those with straight ileal–anal anastomosis. During the day, among both groups of patients about 60% had absolutely no leakage, while about one third had a minor degree of leakage, which was not of great concern. However, among the patients with straight ileal–anal anastomosis there were 7% who had major leakage (soiling of clothing) that was bothersome and embarrassing. Whereas, among the ileal pouch–anal patients, none experienced such leakage. The degree of continence at night was also better among the ileal pouch–anal patients than among the straight ileal–anal patients. The percent of patients with no leakage or minor leakage was similar in the two groups, but none of the patients with ileal pouch–anal anastomosis had major leakage that soiled the bedclothes or pajamas. Among the straight ileal–anal patients, about 20% had such leakage.

We asked the patients to grade subjectively the result of their operation, with 1 being the worst result (a failure) and 10 being the best possible result (a perfect result). The average patient with straight ileal–anal anastomosis graded himself as a 6, while the average patient with an ileal pouch–anal anastomosis graded himself as a 9. We also asked the patients to compare their present situation to the situation when they had a Brooke ileostomy in the immediate postoperative period. Seventy-five percent of the patients with the straight ileal–anal anastomosis said that they preferred their anastomosis to the Brooke ileosotomy, whereas among the patients with ileal pouch–anal anastomosis, 100% preferred their anastomosis to a Brooke ileostomy.

Conclusions

We concluded that construction of a terminal ileal pouch with ileal–anal anastomosis decreased stooling, reduced the need for medication, improved continence, and enhanced patient satisfaction compared with straight ileal–anal anastomosis. Further improvement of this operation is likely to come from improvements with ileal pouch–anal anastomosis rather than with straight ileal–anal anastomosis. The endorectal ileal pouch–anal anastomosis, thus, is an attractive alternative to the Brooke ileostomy and to the continent ileal pouch, but it, too, is not a perfect procedure. The patients have more bowel movements/day than a healthy person and they do not have perfect control of fecal discharge. Some patients require medication long-term, and some with diarrhea and leakage have perineal irritation. Alternate techniques to provide continence should be pursued. We are currently exploring two newer options.

NEWER APPROACHES

Ileostomy occlusion

We wondered whether an ileostomy might be occluded with an artificial obstructing device to achieve continence. We reasoned that an ileostomy could be occluded if it were done by gradually lengthening the intervals of occlusion over weeks or months. The occlusion might then achieve fecal continence without impairing intestinal function.

The device. We developed an indwelling occlusive device that could be inserted into the stoma of the subject (Fig. 3). A balloon was fixed to the

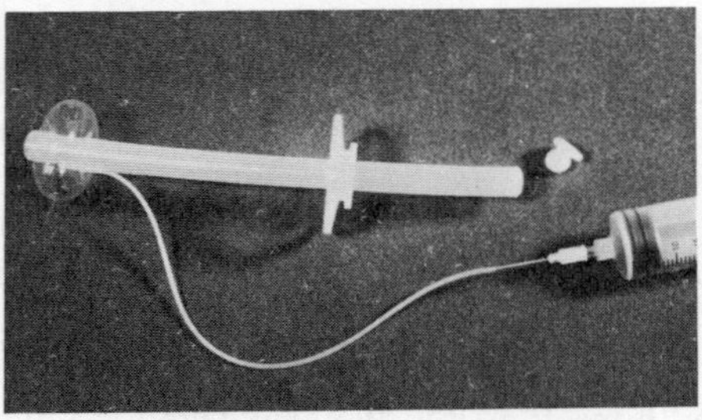

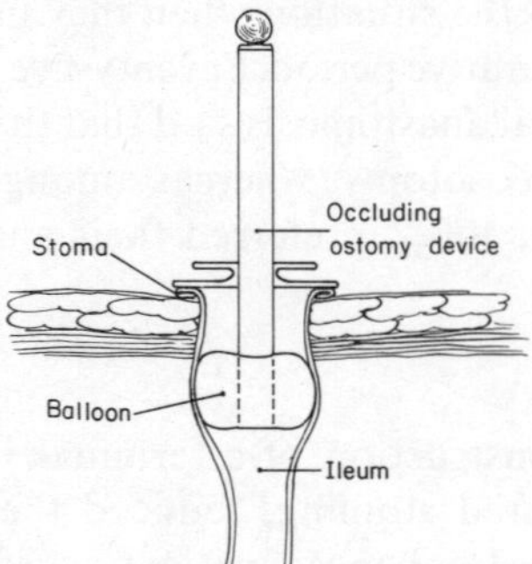

FIG. 3. Ileostomy-obstructing device (upper). Device in place in stoma and terminal ileum (lower). (From Pemberton, J. H., Kelly, K. A., and Phillips, S. F.[14])

end of a No. 28 French silastic tube. The end of the tube and the balloon were passed through the stoma into the intra-abdominal ileal lumen. The balloon was then inflated and drawn up against the anterior abdominal wall to occlude the outflow of the ileostomy. The device was kept in place and the balloon kept pulled up against the abdominal wall by slipping a retaining disc over the external end of the tube and snugging it up against the skin. The tubing leading from the ileal lumen to the outside was occluded by folding the tubing and fixing it to the retaining disc outside the body. With the device in place the ileostomy was continent.

Canine tests. We tested the device in dogs with ileostomies.[14] An initial group of seven dogs were divided into a group of four that received occlusion, while the other group of three were kept as controls. The occluded group underwent repeated occlusion of gradually lengthening intervals over a duration of 20 weeks. By 20 weeks, they were tolerating the occlusion for periods of 6–8 hours. The animals were tested initially before any occlusion and then again at 20 weeks. The controls similarly were tested initially and then again at 20 weeks.

All animals lost weight in the first six weeks after operation and then gradually regained weight up to and often exceeding that noted preoperatively. There was no difference between the control animals and the occluded animals, suggesting that the occlusion by itself did not impair the health of the dogs. By 20 weeks, marked changes were noted in the ileum of the dogs with the stomal occluding device in place. The ileum had greatly dilated compared with the controls and had formed a functional reservoir. With the device in place, the animals were completely continent. For example, none of a $BaSO_4$ suspension placed into the terminal ileum leaked out the stoma onto the skin in the occluded dogs. In contrast, in the control animals, ileal content flowed freely from the terminal ileum through the stoma and onto the skin.

The increased capacity of the terminal ileum in the occluded dogs was demonstrated by comparing the pressure–volume curves of the terminal ileum in the two groups of animals. In the occluded group, at 20 weeks, little increase in pressure occurred as 250 ml of fluid were instilled into a flaccid balloon placed into the terminal ileum. The rather flat pressure–volume curve in the occluded dogs at 20 weeks was in contrast to the steeply rising curve before the occlusions were started. The pressure–volume curves of the control dogs changed little over the 20-week period. Sharp increases in pressure occurred with small increases in volume both initially and after 20 weeks. The ileal occluded dogs did have a slower transit of intestinal content through the terminal ileum than did the control dogs, whose transit was not changed 20 weeks later. However, the absorption of fat, an index of digestion and absorption in the small bowel, was not impaired in the dogs that received occlusion compared with the controls. In both groups, about 12 to 14% of digested fat was recovered in the ileal content.

Thus, chronic intermittent stomal occlusion of the conventional Brooke ileostomy achieved fecal continence; resulted in a dilated, compliant, distal ileum; slowed ileal transit; and yet did not impair intestinal absorption in dogs. These encouraging canine tests prompted us to conduct similar tests in patients.

Human tests. Four patients with a conventional Brooke ileostomy in place for 3 to 16 years were studied.[15] All had had chronic ulcerative colitis and currently had well-functioning Brooke ileostomies. Tests similar to those performed in dogs were done, including ileal contrast X-rays, ileal compliance, endoscopy, ileal absorption and motility, daily fecal outputs, Schilling tests, and transit times. The results in man were nearly identical to those in dogs. The humans occluded intermittently for 10 to 16 weeks showed terminal ileal dilatation and enhanced ileal compliance without endoscopic or anatomic evidence of ulceration or necrosis produced by the device. Ileal absorption remained normal and ileal motility was little changed from controls. The daily fecal outputs, Schilling tests, and ileal transit times were similar in the occluded patients to the pre-occlusion values. Thus, patients with Brook ileostomy were made continent with the ileostomy-obstructing device without impairing intestinal function.

An initial period of cramping, abdominal pain, and stomal discomfort did occur in the patients. These symptoms likely resulted from stretching of the terminal ileum in the early weeks of adapting to the device. To obviate these symptoms, we have in certain selected patients created a pre-stomal ileal pouch without a valve at the time of the proctocolectomy. The artificial device is inserted in the operating room. These patients adapt more rapidly to the ileal occlusion brought about by the device than do those with a straight, conventional Brooke ileostomy. The ileal pouch provides an immediate reservoir which quickly expands without a period of adaptation as is required when a conventional ileostomy is obstructed.

Electrical pacing

We have also explored electrical pacing as a means of augmenting continence and decreasing output in patients with ileostomy. The motility of the small intestine is controlled by a pacemaker located within the first centimeter of duodenum.[16] The pacemaker generates electrical cycles, called the pacesetter potentials, which propagate from the pacemaker in a distal direction down the small intestine. The pacesetter potentials phase the onset of action potentials, and hence contractions, and in this way determine the frequency of contractions, their velocity of distal propagation, and their direction of propagation.

Technique and results. The canine small intestinal pacesetter potentials can be entrained or paced by electrical stimulation.[17)] Using a stimulating frequency slightly faster than the frequency of the natural pacemaker, the pacesetter potentials of the small bowel can be captured and then driven to the faster frequency of the pacing unit. Electrical pacing can be done either at a site in the proximal bowel or at a site in the distal bowel. Pacing at proximal sites allows the generated pacesetter potentials to propagate in the normal or aboral direction. In contrast, pacing at distal sites allows the experimenter to pace the small bowel in a backward or orad direction (Fig. 4). When pacesetter potentials are driven in a backward or orad direction, contractions, whose onset is phased in by the potentials, also move in a backward or orad direction toward the stomach. Such backward pacing markedly slows aboral transit and may even reverse the direction of transit of content from aboral to orad. This means that intestinal content is exposed to the absorbing epithelium of the small intestine for a longer period. Hence, a greater amount of water, nutrients, and electrolytes are absorbed compared with the control when there is no pacing.[18)]

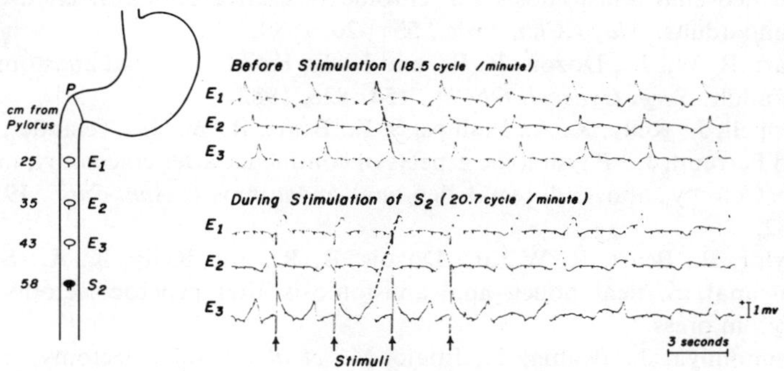

FIG. 4. Pacing the canine small intestinal pacesetter potentials with electrical stimuli. (From Akwari, O. E., Kelly, K. A., Steinbach, J. H., and Code, C. F.[17)])

Possible uses. The increased absorption with backward pacing could benefit patients with ileostomy. It might be possible using electrical pacing to decrease ileostomy output from the usual volume of 625 g/day to perhaps 300 g/day or less. Such a decrease would make the output easier to manage. Thus, electrical pacing may prove a useful adjunct to other techniques of management of patients with ileostomy.

REFERENCES

1. Roy, R. H., Sauer, W. G., Beahrs, O. H., and Farrow, G. M.: Experience with ileostomies: Evaluation of long-term rehabilitation in 497 patients. *Am. J. Surg.*, **119**: 77, 1970.
2. Kock, N. G.: Continent ileostomy. *Prog. Surg.*, **12**: 180, 1973.
3. Beahrs, O. H., Kelly, K. A., Adson, M. A., and Chong, G. C.: Ileostomy with ileal reservoir rather than ileostomy alone. *Ann. Surg.*, **179**: 634, 1974.
4. Dozois, R. R., Kelly, K. A., Ilstrup, D., Beart, R, W., Jr., and Beahrs, O. H.: Factors affecting revision rate after continent ileostomy. *Arch. Surg.*, **116**: 610, 1981.
5. Dozois, R. R., Kelly, K. A., Beart, R. W., Jr., and Beahrs, O. H.: Improved results with continent ileostomy. *Ann. Surg.*, **192**: 319–324, 1980.
6. Kelly, D. G., Branon, M. E., Phillips, S. F., and Kelly, K. A.: Diarrhea after continent ileostomy. *Gut*, **21**: 711, 1980.
7. Schjønsby, H., Halvorsen, J. F., Hofstad, T., and Hovdenak, N.: Stagnant loop syndrome in patients with continent ileostomy (intra-abdominal ileal reservoir). *Gut*, **18**: 795, 1977.
8. Kelly, D. G., Phillips, S. F., Kelly, K. A., Weinstein, W. M., and Gilchrist, M. J. R.: Bacterial overgrowth in the jejunum of patients with ileal pouches. *Gastroenterology*, **78**: 1193, 1980.
9. Telander, R. L. and Perrault, J.: Total colectomy with rectal mucosectomy and ileo-anal anastomosis for chronic ulcerative colitis in children and young adults. *Mayo Clin. Proc.*, **55**: 420, 1980.
10. Beart, R. W., Jr., Dozois, R. R., and Kelly, K. A.: Ileoanal anastomosis in the adult. *Surg. Gynecol. Obstet.*, **154**: 826, 1982.
11. Heppell, J., Kelly, K. A., Phillips, S. F., Beart, R. W., Jr., Telander, R. L., and Perrault, J.: Physiologic aspects of continence after colectomy, mucosal proctectomy, and endorectal ileo-anal anastomosis. *Ann. Surg.*, **195**: 435, 1982.
12. Taylor, B., Beart, R. W., Jr., Dozois, R. R., and Kelly, K. A.: Straight ileal–anal vs. ileal pouch–anal anastomosis after proctocolectomy. *Ann. Surg.*, in press.
13. Utsunomiya, J., Iwama, T., Imajo, M., *et al.*: Total colectomy, mucosal proctectomy, and ileoanal anastomosis. *Dis. Colon Rectum*, **23**: 459, 1980.
14. Pemberton, J. H., Kelly, K. A., and Phillips, S. F.: Achieving ileostomy continence with an indwelling stomal device. *Surgery*, **90**: 336, 1981.
15. Pemberton, J. H., van Heerden, J. A., Beart, R. W., Jr., Kelly, K. A., and Phillips, S. F.: Achieving ileostomy continence in man with an indwelling stomal device. *Gastroenterology*, **82**: 1148, 1982.
16. Hermon-Taylor, J. and Code, C. F.: Localization of the duodenal pacemaker and its role in the organization of duodenal myoelectric activity. *Gut*, **12**: 40, 1971.
17. Akwari, O. E., Kelly, K. A., Steinbach, J. H., and Code, C. F.: Electric pacing of intact and transected canine small intestine and its computer model. *Am. J. Physiol.*, **229**: 1188, 1975.

18. Collin, J., Kelly, K. A., and Phillips, S. F.: Enhancement of absorption from the intact and transected canine small intestine by electrical pacing. *Gastroenterology*, **76**: 1422, 1979.

Ileorectal Anastomosis Overview

David G. Jagelman

None of the surgical options available to patients with ulcerative colitis are ideal. Proctocolectomy and ileostomy is curative for the disease but at a price. The nuisance of an ileostomy and its psychological and sexual disadvantages have tended to be overlooked in the past. The physical problems following proctocolectomy have been well documented by Rhodes and Kirsner in 1965[1] and by Goligher in 1966.[2] They included skin excoriation, ileostomy prolapse and recession, impotence, and a high incidence of failure of healing of the perineal wound in over half the cases. A greater realization that proctocolectomy and ileostomy is not as satisfactory as has been previously thought has spurred the development of alternative procedures such as the continent ileostomy and ileoanal pull-through procedure with and without an accompanying pouch. They indeed also have their problems both from a surgical viewpoint and from the postoperative functional result.

Ileorectal anastomosis (IRA) has always been a controversial procedure acclaimed by many as giving excellent results and condemned by others as being like an anal ileostomy with a high risk of subsequent cancer in the residual rectum. It is difficult to discern why this difference of opinion has arisen especially to those of us who have had a good experience with the procedure.

Let us assume for a moment that ileorectal anastomosis is compatible with a good functional result, and that the long-term complications are either controllable or of acceptably low incidence as to make the procedure acceptable. Specifically, we are considering the symptomatology of residual proctitis and later cancer risk in the rectal stump. Ileorectal anastomosis then avoids most of the side effects related to ileostomy both of a physical and sexual nature and would seem to be technically less demanding and

Department of Colon and Rectal Surgery, Cleveland Clinic Foundation, Cleveland, Ohio, U.S.A.

time consuming for surgeon and patient alike. Of course not all patients undergoing ileorectal anastomosis will have excellent results, but it has been our experience that sufficient numbers are successful that we regard the procedure as a viable alternative. We believe the short-term complications of residual proctitis and the long-term complications of rectal cancer are less troublesome and frequent than previously thought. To justify this concept let us review the following features regarding ileorectal anastomosis: surgical complications, functional results, failure rate, and cancer risk.

SURGICAL COMPLICATIONS

The main concern in performing ileorectal anastomosis has been the problems associated with performing an anastomosis in diseased bowel. Some protagonists of IRA have recommended the use of a temporary loop ileostomy on every occasion. It would seem nowadays that the use of such a diverting ileostomy should be individualized for each patient based on his or her nutritional state and the degree of activity of the rectal inflammation. Fazio *et al.*[3] in 1975 reported 157 patients undergoing IRA at the Cleveland Clinic for various conditions. One hundred three patients were suffering from ulcerative colitis or Crohn's disease. The operative mortality was 1.9% and the anastomotic leak rate was 1.2%. Aylett[4] in 1966 reported 300 cases of IRA for ulcerative colitis and had an operative mortality of 5.7% and an anastomotic leak rate of 12.4%. Baker[5] in 1970 in reviewing the results from St. Mark's Hospital reported an operative mortality of 5% and an anastomotic leak rate of 14%. More recently Khubchandani *et al.*[6] in 1978 reviewed 56 cases with a zero operative mortality and an anastomotic dehiscence rate of 1.8%. The complications therefore are or were significant but it would seem that with careful technique and utilization of appropriate temporary ileostomy on occasion they are not prohibitive.

FUNCTIONAL RESULTS

There has always been great debate regarding the functional results following IRA. The suggestion by some has been that the frequency of bowel action was so frequent as to be incompatible with a normal existence. On the other hand Aylett (1966)[4] claimed successful results in over 90% of patients. I had the good fortune to see a large number of these patients at first hand and could not help but be impressed with the well being and good results he obviously achieved. We published the results of a postal questionnaire sent to 200 of Aylett's patients selected at random from his series of over 300 cases.[7)] One hundred seventy-four patients replied to the inquiry and the vast majority were leading normal working and social lives. Forty percent had three or fewer stools in 24 hours and in fact 90% had six or fewer stools in the same period. In another more detailed study, Newton and Baker[8)] in 1975 reviewed 92 patients. Bowel frequency ranged from 1.7 to 8.7 stools with a mean of 4.5 per 24 hours. Only 4% had to get up at night. Dietary restrictions were minimal and about half the patients took an occasional antidiarrheal medication. The physical well being of these patients and the results of the study do not suggest inferior results, in fact just the reverse.

Aylett has always contended that the appearance of the rectal mucosa and degree of activity does not influence the end functional result. There is a tendency for the rectal inflammation to subside postoperatively in most patients and to get worse in others. This feature has always been well documented by others (Aylett, 1970[9)]; Sprechler and Baden, 1971[10)]; Watts and Hughes, 1977[11)]). This is of course important as it opens up the availability of IRA to nearly all patients rather than those with so-called rectal sparing, an infrequent event in ulcerative colitis. It also explains the wide variations in utilization of IRA in various series of patients undergoing surgery for ulcerative colitis, from less than 10% as reported by Veidenheimer in 1970[12)] to over 90% as reported by Aylett.[4)] Well documented features that tend to lead to inferior results in all series are rectal stricturing and perianal fistulous disease—the latter being unusual in ulcerative colitis.

ILEORECTAL ANASTOMOSIS——FAILURE RATE

Aylett[4)] reported 300 cases in which only 14 patients (5%) had required proctectomy and ileostomy due to the development of stricture, incontinence, or rectal carcinoma. Watts, de Dombal, and Goligher[2)] in 1966, with a limited experience of 14 patients, had four failures requiring ileostomy but also recommended conversion to two other patients who declined their offer. Farnell *et al.*[13)] in 1980 in reviewing 63 patients from Mayo Clinic stated that 24% required proctectomy and ileostomy for proctitis and general poor function. Khubchandani *et al.*[6)] in 1978 reported on 56 patients and only three required conversion over an eight-year follow-up. Sprechler and Baden[10)] in 1971 had 48 patients and only two required take-down of IRA and ileostomy. Allowing for some variation of failure rates, the vast majority of patients in fact do well, are satisfied with their results, and able to resume normal working and social lives, and this in fact has been my own personal experience. Over the past eight years, I have performed 39 IRAs and none have required conversion to ileostomy.

RECTAL CANCER RISK

One of the main arguments against IRA for ulcerative colitis has been the uncertainty as to the risk of developing rectal cancer. I believe that this risk has been overstated in the past but that is not to dismiss the risk as trivial, as it most certainly is not. Most of the predictions (and they were predictions as it is only comparatively recently that we have had any hard data) were based on the risk involved if the whole colon was involved and not removed. The risk of course is not necessarily the same if only the rectum remains. Goligher[14)] in 1968 estimated the cumulative incidence to reach 42% after 25 years of the disease. Devroede[15)] in 1971 and more recently Kewenter[16)] in 1978 estimated the cumulative incidence to be 34% for total colitis. Is the risk the same after IRA, as has been suggested, or is it different? Does colectomy and IRA decrease the risk by removal of most of the large intestine? There are a large number of reports of series of patients followed for many years with a zero incidence of rectal cancer. However, most of these reports are of comparatively few cases followed for short periods. A review of Aylett's series of 384 cases as reported by Baker *et al.*[17)] in 1978 is very significant as it describes the results of the largest series of patients subjected to IRA and followed for the longest period of time. Three hundred eighty-four patients were operated upon between 1952 and 1976; 374 left hospital with a functioning IRA. They have been followed for periods up to 23 years. Twenty-two patients are known to have developed rectal cancer (6%). Within 10 years of onset of disease no rectal cancers were found in 3,534 patient years. The cumulative risk of developing rectal cancer was 6% (± 2%) at 20 years; 15% (± 4%) at 30 years; and 18% (± 5%) at 35 years. These figures are significantly less than when compared to the estimates related to total residual colitis period by period. Of the 22 patients who developed cancer, 13 were dead and nine alive and well. Eighteen were poorly differentiated, and 12 were found to be Dukes' C cancers. Although the risk seems less than anticipated, when the cancers do arise they tend to be aggressive. It should be pointed out, however, that most of the patients in this study were not subjected to regular rectal mucosal biopsy surveillance for dysplasia as the histological changes had not been described by Morson and Pang[18)] in 1967. It has become accepted clinical practice to subject patients with ulcerative colitis who have not required surgery to annual colonoscopy and multiple biopsy for dysplasia. It would seem reasonable to assume that similar surveillance following IRA is easier, less time consuming, and as safe, and can be justified on those grounds. Grundfest *et al.*[19)] in 1981 reviewed our experience at the Cleveland Clinic. Eighty-nine patients underwent IRA between 1957 and 1977. Eighty-four patients were available for follow-up. Four patients (4.8%) developed rectal cancer. The cumulative risk at 10 years of disease was 0%; at 15 years 2.1% (± 2.1%); at 20 years 5% (± 3.5%); and at 25 years 12.9% (± 8.3%). The follow-up at the 25-year level was based on only a small number of cases. Two patients died of their cancer and two survived. An important point described that five of seven patients having cancer or pre-cancer in the original colectomy specimen subsequently developed cancer or pre-cancer in the rectum.

The risk of developing rectal cancer is obviously increased but does not appear to be excessively high. It is hoped that with regular biopsy surveillance the risk and mortality can be further reduced.

CURRENT SELECTION OF PATIENTS AND FOLLOW-UP

Almost all patients with ulcerative colitis may be suitable for IRA. The appearance of the rectal mucosa does not predict outcome. Rectal distensibility appears important to function after IRA, and rectal stricturing and perianal disease would be contraindications. The presence of colonic carcinoma or dysplasia in association with ulcerative colitis would be relative contraindications.

The follow-up has to be meticulous and thorough and we have established a registry of these cases. They are automatically notified at least on an annual basis if they fail to attend for follow-up. This we hope will improve patient compliance and make the procedure even safer. Proctosigmoidoscopy and three to four random rectal mucosal biopsies are taken and subjected to histological examination for pre-malignant change. The presence of persistent moderate or severe dysplasia is judged as an indication for proctectomy.

In conclusion we believe IRA is a viable alternative to proctocolectomy and ileostomy. It is suitable for most patients with ulcerative colitis and is compatible with a good functional result in most cases. The rectal cancer risk is real but we believe overemphasized. The need for regular examination and biopsy surveillance is stressed for the patient's whole life.

REFERENCES

1. Rhodes, J. B. and Kirsner, J. B.: The early and later course of patients with ulcerative colitis after ileostomy and colectomy. *Surg. Gynecol. Obstet.*, **121**: 1303, 1965.
2. Watts, McK. J., de Dombal, F. T., and Goligher, J. C.: Long term complications and prognosis following major surgery for ulcerative colitis. *Br. J. Surg.*, **53**: 1014, 1966.

3. Fazio, V., Turnbull, R. B., and Goldsmith, M. G.: Ileorectal anastomosis. A safe surgical technique. *Dis. Colon Rectum*, **18**: 107, 1975.
4. Aylett, S. O.: Three hundred cases of diffuse ulcerative colitis treated by colectomy and ileorectal anastomosis. *Br. Med. J.*, **1**: 1001, 1966.
5. Baker, W. N. W.: The results of ileorectal anastomosis at St. Mark's Hospital from 1953–1968. *Gut*, **11**: 235, 1970.
6. Khubchandani, I. T., Trimpi, H. D., Sheets, T. A., Stasik, J. J., and Kleckner, F. S.: Ileorectal anastomosis for ulcerative colitis and Crohn's colitis. *Am. J. Surg.*, **135**: 751, 1978.
7. Jagelman, D. G., Lewis C. B., and Rowe-Jones D. C.: Ileorectal anastomosis: appreciation by patients. *Br. Med. J.*, **1**: 756, 1969.
8. Newton, C. R. and Baker, W. N. W.: Comparison of bowel function after ileorectal anastomosis for ulcerative colitis and colonic polyposis. *Gut*, **16**: 785, 1975.
9. Aylett, S. O.: Delayed ileorectal anastomosis in the surgery of ulcerative colitis. *Br. Med. J.*, **57**: 812, 1970.
10. Sprechler, M. and Baden, H.: Ileorectal anastomosis for ulcerative colitis. *Br. Med. J.*, **2**: 527, 1971.
11. Watts, McK. J. and Hughes, E. S. R.: Ulcerative colitis and Crohn's disease: results after colectomy and ileorectal anastomosis. *Br. J. Surg.*, **64**: 77, 1977.
12. Veidenheimer, M. C., Dailey, T. H., and Meisner, W. A.: Ileorectal anastomosis for inflammatory bowel disease. *Am. J. Surg.*, **119**: 375, 1970.
13. Farnell, M. B., Van Heerden, J. A., Beart, R. W., and Weiland L. H.: Rectal preservation in nonspecific inflammatory disease of the colon. *Ann. Surg.*, **192**: 249, 1980.
14. Goligher, J. C., de Dombal, F. T., Watts, McK. J., and Watkinson, G.: Ulcerative Colitis. Williams and Wilkins, Baltimore, 1968.
15. Devroede, G. J., Taylor, W. F., and Sauer, W. G.: Cancer risk and life expectancy of children with ulcerative colitis. *N. Eng. J. Med.*, **285**: 17, 1971.
16. Kewenter, J., Ahlman, H., and Hultein, L.: Cancer risk in extensive ulcerative colitis. *Ann. Surg.*, **188**: 824, 1978.
17. Baker, W. N. W., Glass, R. E., Ritchie, J. K., and Aylett, S. O.: Cancer of the rectum following colectomy and ileorectal anastomosis for ulcerative colitis. *Br. J. Surg.*, **65**: 862, 1978.
18. Morson, B. C. and Pang, L. S. C.: Rectal biopsy as an aid to cancer control in ulcerative colitis. *Gut*, **8**: 423, 1967.
19. Grundfest, S. F., Fazio, V., Weiss, R. A., Jagelman, D., Lavery, I., Weakley, F. L., and Turnbull, R. B.: The risk of cancer following colectomy and ileorectal anastomosis for extensive mucosal ulcerative colitis. *Ann. Surg.*, **193**: 9, 1981.

Discussion: Surgical Treatment

Keith A. Kelly and Shuji Tsuchiya, Chairmen

Dr. Kelly: I note that the type of the patients and the spectrum of the disease Dr. Nakano and co-workers are seeing are very similar to what we see in Rochester. It also appears that when the disease is entirely removed the patients do better than when the disease is left. The operative mortality in Japan is higher than one would like it to be. The comment to that here is that for benign diseases like colitis and Crohn's disease the operative mortality should be less than 1% in elective cases and less than 10% in emergency. I think you need to work on lowering your mortality rates.

Dr. Tsuchiya: The Japanese cases presented by Dr. Nakano include many cases operated on many years ago. This is one reason why our total mortality is higher. We have much lower mortality in recent years because supportive therapy has generally improved greatly, and particularly in emergency cases, surgeons are called in much earlier than before.

Dr. Kelly: It is more difficult to deal with acutely ill patients with toxic megacolon. It is not only surgeons who are involved in this, but also gastroenterologists. They cannot keep the patient too long and call the surgeon at the last minute and expect a cure. Both the internists and the surgeons have to observe patients very carefully, not delaying operation. Whether rectoileostomy or complete excision is done depends on the situation at the time, but generally speaking the worse the patient the more inclined I am to take the entire disease process out and not to rely on anastomosis.

Dr. Jagelman: It is true that fecal diversion is very effective in dealing with even severe acute toxic ulcerative colitis. As shown by Dr. Farmer, these patients can become extremely well.

I have one small question for Dr. Shiratori. The majority of patients coming to surgery for ulcerative colitis have total colitis. It is very unusual or comparatively unusual to be operating on just left-sided colitis or proctosigmoiditis, so we are talking about the total colonic disease. My own personal preference for diversion has always been ileostomy, inasmuch as it is easier to manage than colostomy which is done on the disease site and is more difficult to manage. But fecal diversion is apparently a simple, effective, and quick way to manage patients in an otherwise difficult situation and it allows them get well without long-term hospitalization and hyperalimentation. Then we do the elective procedure when they are well.

Dr. Shiratori: In the earlier period we did ileostomy for fecal diversion, but we had difficulty managing the frequent stools. Then we tried cecostomy which proved to be easier for managing stools. Finally, we did ascendicostomy despite the presence of disease at the site of the stoma and got satisfactory results. Our policy is to do colectomy with preservation of the anal sphincter at the time when the general condition is ameliorated by ascendicostomy or something similar.

Dr. Kelly: We have not used these diverting procedures at Mayo very often. As you pointed out, when the bowel is left in place, the disease still disturbs the stoma with continuing bleeding, losing protein, fluid, and electrolytes, and the patients continued to be ill. So we rather attempted to resect the diseased bowel and establish the stoma. Our possible exception is the patient with toxic megacolon. But even there, if the surgeon can remove the entire disease, the patient is very apt to get well.

Dr. Shiratori: In acutely ill cases, I believe most surgeons do colectomy without removing the rectum. I would like to prove clinically if the ascendicostomy alone with the diseased bowel left in place might keep the patients well for a long period of time.

Dr. Kelly: I do proctocolectomy and ileostomy in very severe cases in that this operation does cure the disease, it is safe, and patients generally have a rapid recovery, return to good health, and return to work, as Dr. Sekine pointed out. Also, since the disease is removed, there are usually few complications from it. One major disadvantage of this operation is that it leaves the patient with abdominal stoma and difficulties in managing that. I would ask whether patients have difficulties in managing ileostomy in Japan.

Dr. Sekine: Sometimes there are difficulties, particulary concerning peristomal dermatitis, but we can apply drugs which are sometimes effective. Convenient devices newly developed in many countries are also available here.

Dr. Kelly: The ileorectal anastomosis or ileoproctostomy has been used at Mayo, but not very often. We use it in cases of mild rectal disease because anastomosis is generally done safely. We have generally done it in a one-stage operation. The patient in general might be well, although after five to eight years about half of the cases had to have their rectum removed. The problem is that the mucosa of the rectum leads to continuous symptoms with continued need for treatment and also possible risk of cancer. Thus half of them eventually have to come for resection of the rectum. The other thing is that mild rectal disease is most suitable for ileoanal anastomosis because the resection of the rectal mucosa is the easiest. I think because of that we are not doing much in the way of ileorectostomy today. As to the report of Dr. Utsunomiya, the method is exciting and most stimulating and the evolution of our approach has been similar for years using a shorter rectal cuff and J-pouch. One difference in our approach is that we evert the rectum onto the perineum to do the mucosal resection, while he dissects up within the rectal canal. I believe his method has some theoretical advantage, but ours is easier and still maintains a good sphincter.

We have also seen the complication after colectomy with urinary stones and gallstones at Mayo. Patients with ileostomy are in a state of chronic water and salt depletion and secrete small amounts of urine with high acidic pH. They are prone to the development of urinary stones especially the uric-acid type, as has been demonstrated nicely by the Yokohama group. To get oxalate stones, we think that the patient develops diarrhea which binds calcium, and oxalate in the lumen comes down into the colon and is broken apart by bacteria, absorbed, and excreted in the urine, and the patient gets oxalate stones. Gallstones are probably the result of some ileum being resected or diseased so there is failure to properly absorb bile salts and the bile gets lithogenic. Orally ingesting bile salt is a very good idea, which we have not done, but which will be evaluated in the future.

Dr. Tsuchiya: I have the feeling that there is some difference in what Dr. Kelly and Dr. Jagelman are doing and thinking about the surgical policy of treating IBD. I would like to hear their comments.

Dr. Kelly: These are quite different approaches. We are doing both operations, but mainly the pull-through operation at Mayo and I think that Dr. Jagelman will agree that he doesn't use IRA in every case.

Dr. Jagelman: It seems to me that one has to favor a procedure which is good for rehabilitation and function based on the patients' needs rather than on the philosophical need to eradicate the disease. I don't use IRA for unsuitable cases such as cancer or dysplasia.

Dr. Muto: I think it is important to reduce the failure rate of IRA. But why are there so many differences in failure rate in the reports from various institutions?

Dr. Kelly: This is a key point. What some doctors or patients accept as a success is to other patients or doctors a failure. There is no objective standard, and there must be a discussion as to what is a failure and what is a success. It is true that the patients having rectal distress postoperatively have found it unacceptable, and their doctors as well. On the other hand, some patients may get along with a lesser degree of symptoms in spite of the bowel disease and may regard this as acceptable. But after the total excision of the bowel, the patients have a sense of freedom from it even though they have frequent bowel movements. In general they can control it quite well with an ileoanal anastomosis and they don't have much distress or disability with it. Moreover, doctors don't have to keep the patient to examine the rectum for cancer surveillance. I think that Dr. Jagelman's operation is a simple operation and one which has fewer complications. Perhaps from the worldwide point of view, it can be used from case to case.

Dr. Jagelman: What makes a failure belongs to preoperative selection or prediction. If the rectum is retained for 20 cm, the function is good. But if only 2 cm is retained, it is like a straight ileoanal anastomosis and the function is not good. The evaluation is a patient's evaluation, and failure requiring ileostomy is very rare. I think ileoanal anastomosis is time consuming and complex with unpredictable functional results. If you have an IRA, you can leave the hospital in 7–10 days and go back to work within 6 weeks. The pouch patients still have an ileostomy, and in two-stage operations six months are required and still need a year for rehabilitation. What operation to have is the patient's option, and none of the operations is 100% ideal.

Dr. Matsueda: I think the etiology of cancer occurring in the retained rectum is similar to that of gastric cancer in the partially resected stomach in that both may be exposed bile acids or contents of the small bowel.

Dr. Kelly: I think it may be possible, and bacteria may play a role as well.

Dr. Jagelman: The incidence of dysplasia and cancer in ulcerative colitis will increase overall with time, but IRA is still not prohibitive and it is hoped that cancer will be controlled by regular rectal biopsy surveillance.

Dr. Tsuchiya: Are there any comments on the surgical problems discussed from the side of internal medicine?

Dr. Jewell: Panproctocolectomy with a Brooke ileostomy is still the favored operation in the U.K., although I think there is less antagonism to ileorectal anastomosis than existed a few years ago. As a physician, I prefer all the diseased mucosa to be resected if a surgical procedure is to be performed. I think the new developments of ileoanal anastomosis with a pouch or an ileostomy occlusive device are exciting possibilities.

Dr. Farmer: The value of the newer operations is increasingly apparent, despite the problems encountered. Despite the problems, there is value in pursuing ileorectal or ileoanal anastomosis and cancer surveillance techniques. Although I am from the institution of Dr. Turnbull's pioneering ileostomy techniques and the famous enterostomal therapist, I think surgical techniques which avoid stoma are more desirable for surgical patients. I think the surgical experience in Japan is in the state found in the U.S.A. 20 years ago because of the incidence of the disease. But Japanese surgeons have gone to the non-stoma or anastomotic procedure much earlier than I saw in the U.S.A. and this is a favorable trend.

Executive Members of Japan Medical Research Foundation